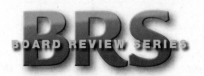

BRS
BOARD REVIEW SERIES

Cell Biology and Histology

SEVENTH EDITION

Leslie P. Gartner, PhD
Professor of Anatomy (Retired)
Department of Biomedical Sciences
University of Maryland Dental School
Baltimore, Maryland

James L. Hiatt, PhD
Professor Emeritus
Department of Biomedical Sciences
University of Maryland Dental School
Baltimore, Maryland

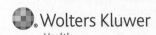
. Wolters Kluwer
Health

Philadelphia · Baltimore · New York · London
Buenos Aires · Hong Kong · Sydney · Tokyo

Acquisitions Editor: Crystal Taylor
Product Development Editor: Amy Weintraub
Production Project Manager: Priscilla Crater
Design Coordinator: Holly Reid McLaughlin
Manufacturing Coordinator: Margie Orzech
Compositor: S4Carlisle Publishing Services

Library of Congress Cataloging-in-Publication Data
Gartner, Leslie P., 1943- author.
  Cell biology and histology / Leslie P. Gartner, James L. Hiatt. — Seventh edition.
     p. ; cm. — (Board review series)
  Includes bibliographical references and index.
  ISBN 978-1-4511-8951-3 (paperback : alk. paper)
  I. Hiatt, James L., 1934- author. II. Title. III. Series: Board review series.
  [DNLM: 1. Histological Techniques—Outlines.   2. Cytological Techniques—Outlines. QS 18.2]
  QM553
  611'.018—dc23

                                                                2014018636

DISCLAIMER
Care has been taken to confirm the accuracy of the information present and to describe generally accepted practices. However, the authors, editors, and publisher are not responsible for errors or omissions or for any consequences from application of the information in this book and make no warranty, expressed or implied, with respect to the currency, completeness, or accuracy of the contents of the publication. Application of this information in a particular situation remains the professional responsibility of the practitioner; the clinical treatments described and recommended may not be considered absolute and universal recommendations.

The authors, editors, and publisher have exerted every effort to ensure that drug selection and dosage set forth in this text are in accordance with the current recommendations and practice at the time of publication. However, in view of ongoing research, changes in government regulations, and the constant flow of information relating to drug therapy and drug reactions, the reader is urged to check the package insert for each drug for any change in indications and dosage and for added warnings and precautions. This is particularly important when the recommended agent is a new or infrequently employed drug.

Some drugs and medical devices presented in this publication have Food and Drug Administration (FDA) clearance for limited use in restricted research settings. It is the responsibility of the health care provider to ascertain the FDA status of each drug or device planned for use in their clinical practice.

To purchase additional copies of this book, call our customer service department at **(800) 638-3030** or fax orders to **(301) 223-2320**. International customers should call **(301) 223-2300**.
Visit Lippincott Williams & Wilkins on the Internet: http://www.lww.com. Lippincott Williams & Wilkins customer service representatives are available from 8:30 am to 6:00 pm, EST.

Preface

We were very pleased with the reception of the sixth edition of this book, as well as with the many favorable comments we received from students who used it in preparation for the USMLE Step 1 or as an outline and study guide for their histology and/or cell biology courses in professional schools or undergraduate colleges.

Many of the chapters have been extensively revised and updated to incorporate current information, and we have attempted to refine the content of the text to present material emphasized on National Board Examinations as succinctly as possible while still retaining the emphasis on the relationship between cell structure and function through the vehicle of cell and molecular biology. A tremendous amount of material has been compressed into a concise but highly comprehensive presentation, using some new and revised illustrations. The relevancy of cell biology and histology to clinical practice is illustrated by the presence of clinical considerations within each chapter as appropriate.

The greatest changes that occurred in the evolution of this book from its previous edition are that we have added many more clinical considerations and compressed information into tabular form. We believe that these changes make this board review book more interesting and pertinent and the presentation of material in tables conserves time in the review process for medical students in their preparation for the USMLE Step 1.

We are sad to announce that Judy Strum, our coauthor throughout the first six editions of this review book, decided to complete her retirement from the faculty of the University of Maryland School of Medicine thereby withdrawing her participation in the preparation of the current edition of this textbook.

As always, we welcome comments, suggestions, and constructive criticism of this book. Please address all comments to LPG21136@yahoo.com

Leslie P. Gartner, PhD
James L. Hiatt, PhD

Acknowledgments

We thank the following individuals for their help and support during the preparation of this book: Crystal Taylor, our Acquisitions Editor; and Dana Battaglia and Amy Weintraub, our product Development Editor(s), who helped us weave all of the loose ends into a seamless whole.

Contents

21. SPECIAL SENSES   366

chapter 1

Plasma Membrane

I. OVERVIEW—THE PLASMA MEMBRANE (PLASMALEMMA; CELL MEMBRANE)

A. **Structure**. The plasma membrane is approximately 7.5 nm thick and consists of two leaflets, known as the **lipid bilayer** that houses associated **integral** and **peripheral proteins**.
   1. The **inner leaflet** of the plasma membrane faces the cytoplasm, and the **outer leaflet** faces the extracellular environment.
   2. When examined by transmission electron microscopy, the plasma membrane displays a trilaminar (**unit membrane**) structure.

B. **Function**
   1. The plasma membrane envelops the cell and maintains its structural and functional integrity.
   2. It acts as a **semipermeable** membrane between the cytoplasm and the external environment.
   3. It permits the cell to recognize macromolecules and other cells as well as to be recognized by other cells.
   4. It participates in the transduction of extracellular signals into intracellular events.
   5. It assists in controlling interaction between cells.
   6. It maintains an electrical potential difference between the cytoplasmic and extracellular sides.

II. FLUID MOSAIC MODEL OF THE PLASMA MEMBRANE

A. **The lipid bilayer** (Figures 1.1, 1.2, and 1.3) is freely permeable to small, lipid-soluble, nonpolar molecules but is impermeable to charged ions.
   1. **Molecular structure.** The lipid bilayer is composed of phospholipids, glycolipids, and cholesterol, of which, in most cells, phospholipids constitute the highest percentage.
      a. **Phospholipids** are **amphipathic** molecules, consisting of one **polar** (**hydrophilic**) head and two **nonpolar** (**hydrophobic**) fatty acyl tails, one of which is usually unsaturated.
      b. The two leaflets are not identical; instead the distribution of the various types of phospholipids is asymmetrical.
         (1) The **polar head** of each molecule faces the membrane surface, whereas the **tails** project into the interior of the membrane, facing each other.
         (2) The **tails** of the two leaflets are mostly 16 to 18 carbon chain fatty acids, and they form weak **noncovalent** bonds that attach the two leaflets to each other.

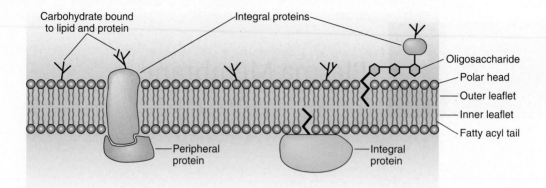

FIGURE 1.1. The plasma membrane showing the outer (*top*) and inner (*bottom*) leaflets of the unit membrane. The hydrophobic fatty acyl tails and the polar heads of the phospholipids constitute the lipid bilayer. Integral proteins are embedded in the lipid bilayer. Peripheral proteins are located primarily on the cytoplasmic aspect of the inner leaflet and are attached by noncovalent interactions to integral proteins.

   c. Glycolipids are restricted to the extracellular aspect of the outer leaflet. **Polar carbohydrate residues** of glycolipids extend from the outer leaflet into the extracellular space and form part of the **glycocalyx**.
   d. Cholesterol, constituting 2% of plasmalemma lipids, is present in both leaflets, and helps maintain the structural integrity of the membrane.

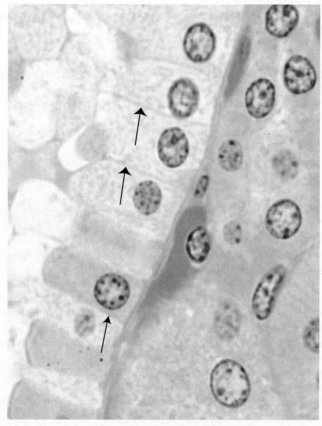

FIGURE 1.2. Photomicrograph of a collecting duct of the kidney displaying tall columnar cells. The *arrows* indicate the cell membranes where two cells contact each other (×1,323).

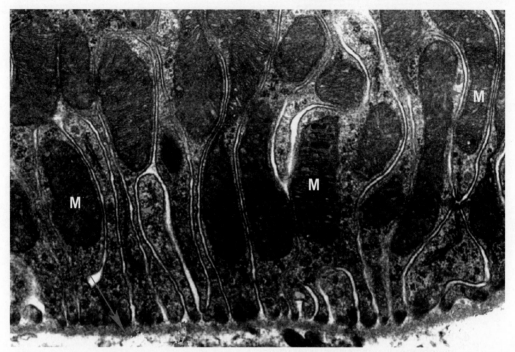

FIGURE 1.3. Transmission electron micrograph of the basal region of a columnar cell from a kidney-collecting tubule. The basal cell membrane forms numerous complex folds to increase its surface area. M, mitochondria; *red arrowheads*, plasmalemma; *red arrow*, basal lamina (×28,435).

     e. Microdomains of the cell membrane rich in **cholesterol** and **glycosphingolipids** are less fluid and thicker than the surrounding cell membrane, and are known as **lipid rafts**.

  2. **Fluidity** of the lipid bilayer is crucial to **exocytosis, endocytosis, membrane trafficking**, and **membrane biogenesis**.

     a. Fluidity **increases** with increased temperature and with decreased saturation of the fatty acyl tails.

     b. Fluidity **decreases** with an increase in the membrane's cholesterol content.

B. **Membrane proteins** (see Figure 1.1) include integral proteins and peripheral proteins and, in most cells, constitute approximately 50% of the plasma membrane composition.

  1. **Integral proteins** are dissolved in the lipid bilayer.

     a. **Transmembrane proteins** span the entire thickness of the plasma membrane and **may** function as membrane **receptors, enzymes, cell adhesion molecules, cell recognition proteins**, molecules that function in message **transduction**, and **transport proteins**.

       (1) Most transmembrane proteins are **glycoproteins**.

       (2) Transmembrane proteins are **amphipathic** and contain **hydrophilic** and **hydrophobic** amino acids, some of which interact with the hydrocarbon tails of the membrane phospholipids.

       (3) Most transmembrane proteins are folded, so that they pass back and forth across the plasmalemma; therefore, they are also known as **multipass proteins**.

     b. Integral proteins may also be anchored to the inner (or occasionally outer) leaflet via fatty acyl or prenyl groups.

     c. In freeze-fracture preparations, integral proteins remain preferentially attached to the **P-face**, the outer (**p**rotoplasmic face) surface of the inner leaflet, rather than the **E-face** (**e**xtracellular face) (Figure 1.4).

  2. **Peripheral proteins** do not extend into the lipid bilayer.

     a. These proteins are located on the cytoplasmic as well as on the extracellular aspects of the cell membrane.

     b. The outer leaflets of some cells possess covalently linked glycolipids to which peripheral proteins are anchored; these peripheral proteins thus project into the **extracellular space**.

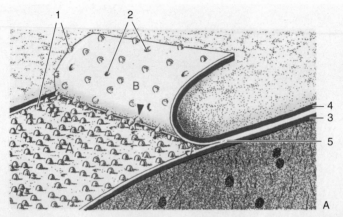

FIGURE 1.4. Freeze-fracturing cleaves the plasma membrane (5). The impressions (2) of the transmembrane proteins are evident on the E-face between the inner (3) and outer leaflets (4). The integral proteins (1) remain preferentially attached to the P-face **(A)**, the external surface of the inner leaflet; fewer proteins remain associated with the E-face **(B)**, the internal surface of the outer leaflet. The *arrowhead* indicates a transmembrane protein attached to both E-face and P-face. (Reprinted with permission from Krstic RV. *Ultrastruktur der Saugertierzelle.* Berlin, Germany: Springer Verlag; 1976:177.)

     c. Frequently, carbohydrates may bind to the peripheral proteins on the extracellular aspect of the plasmalemma; these glycogen groups are referred to as **glycoproteins**.

     d. Peripheral proteins bind to the phospholipid polar groups or integral proteins of the membrane via noncovalent interactions.

     e. They usually function as electron carriers (e.g., cytochrome c) part of the **cytoskeleton** or as part of an **intracellular second messenger system**.

     f. They include a group of anionic, calcium-dependent, lipid-binding proteins known as **annexins**, which act to modify the relationships of other peripheral proteins with the lipid bilayer and also to function in membrane trafficking and the formation of ion channels; **synapsin I**, which binds synaptic vesicles to the cytoskeleton; and **spectrin**, which stabilizes cell membranes of erythrocytes.

  3. Functional characteristics of membrane proteins

     a. The lipid-to-protein ratio (by weight) in plasma membranes ranges from 1:1 in most cells to as much as 4:1 in myelin.

     b. Some membrane proteins **diffuse laterally** in the lipid bilayer; others are **immobile** and are held in place by cytoskeletal components.

C. Glycocalyx (cell coat), located on the outer surface of the outer leaflet of the plasmalemma, varies in appearance (fuzziness) and thickness (up to 50 nm).

  1. Composition. The glycocalyx consists of polar oligosaccharide side chains linked covalently to most proteins and some lipids (glycolipids) of the plasmalemma. It also contains **proteoglycans** (**glycosaminoglycans** bound to integral proteins).

  2. Function

     a. The glycocalyx aids in **attachment** of some cells (e.g., fibroblasts but not epithelial cells) to extracellular matrix components.

     b. It **binds** antigens and enzymes to the cell surface.

     c. It facilitates **cell–cell recognition** and **interaction**.

     d. It **protects cells** from injury by preventing contact with inappropriate substances.

     e. It assists T cells and antigen-presenting cells in **aligning** with each other in proper fashion and aids in preventing inappropriate enzymatic cleavage of receptors and ligands.

     f. In blood vessels, it lines the endothelial surface to decrease frictional forces as the blood rushes by and it also diminishes loss of fluid from the vessel.

D. Lipid rafts, as mentioned above, are microdomains of the plasma membrane that are thicker than the surrounding plasma membrane, and for this reason they protrude slightly into the extracellular space. Because of their higher cholesterol concentration and because they are rich in glycosphingolipids, they are less fluid than the surrounding cell membrane. Some of these lipid rafts have integral and peripheral proteins associated with them and they function in **cell signaling**. Different lipid rafts may specialize as specific signaling processes, thus separating the various signaling modalities and enhancing the possibility of the occurrence of specific signaling events.

III. PLASMA MEMBRANE TRANSPORT PROCESSES

These processes include transport of a single molecule (**uniport**) or cotransport of two different molecules in the same (**symport**) or opposite (**antiport**) direction.

A. **Passive transport** (Figure 1.5) includes **simple** and **facilitated diffusion**. Neither of these processes requires energy because molecules move across the plasma membrane **down a concentration or electrochemical gradient**.
   1. **Simple diffusion** transports small nonpolar molecules (e.g., O_2 and N_2) and small, uncharged, polar molecules (e.g., H_2O, CO_2, and glycerol). It exhibits little specificity, and the diffusion rate is proportional to the concentration gradient of the diffusing molecule.
   2. **Facilitated diffusion** occurs via **ion channels** and/or **carrier proteins**, structures that exhibit **specificity** for the transported molecules. Not only is it faster than simple diffusion but it is also responsible for providing a pathway for ions and large polar molecules to traverse membranes that would otherwise be impermeable to them.
      a. **Ion channel proteins** are multipass transmembrane proteins that form small aqueous pores across membranes through which specific small water-soluble molecules and ions, such as Cl^-, pass down an electrochemical gradient (**passive transport**).
      b. **Aquaporins** are channels designed for the rapid transport of water across the cell membrane without permitting an accompanying flow of protons to pass through the channels. They accomplish this by forcing the water molecules to flip-flop halfway down the channel, so that water molecules enter aquaporins with their oxygen leading into the channel and leave with their oxygen trailing the hydrogen atoms.
      c. **Carrier proteins** are multipass transmembrane proteins that undergo reversible conformational changes to transport specific molecules across the membrane; these proteins function in both passive transport and **active transport**.

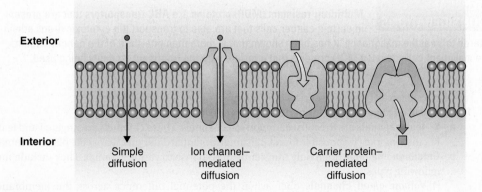

FIGURE 1.5. Passive transport of molecules across plasma membranes by simple diffusion (*left*) and by either of the two types of facilitated diffusion mediated by ion channel proteins (*center*) and carrier proteins (*right*).

Cystinuria is a hereditary condition caused by abnormal carrier proteins that are unable to remove cystine from the urine, resulting in the formation of kidney stones.

     Cystic fibrosis is a hereditary disease involving a mutation in the *cystic fibrosis transmembrane conductance regulator* **(CFTR) gene** that produces malformed **chloride channel proteins** that are unable to transport chloride ions, causing an increase in the entry of Na^+ ions into the cell. The higher intracellular concentration of NaCl increases the flow of water into the cell, and the mucin that is released into the extracellular environment cannot become normally hydrated, thus making the mucus thicker than normal, which obstructs the very small bronchiolar passageways of the lungs. As the disease progresses, infections result, the lungs become unable to function properly, and the individual succumbs to the disease and dies.

B. **Active transport** is an **energy-requiring process** that transports a molecule **against** an electrochemical gradient via carrier proteins.
 1. **Na^+–K^+ pump**
    a. **Mechanism.** The Na^+–K^+ pump involves the **antiport** transport of Na^+ and K^+ ions mediated by the carrier protein, **Na^+–K^+ adenosine triphosphatase (ATPase)**.
       (1) Three Na^+ ions are pumped **out** of the cell and two K^+ ions are pumped **into** the cell.
       (2) The hydrolysis of a single adenosine triphosphate (ATP) molecule by the Na^+–K^+ ATPase is required to transport five ions.
    b. **Function**
       (1) The primary function is to **maintain constant cell volume** by decreasing the intracellular ion concentration (and thus the osmotic pressure) and increasing the extracellular ion concentration, thus decreasing the flow of water into the cell.
       (2) The Na^+–K^+ pump also plays a minor role in the maintenance of a **potential difference** across the plasma membrane.
 2. **Glucose transport** involves the **symport** movement of glucose across an epithelium (**transepithelial transport**). Transport is frequently powered by an electrochemical Na^+ gradient, which drives carrier proteins located at specific regions of the cell surface.
 3. **ATP-binding cassette transporters (ABC transporters)** are transmembrane proteins that have two domains, the intracellularly facing **nucleotide-binding domain (ATP-binding domain)** and the **membrane-spanning domain (transmembrane domain)**. In eukaryotes, ABC transporters function in exporting materials, such as toxins and drugs, from the cytoplasm into the extracellular space, using ATP as an energy source. ABC transporters may have additional functions, such as those of the placenta, which presumably protect the developing fetus from **xenobiotics**, macromolecules such as antibiotics, not manufactured by cells of the mother.

Multidrug-resistant (MDR) proteins are **ABC transporters** that are present in certain cancer cells that are able to transport the cytotoxic drugs administered to treat the malignancy. It has been shown that in more than one-third of the cancer patients, the malignant cells develop MDR proteins that interfere with the treatment modality being used.

C. **Facilitated diffusion of ions** can occur via ion channel proteins or ionophores.
 1. Selective ion channel proteins permit only certain ions to traverse them.
    a. **K^+ leak channels** are the most common ion channels. These channels are ungated and leak K^+, the ions most responsible for establishing a potential difference across the plasmalemma.
    b. **Gated ion channels** open only transiently in response to various stimuli. They include the following types:
       (1) **Voltage-gated channels** open when the potential difference across the membrane changes (e.g., voltage-gated Na^+ channels, which function in the generation of action potentials; see Chapter 9 VIII B 1 e).
       (2) **Mechanically gated channels** open in response to a mechanical stimulus (e.g., the tactile response of the hair cells in the inner ear).

(3) Ligand-gated channels open in response to the binding of a **signaling molecule** or **ion**. These channels include neurotransmitter-gated channels, nucleotide-gated channels, and G protein–gated K^+ channels of cardiac muscle cells.

CLINICAL CONSIDERATIONS **Ligand-gated ion channels** are probably the location where anesthetic agents act to block the spread of action potentials.

2. **Ionophores** are lipid-miscible molecules that form a complex with ions and insert into the lipid bilayer to transport those ions across the membrane. There are two ways in which they perform this function:

   a. They enfold the ion and pass through the lipid bilayer.

   b. They insert into the cell membrane to form an ion channel whose lumen is hydrophilic. Ionophores are frequently fed to cattle and poultry as antibiotic agents and growth-enhancing substances.

IV. CELL-TO-CELL COMMUNICATION

A. **Signaling molecules,** secreted by signaling cells, bind to receptor molecules of target cells, and in this fashion, these molecules function in cell-to-cell communication in order to coordinate cellular activities. Examples of such signaling molecules that effect communications include neurotransmitters, which are released into the synaptic cleft (see Chapter 8 IV A 1 b; Chapter 9 IV B 5); endocrine hormones, which are carried in the bloodstream and act on distant target cells; and hormones released into the intercellular space, which act on nearby cells (**paracrine hormones**) or on the releasing cell itself (**autocrine hormones**).

1. **Lipid-soluble signaling molecules** penetrate the plasma membrane and bind to *receptors within the cytoplasm* or inside the **nucleus**, activating intracellular messengers. Examples include hormones that influence gene transcription.

2. **Hydrophilic signaling molecules** bind to and activate **cell-surface receptors** (as do some lipid-soluble signaling molecules) and have diverse physiologic effects (see Chapter 13). Examples include neurotransmitters and numerous hormones (e.g., serotonin, thyroid-stimulating hormone, insulin).

B. **Membrane receptors** are primarily integral membrane glycoproteins. They are embedded in the lipid bilayer and have three domains: an **extracellular domain** that protrudes into the extracellular space and has binding sites for the signaling molecule, a **transmembrane domain** that passes through the lipid bilayer, and an **intracellular domain** that is located on the cytoplasmic aspect of the lipid bilayer and contacts either peripheral proteins or cellular organelles, thereby **transducing** the extracellular contact into an intracellular event.

CLINICAL CONSIDERATIONS **Venoms,** such as those of some poisonous snakes, inactivate acetylcholine receptors of skeletal muscle sarcolemma at neuromuscular junctions.
   Autoimmune diseases may lead to the production of antibodies that specifically **bind to and activate certain plasma membrane receptors**. An example is **Graves disease** (hyperthyroidism) (see Chapter 13 IV B).

1. **Function**

   a. Membrane receptors **control plasmalemma permeability** by regulating the conformation of ion channel proteins.

   b. They **regulate the entry of molecules** into the cell (e.g., the delivery of cholesterol via low-density lipoprotein receptors).

   c. They **bind extracellular matrix molecules** to the cytoskeleton via **integrins**, which are essential for cell–matrix interactions.

    d. They **act as transducers** to translate extracellular events into an intracellular response via the second messenger systems.

    e. They permit pathogens that mimic normal ligands to enter cells.

2. Types of membrane receptors (See Table 1.2).

    a. Channel-linked receptors bind a signaling molecule that temporarily opens or closes the gate, permitting or inhibiting the movement of ions across the cell membrane. Examples include **nicotinic acetylcholine receptors** on the muscle-cell sarcolemma at the myoneural junction (see Chapter 8 IV A).

    b. Catalytic receptors are single-pass transmembrane proteins.

      (1) Their extracellular moiety is a receptor and their **cytoplasmic component** is a protein kinase.

      (2) Some catalytic receptors lack an extracytoplasmic moiety and, as a result, are continuously activated; such defective receptors are coded for by some **oncogenes**.

      (3) Examples of catalytic receptors include the following:

        (a) Insulin binds to its receptor, which **autophosphorylates**. The cell then takes up the insulin–receptor complex by **endocytosis**, enabling the complex to function within the cell.

        (b) Growth factors (e.g., epidermal growth factor, platelet-derived growth factor) bind to specific catalytic receptors and induce mitosis.

    c. G protein–linked receptors are transmembrane proteins associated with an ion channel or with an enzyme that is bound to the cytoplasmic surface of the cell membrane.

      (1) These receptors interact with **heterotrimeric G protein** (guanosine triphosphate [GTP]-binding regulatory protein) after binding of a signaling molecule. The heterotrimeric G protein is composed of three subunits: α, β, and γ **complex.** The binding of the signaling molecule causes either

        (a) the dissociation of the α subunit from the β and γ complex where the α subunit interacts with its target or

        (b) the three subunits do not dissociate, but either the α subunit and/or the β and γ **complex** become activated and can interact with their targets.

      This interaction results in the activation of **intracellular second messengers**, the most common of which are cyclic adenosine monophosphate **(cAMP)**, Ca^{2+}, and the **inositol phospholipid–signaling pathway.**

      (2) Examples include the following:

        (a) Heterotrimeric G proteins (Table 1.1), which are folded in such a fashion that they make seven passes as they penetrate the cell membrane. These are stimulatory G protein (G_s) (Figure 1.6); inhibitory G protein (G_i); phospholipase C activator G protein (G_q); olfactory-specific G protein (G_{olf}); transducin (G_t); G_o, which acts to open K^+ channels and close Ca^{2+} channels; and $G_{12/13}$, which controls the formation of the actin component of the cytoskeleton and facilitates migration of the cell.

        (b) Monomeric G proteins (low-molecular-weight G proteins) are small single-chain proteins that also function in signal transduction.

          1. Various subtypes resemble Ras, Rho, Rab, and ARF proteins.

          2. These proteins are involved in pathways that regulate cell proliferation and differentiation, protein synthesis, attachment of cells to the extracellular matrix, exocytosis, and vesicular traffic.

CLINICAL CONSIDERATIONS   **Cholera toxin** is an exotoxin produced by the bacterium *Vibrio cholerae* that alters G_s protein, so that it is unable to hydrolyze its GTP molecule. As a result, cAMP levels increase in the surface-absorptive cells of the intestine, leading to excessive loss of electrolytes and water and severe diarrhea.

    Pertussis toxin, the product of the bacterium that causes whooping cough, inserts ADP-ribose into the α subunits of trimeric G proteins, causing the accumulation of the inactive form of G proteins resulting in irritation of the mucosa of the bronchial passages.

    Defective G_s proteins may lead to mental retardation, diminished growth and sexual development, and decreased responses to certain hormones.

t a b l e **1.1**		Functions and Examples of Heterotrimeric G Proteins	
Type	Function	Result	Examples
G_s	Activates adenylate cyclase, leading to formation of cAMP	Activation of protein kinases	Binding of epinephrine to β-adrenergic receptors increases cAMP levels in cytosol
G_i	Inhibits adenylate cyclase, preventing formation of cAMP	Protein kinases remain inactive	Binding of epinephrine to α_2-adrenergic receptors decreases cAMP levels in cytosol
G_q	Activates phospholipase C, leading to formation of inositol triphosphate and diacylglycerol	Influx of Ca^{2+} into cytosol and activation of protein kinase C	Binding of antigen to membrane-bound IgE causes the release of histamine by mast cells
G_o	Opens K^+ channels and closes Ca^{2+} channels	Inhibits adenylate cyclase Influx of K^+ and limits Ca^{2+} movement	Inducing contraction of smooth muscle
G_{olf}	Activates adenylate cyclase in olfactory neurons	Opens cAMP-gated Na^+ channels	Binding of odorant to G protein–linked receptors initiates generation of nerve impulse
G_t	Activates cGMP phosphodiesterase in rod cell membranes, leading to hydrolysis of cGMP	Hyperpolarization of rod cell membrane	Photon activation of rhodopsin causes rod cells to fire
$G_{12/13}$	Activates Rho family of guanosine triphosphatases	Regulates cytoskeleton assembly by controlling actin formation	Facilitating cellular migration

cAMP, cyclic adenosine monophosphate; cGMP, cyclic guanosine monophosphate; IgE, immunoglobulin E.

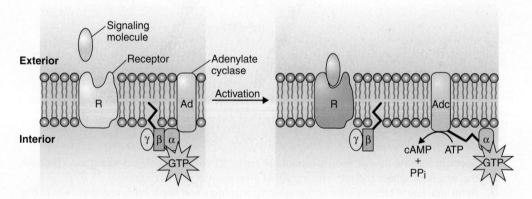

FIGURE 1.6. Functioning of G_s protein–linked receptors. The signaling molecule binds to the receptor, which causes the α-subunit of the G_s protein to bind guanosine triphosphate (GTP) and dissociate from the β and γ subunits. Activation of adenylate cyclase by the GTP–α-subunit complex stimulates synthesis of cyclic adenosine monophosphate (cAMP), one of the most common intracellular messengers.

V. PLASMALEMMA–CYTOSKELETON ASSOCIATION

The plasmalemma and cytoskeleton associate through **integrins**. The extracellular domain of integrins binds to extracellular matrix components, and the intracellular domain binds to cytoskeletal components. Integrins stabilize the plasmalemma and determine and maintain cell shape.

A. **Red blood cells** (Figure 1.7A) have integrins, called **band 3 proteins**, which are located in the plasmalemma. The cytoskeleton of a red blood cell consists mainly of spectrin, actin, band 4.1 protein, and ankyrin.

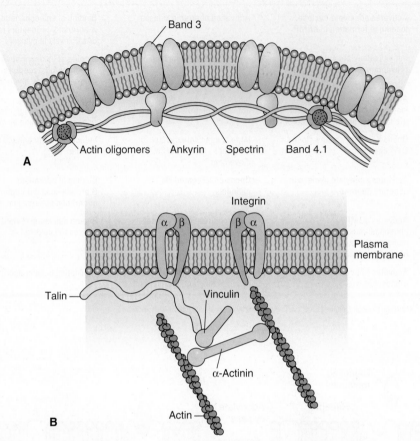

FIGURE 1.7. Plasmalemma–cytoskeleton association in red blood cells **(A)** and nonerythroid cells **(B)**. (Adapted with permission from Widnell CC, Pfenninger KH. *Essential Cell Biology*. Baltimore, MD: Williams & Wilkins; 1990:82.)

1. **Spectrin** is a long, flexible protein (about 110 nm long), composed of an **α-chain** and a **β-chain**, that forms **tetramers** and provides a scaffold for structural reinforcement.
2. **Actin** attaches to binding sites on the spectrin tetramers and holds them together, thus aiding in the formation of a hexagonal spectrin latticework.
3. **Band 4.1 protein** binds to and stabilizes spectrin–actin complexes.
4. **Ankyrin** is linked to both band 3 proteins and spectrin tetramers, thus attaching the spectrin–actin complex to transmembrane proteins.

B. The cytoskeleton of **nonerythroid cells** (Figure 1.7B) consists of the following major components:
   1. **Actin** (and perhaps **fodrin**), which serves as a nonerythroid spectrin.
   2. **α-Actinin**, which cross-links actin filaments to form a meshwork.
   3. **Vinculin**, which binds to α-actinin and to another protein, called **talin**, which, in turn, attaches to the integrin in the plasma membrane.

CLINICAL CONSIDERATIONS

1. **Hereditary spherocytosis** results from a **defective spectrin** that has a decreased ability to bind to band 4.1 protein. The disease is characterized by fragile, misshapen red blood cells, or spherocytes; destruction of these **spherocytes** in the spleen leads to anemia.

2. During high-speed car accidents and often in shaken baby syndrome, the sudden accelerating and decelerating forces applied to the brain cause shearing damage to axons, especially at the interface between white matter and gray matter. The stretching of the axons results in **diffuse axonal injury**, a widespread lesion whose consequence is the onset of a persistent coma from which only 10% of the affected individuals regain consciousness. Examination of the affected tissue displays irreparable cleavage of **spectrin**, with an ensuing destruction of the neuronal cytoskeleton, leading to loss of plasma membrane integrity and eventual cell death.

t a b l e   1.2   Major Classes of Membrane Proteins

Major Class	Functions
Receptor protein	Recognizes and binds signaling molecule on the extracellular surface of the cell membrane
Enzyme	Functions differ depending on the enzyme (e.g., energy utilization and digestion)
Pump	Transports ions and small molecules across the cell membrane by the expenditure of energy
Channel	Transports ions and small molecules across the cell membrane without the expenditure of energy
Linker protein	Functions in the attachment of the cell to the extracellular matrix
Structural protein	Functions in attaching neighboring cells to each other

Review Test

Directions: Each of the numbered items or incomplete statements in this section is followed by answers or by completions of the statement. Select the ONE lettered answer or completion that is BEST in each case.

1. A herpetologist is bitten by a poisonous snake and is taken to the emergency department with progressive muscle paralysis. The venom is probably incapacitating his

(A) Na^+ channels.
(B) Ca^{2+} channels.
(C) phospholipids.
(D) acetylcholine receptors.
(E) spectrin.

2. Cholesterol functions in the plasmalemma to

(A) increase fluidity of the lipid bilayer.
(B) decrease fluidity of the lipid bilayer.
(C) facilitate the diffusion of ions through the lipid bilayer.
(D) assist in the transport of hormones across the lipid bilayer.
(E) bind extracellular matrix molecules.

3. The cell membrane consists of various components, including integral proteins. These integral proteins

(A) are not attached to the outer leaflet.
(B) are not attached to the inner leaflet.
(C) include transmembrane proteins.
(D) are preferentially attached to the E-face.
(E) function in the transport of cholesterol-based hormones.

4. Which one of the following transport processes requires energy?

(A) Facilitated diffusion
(B) Passive transport
(C) Active transport
(D) Simple diffusion

5. Which one of the following substances is unable to traverse the plasma membrane by simple diffusion?

(A) O_2
(B) N_2
(C) Na^+
(D) Glycerol
(E) CO_2

6. Symport refers to the process of transporting

(A) a molecule into the cell.
(B) a molecule out of the cell.
(C) two different molecules in opposite directions.
(D) two different molecules in the same direction.
(E) a molecule between the cytoplasm and the nucleus.

7. One of the ways that cells communicate with each other is by secretion of various molecules. The secreted molecule is known as

(A) a receptor molecule.
(B) a signaling molecule.
(C) a spectrin tetramer.
(D) an integrin.
(E) an anticodon.

8. Adrenocorticotropic hormone (ACTH) travels through the bloodstream, enters connective tissue spaces, and attaches to specific sites on target-cell membranes. These sites are

(A) peripheral proteins.
(B) signaling molecules.
(C) G proteins.
(D) G protein–linked receptors.
(E) ribophorins.

9. Examination of the blood smear of a young patient reveals misshapen red blood cells, and the pathology report indicates hereditary spherocytosis. Defects in which one of the following proteins cause this condition?

(A) Signaling molecules
(B) G proteins
(C) Spectrin
(D) Hemoglobin
(E) Ankyrin

10. Which of the following statements concerning plasma membrane components is TRUE?

(A) All G proteins are composed of three subunits.
(B) The glycocalyx is usually composed of phospholipids.
(C) Ion channel proteins are energy dependent (require adenosine triphosphate).
(D) Gated channels are always open.
(E) Ankyrin binds to band 3 of the red blood cell plasma membrane.

Answers and Explanations

1. **D.** Snake venom usually blocks acetylcholine receptors, preventing depolarization of the muscle cell. The Na^+ and Ca^{2+} channels are not incapacitated by snake venoms (see Chapter 1 IV B).

2. **B.** The fluidity of the lipid bilayer is decreased in three ways: (1) by lowering the temperature, (2) by increasing the saturation of the fatty acyl tails of the phospholipid molecules, and (3) by increasing the membrane's cholesterol content (see Chapter 1 II A 2).

3. **C.** Integral proteins are not only closely associated with the lipid bilayer but also tightly bound to the cell membrane. These proteins frequently span the entire thickness of the plasmalemma and are thus termed transmembrane proteins (see Chapter 1 II B 1).

4. **C.** Active transport requires energy. Facilitated diffusion, which is mediated by membrane proteins, and simple diffusion, which involves passage of material directly across the lipid bilayer, are types of passive transport (see Chapter 1 III B).

5. **C.** Na^+ and other ions require channel (carrier) proteins for their transport across the plasma membrane. The other substances are small nonpolar molecules and small uncharged polar molecules. The molecules can traverse the plasma membrane by simple diffusion (see Chapter 1 III A 2).

6. **D.** The coupled transport of two different molecules in the same direction is termed "symport" (see Chapter 1 III B).

7. **B.** Cells can communicate with each other by releasing signaling molecules, which attach to receptor molecules on target cells (see Chapter 1 IV A).

8. **D.** G protein–linked receptors are sites where ACTH and some other signaling molecules attach. Binding of ACTH to its receptor causes G_s protein to activate adenylate cyclase, setting in motion the specific response elicited by the hormone (see Chapter 1 IV B 2 c).

9. **C.** Hereditary spherocytosis is caused by a defect in spectrin that renders the protein incapable of binding to band 4.1 protein, thus destabilizing the spectrin–actin complex of the cytoskeleton. Although defects in hemoglobin (the respiratory protein of erythrocytes) also cause red blood cell anomalies, hereditary spherocytosis is not one of them (see Chapter 1 V A).

10. **E.** Ankyrin is linked both to band 3 proteins and to spectrin tetramer, thus attaching the spectrin–actin complex to transmembrane proteins of the erythrocyte. There are two types of G proteins: trimeric and monomeric; glycocalyx (the sugar coat on the membrane surface) is composed mostly of polar carbohydrate residues; only carrier proteins can be energy requiring; gated channels are open only transiently (see Chapter 1 V A).

I. OVERVIEW—THE NUCLEUS (Figure 2.1)

A. **Structure.** The nucleus, the largest organelle of the cell, includes the **nuclear envelope, nucleolus, nucleoplasm**, and **chromatin** and contains the genetic material encoded in the **deoxyribonucleic acid (DNA)** of chromosomes.

B. **Function.** The nucleus directs protein synthesis in the cytoplasm via **ribosomal ribonucleic acid (rRNA), messenger RNA (mRNA)**, and **transfer RNA (tRNA)**. All types of RNAs, including **regulatory RNAs (noncoding RNAs)**, are synthesized in the nucleus.

II. NUCLEAR ENVELOPE

The nuclear envelope surrounds the nuclear material and consists of two parallel membranes separated from each other by a narrow perinuclear cisterna. These membranes fuse at intervals, forming openings called nuclear pores in the nuclear envelope.

A. **Outer nuclear membrane**
  1. This membrane is about 6 nanometers (nm) thick.
  2. It faces the cytoplasm and is continuous at certain sites with the rough endoplasmic reticulum (RER).
  3. A loosely arranged mesh of intermediate filaments (**vimentin**) surrounds the outer nuclear membrane on its cytoplasmic aspect.
  4. **Ribosomes** stud the cytoplasmic surface of the outer nuclear membrane. These ribosomes synthesize proteins that enter the perinuclear cisterna.

B. **Inner nuclear membrane**
  1. The inner nuclear membrane is also about 6 nm thick.
  2. It faces the nuclear material but is separated from it and is supported on its inner surface by the **nuclear lamina**, fibrous lamina that is 80 to 300 nm thick and composed primarily of **lamins A, B1, B2, and C**. These intermediate filament proteins form an orthogonal trellis that binds to transmembrane receptor molecules, such as **emerin** and various **lamina-associated polypeptides** traversing the inner nuclear membrane. The various lamins assist in organizing the nuclear envelope, directing the formation of nuclear pore complexes (NPCs), and the

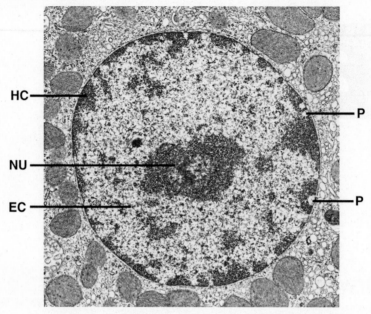

FIGURE 2.1. Electron micrograph of the cell nucleus. The nuclear envelope is interrupted by nuclear pores (P). The inactive heterochromatin (HC) is dense and mostly confined to the periphery of the nucleus. Euchromatin (EC), the active form, is less dense and is dispersed throughout. The nucleolus (NU) contains fibrillar and granular portions.

organization of perinuclear chromatin. In addition, they are essential during the mitotic events, when they are responsible for the ordered disassembly and reassembly of the nuclear envelope. Phosphorylation of lamins leads to disassembly, and dephosphorylation results in reassembly of the nuclear envelope.

C. Perinuclear cisterna
1. The **perinuclear cisterna** is located between the inner and outer nuclear membranes and is 20 to 40 nm wide.
2. It is continuous with the cisterna of the RER.
3. It is perforated by nuclear pores at various locations.

D. Nuclear pores
1. Nuclear pores average 80 nm in diameter and number from dozens to thousands, depending upon metabolic activity of the cell; they are associated with the NPC.
2. They are formed by fusion of the inner and outer nuclear membranes.
3. They permit passage of certain molecules in either direction between the nucleus and the cytoplasm via a 9-nm channel opening.
4. NPCs are aided in communicating with each other by the nuclear lamina.

E. The **NPC** represents protein subunits surrounding the nuclear pore (Figure 2.2).
1. **Structure.** The NPC is composed of nearly 100 proteins (jointly known as **nucleoporins**), some of which are arranged in eightfold symmetry around the margin of the pore. The nucleoplasmic side of the pore exhibits a nuclear basket, whereas the cytoplasmic side displays fibers extending into the cytoplasm. A transporter protein is located in the central core and is believed to be responsible for transporting proteins into and out of the nucleus via **receptor-mediated transport.**
    a. The **cytoplasmic ring**, located around the cytoplasmic margin of the nuclear pore, is composed of eight subunits, each possessing a **cytoplasmic filament** composed of a

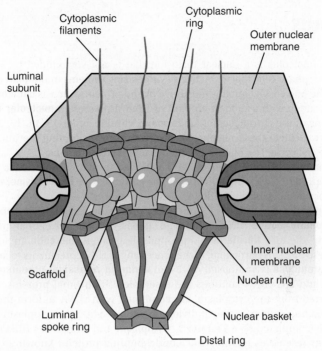

Cytoplasmic filaments

Cytoplasmic ring

Outer nuclear membrane

Luminal subunit

Inner nuclear membrane

Scaffold

Nuclear ring

Luminal spoke ring

Nuclear basket

Distal ring

FIGURE 2.2. The nuclear pore complex. (Copyright 1994 from *Molecular Biology of the Cell*, 3rd ed., by Alberts et al. Adapted with permission from Garland Science/Taylor & Francis LLC.)

Ran-binding protein (guanosine triphosphate [GTP]–binding protein) extending into the cytoplasm. These fibers may serve as a staging area prior to protein transport.

b. The **nucleoplasmic ring** is located around the nucleoplasmic margin of the nuclear pore and is composed of eight subunits. Extending from this ring into the nucleoplasm is a basket-like structure, the **nuclear basket**. Attached to the distal end of the nuclear basket is the **distal ring**. This innermost ring assists in the export of RNA into the cytoplasm.

c. The **luminal ring** is interposed between the cytoplasmic and nucleoplasmic rings. Eight transmembrane proteins project into the lumen of the nuclear pore, anchoring the complex into the pore rim. The lumen may be a gated channel that impedes passive diffusion. A moiety of each of these transmembrane proteins also projects into the perinuclear cistern.

d. A structure described by some as the hourglass-shaped **transporter** or central plug in the center of the luminal ring is believed to be material such as ribosomes or protein complexes that are being transported through the NPC rather than a structural component of the NPC. Thus, the transporter is now referred to as the **central plug**.

2. **Function.** The NPC permits passive movement across the nuclear envelope via a 9- to 11-nm open channel for simple diffusion. Most proteins, regardless of size, pass in either direction only by **receptor-mediated transport**. These proteins have clusters of certain amino acids known as **nuclear localization segments** that act as signals for transport.

3. **Transport mechanisms** involve a group of transporter proteins, **exportins** and **importins**. The function of these transporter proteins is regulated by **Ran**, a group of GTP-binding proteins. Transporter proteins recognize polypeptide sequences on the proteins that are to be transported in one direction or the other. Exportins recognize polypeptide sequences known as **nuclear export sequences** and export molecules bearing them into the cytoplasm, whereas importins recognize **nuclear localization sequences**, and facilitate their import into the nucleus. Transport signals of this type are called **nucleocytoplasmic shuttling signals**.

III. NUCLEOLUS

A. **Structure.** The nucleolus is a nuclear inclusion that is not surrounded by a membrane. It is observed in interphase cells that are actively synthesizing proteins; more than one nucleolus can be present in the nucleus. It contains mostly rRNA and proteins, such as **nucleostemin, nucleolin,** and **fibrillarin,** along with a modest amount of DNA. It possesses **nucleolar organizer regions (NORs),** portions of the chromosomes (in humans, chromosomes 13, 14, 15, 21, and 22) where rRNA genes are located; these regions are involved in reconstituting the nucleolus during the G_1 phase of the cell cycle. The nucleolus contains four distinct regions.

1. **Fibrillar centers** are composed of the NORs of the five chromosomes listed above, the ribonucleoprotein (RNP) **signal recognition particle,** and **RNA polymerase I,** the enzyme required for the transcription of rRNA.

2. The **pars fibrosa** is composed of 5-nm fibrils surrounding the fibrillar centers and contains **transcriptionally active DNA, ribosomal genes,** and a substantial quantity of rRNA. Additionally, the RNP **fibrillarin** and the phosphoproteins **nucleolin** are located in the pars fibrosa; these proteins participate in the processing of rRNA precursors to form mature rRNA.

3. The **pars granulosa** is composed of 15-nm **maturing ribosomal precursor** particles where 18S rRNA and 28S rRNA subunits are assembled. Ribosomal proteins, manufactured in and imported from the cytoplasm, are combined with rRNA to form the small and large ribosomal subunits that are then individually exported into the cytoplasm, where ribosomal assembly is completed (see Chapter 3, Cytoplasm and Organelles IIIB1a). Additionally, a protein that resembles guanine nucleotide–binding protein, known as **nucleostemin,** is located in the pars granulosa. Large quantities of this protein are present in cancer cells and stem cells because it functions in regulating the cell cycle and it also has a direct influence on cell differentiation.

4. **Nucleolar matrix** is a fiber network participating in the organization of the nucleolus.

B. **Function.** The nucleolus is involved in the synthesis of **rRNA** and its preliminary assembly into ribosome subunit precursors as well as in the primary processing of micro RNAs. The nucleolus also sequesters certain nucleolar proteins, such as nucleostemin, that function as cell cycle checkpoint signaling proteins. These cell cycle regulator proteins remain sequestered in the nucleolus until their release is required for targets in the nucleus and/or the cytoplasm. Following prophase of the cell cycle, the nucleolus disintegrates because the NORs of chromosomes 13, 14, 15, 21, and 22 are unavailable for transcription. Subsequent to telophase, the NORs unwind and facilitate the reconstitution of the nucleolus.

IV. NUCLEOPLASM

Nucleoplasm is the protoplasm within the nuclear envelope, in which the chromosomes and nucleoli are embedded. It is a viscous matrix composed mostly of water, whose viscosity is increased by the various types of macromolecules (some from the NPCs) and ions along with transcriptional processing apparatus that are suspended or dissolved in it. It is believed by most authors that the nucleoplasm is ordered by the presence of a cytoskeletal-like framework known as the **nuclear** matrix. Other authors dispute the presence of this structure.

A. **Nuclear matrix** acts as a scaffold that aids in organizing the nucleoplasm.

1. **Structural components** include fibrillar elements, nuclear pore–nuclear lamina complex, residual nucleoli, and a residual RNP network.

2. **Functional components** are involved in the transcription and processing of mRNA and rRNA, steroid receptor-binding sites, carcinogen-binding sites, heat shock proteins, DNA viruses, viral proteins (T antigen), and perhaps many other functions that are as yet not known.

3. A **nucleoplasmic reticulum** is continuous with the endoplasmic reticulum of the cytoplasm and the nuclear envelope. It contains nuclear calcium functioning within the nucleus and possesses receptors for inositol 1,4,5-triphosphate, regulating calcium signals within compartments of the nucleus related to gene transcription, protein transport, and perhaps other functions.

B. **Nuclear particles.**
   1. **Interchromatin granules** are clusters of irregularly distributed particles (20–25 nm in diameter) that contain RNP and various enzymes.
   2. **Perichromatin granules** (Figure 2.1) are single dense granules (30–50 nm in diameter) surrounded by a less dense **halo**. They are located at the periphery of heterochromatin and exhibit a substructure of 3-nm packed fibrils.
      a. Perichromatin granules contain 4.7S RNA and two peptides similar to those found in heterogeneous nuclear RNPs (hnRNPs).
      b. They may represent **messenger RNPs (mRNPs)**.
      c. The number of granules increases in liver cells exposed to carcinogens or temperatures above 37°C.
   3. The **hnRNP particles** are complexes of **precursor mRNA (pre-mRNA)** and proteins and are involved in processing of pre-mRNA.
   4. **Small nuclear RNPs (snRNPs)** are complexes of proteins and **small RNAs** and are involved in hnRNP splicing or in cleavage reactions.

V. CHROMATIN (Figure 2.1)

A. **Structure.** Chromatin consists of DNA double helix complexed with **histones** and **nonhistone proteins**. It resides within the nucleus as heterochromatin and euchromatin. The euchromatin/heterochromatin ratio is higher in malignant cells than in normal cells.
   1. **Heterochromatin** is chromatin that is condensed because it is not being transcribed and comprises approximately 90% of the total chromatin in the cell. It is formed from euchromatin that is folded into 30-nm-thick filaments.
      a. When examined under the light microscope (LM), it appears as basophilic clumps of nucleoprotein.
      b. Although **transcriptionally inactive**, recent evidence indicates that heterochromatin functions in maintaining the integrity of chromosomal centromeres and telomeres and, during meiosis, it also has a role in interchromosomal interactions and chromosomal segregation.
      c. Heterochromatin corresponds to **one of two X chromosomes** and is therefore present in nearly all somatic cells of female mammals. During interphase, the inactive X chromosome, referred to as the **Barr body** (or **sex chromatin**), is visible as a dark-staining body within the nucleus.
   2. **Euchromatin**, constituting approximately 10% of the total chromatin, is **transcriptionally active** and appears in light micrographs as a lightly stained region of the nucleus. Viewed with the transmission electron microscope (TEM), euchromatin appears as electron-lucent regions among heterochromatins and is composed of 10-nm strings of nucleosomes (see Sections VI and VII in this chapter).

B. **Function.** Chromatin has several functions that include
   1. folding of the DNA strand into small enough volume to be able to contain it within the nucleus of the cell;
   2. protecting the DNA from physical damage during and between cell divisions;
   3. controlling the activity of DNA, that is, permitting or preventing its transcription;
   4. controlling the precise duplication of the DNA in preparation for cell division;
   5. facilitating the repair of DNA in case of replication error or due to physical or chemical insult.

VI. CHROMOSOMES

A. **Structure.** Chromosomes consist of chromatin extensively folded into loops; this conformation is maintained by DNA-binding proteins (Figure 2.3). Each chromosome contains a long DNA molecule and associated proteins, assembled into **nucleosomes**, the structural unit of chromatin packaging. Each nucleosome has a **core** of eight **histones** (**histone octamers**) and the **DNA double helix** is wrapped around the histone octamers in such a fashion that it makes two spiral turns. Since the DNA double helix is extremely long, it connects a huge number of histone octamers to each other. The DNA double helix between adjacent histone octamers is not associated with histones and appears as if it were a thin string that connects neighboring histone octamers to each other; therefore, these connecting regions of the DNA double helix are known as **linker DNA**. Chromosomes are visible with the LM only during mitosis and meiosis, when their chromatin **condenses**; otherwise, the chromatin is **extended** and is not visible by light microscopy.

1. **Extended chromatin** is formed by adjacent **nucleosomes**. Each nucleosome core is around which the DNA double helix is wrapped two full turns.

   a. The **nucleosome core** consists of two copies each of **histones H2A, H2B, H3**, and **H4**. Nucleosomes are spaced at intervals of 200 base pairs.

   b. When viewed with TEM, extended chromatin resembles beads on a string; the beads represent **nucleosomes**, and the string between adjacent nucleosomes represents **linker DNA**. Nucleosomes support DNA and regulate its accessibility for replication and transcription as well as for its repair.

2. **Condensed chromatin** contains an additional histone, **H1**, which wraps around groups of nucleosomes, thus forming 30-nm-diameter filaments of helical coils of six nucleosomes per turn, which is the structural unit of the chromosome.

B. **G-banding** is observed in chromosomes during mitosis after staining with Giemsa, which is specific for DNA sequences rich in **adenine** (A) and **thymine** (T). Banding is thought to represent highly

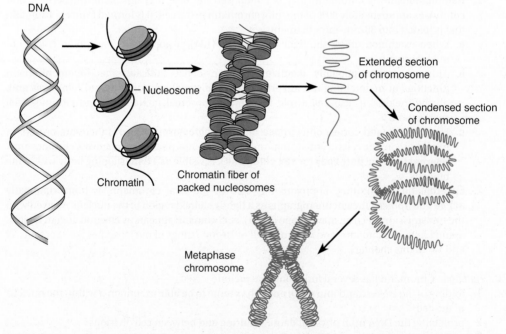

FIGURE 2.3. The packaging of chromatin into the condensed metaphase chromosome. Nucleosomes contain two copies of histones H2A, H2B, H3, and H4 in extended chromatin. An additional histone, H1, is present in condensed chromatin. DNA, deoxyribonucleic acid. (Adapted with permission from Widnell CC, Pfenninger KH. *Essential Cell Biology.* Baltimore, MD: Williams & Wilkins; 1990:47.)

folded DNA loops. G-banding is characteristic for each species and is used to identify particular chromosomes and chromosomal anomalies.

C. **Karyotype** refers to the **number and morphology of chromosomes** and is characteristic for each species.
   1. **Haploid number** (n) is the number of chromosomes in germ cells (23 in humans).
   2. **Diploid number** (2n) is the number of chromosomes in somatic cells (46 in humans).

D. The total genetic complement of an individual is stored in its chromosomes. In humans, the genome consists of 22 pairs of **autosomes** and 1 pair of **sex chromosomes** (either **XX** or **XY**), totaling 23 homologous pairs, or 46 chromosomes.

E. Each chromosome is composed of two **chromatids** joined together at a small point called the centromere.

VII. DNA

DNA is a long double-stranded helical linear molecule composed of multiple nucleotide sequences. It stores the individual's genetic information and acts as a **template for the synthesis of RNA**. The complete nucleotide sequences of a human are located in the 46 chromosomes of each cell and if stretched out and placed end to end it would measure almost 6 ft in length.

A. **Nucleotides** are composed of a base (purine or pyrimidine), a deoxyribose sugar, and a phosphate group.
   1. The **purines** are **adenine** (A) and **guanine** (G).
   2. The **pyrimidines** are **cytosine** (C) and **thymine** (T).

B. The **DNA double helix** consists of **two complementary DNA strands** held together by hydrogen bonds between the base pairs A–T and G–C.

C. **Exons** are regions of the DNA molecule that **code** for specific RNAs.

D. **Introns** are regions of the DNA molecule, between exons, that **do not code** for RNAs.

E. **A codon** is a sequence of **three bases** in the DNA molecule that codes for a **single amino acid**.

F. **A gene** is a segment of the DNA molecule, located in a specific region of a chromosome. It is responsible not only for the formation of a single RNA molecule but also for the regulatory sequences that control the expression of a particular trait. In certain viruses, a gene may be composed of RNA rather than DNA.

G. **A genome** is the complete set of hereditary information that an individual possesses. These are classified into two categories, **genes** and **noncoding segments** of the DNA (or RNA in some viruses). In fact, only about 2% of the genome is composed of genes (which code for proteins/polypeptides), whereas most of the remainder is noncoding, in that they do not code for proteins/polypeptides but possess regulatory or other functions.

CLINICAL CONSIDERATIONS **Oncogenes** are the result of **mutations of certain regulatory genes**, called **proto-oncogenes**, which normally stimulate or inhibit cell proliferation and development.

1. Genetic accidents or viruses may lead to the formation of oncogenes.
2. Whatever be their origin, oncogenes dominate the normal alleles (proto-oncogenes), causing **deregulation** of cell division, which leads to a cancerous state.
3. Bladder cancer and acute myelogenous leukemia are caused by oncogenes.

VIII. RNA

RNA is a linear molecule similar to DNA; however, it is single stranded and contains **riboses** instead of **deoxyribose sugar** and **uracil** (U) instead of **thymine** (T). RNA is synthesized by **transcription** of DNA. Transcription is catalyzed by three **RNA polymerases**: I for rRNA, II for mRNA, and III for tRNA. Some of the noncoding segments of DNA are transcribed to form transfer RNA (tRNA), ribosomal RNA (rRNA), as well as regulatory RNAs. Moreover, other RNAs can act as enzymes, such as ribozymes that catalyze the formation of peptide bonds during protein synthesis.

A. **mRNA** carries the genetic code to the cytoplasm to direct **protein synthesis** (Figure 2.4).
   1. This single-stranded molecule consists of hundreds to thousands of nucleotides.

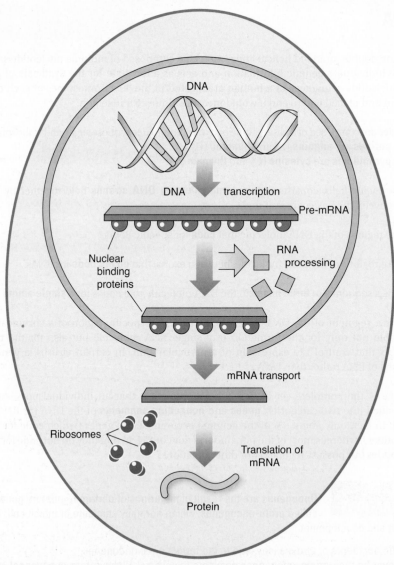

FIGURE 2.4. Steps by which genetic information encoded in deoxyribonucleic acid (DNA) is transcribed into messenger ribonucleic acid (mRNA) and ultimately converted into proteins in the cytoplasm. (Copyright 1994 from *Molecular Biology of the Cell*, 3rd ed., by Alberts et al. Adapted with permission from Garland Science/Taylor & Francis LLC.)

2. mRNA contains codons that are **complementary** to the DNA codons from which it was transcribed, including one **start codon (AUG)** for **initiating** protein synthesis and one of three **stop codons** (**UAA, UAG,** or **UGA**) for **terminating** protein synthesis.

3. mRNA is synthesized in the following series of steps.

   a. **RNA polymerase II** recognizes a **promoter** on a single strand of the DNA molecule and binds tightly to it.

   b. The DNA helix unwinds about two turns, separating the DNA strands and exposing the **codons** that act as the template for synthesis of the complementary RNA molecule.

   c. RNA polymerase II moves along the DNA strand and promotes base pairing between DNA and complementary RNA nucleotides.

   d. When RNA polymerase II recognizes a **chain terminator** (stop codons—**UAA, UAG,** or **UGA**) on the DNA molecule, it terminates its association with the DNA and is released to repeat transcription.

   e. The primary transcript, **pre-mRNA** after the introns are removed, associates with proteins to form **hnRNP**.

   f. Exons are spliced through several steps, involving **spliceosomes** producing an **mRNP**.

   g. Proteins are removed as the mRNP enters the cytoplasm, resulting in **functional mRNA**.

   h. RNA segments remaining from the transcription process as introns were once thought to be degraded and recycled because they were believed to have no function. However, recent evidence shows that these RNA segments may become modified to perform regulatory functions that parallel regulatory proteins related to development, gene expression, and evolution.

B. **tRNA** is folded into a cloverleaf shape and contains approximately 80 nucleotides, terminating in adenylic acid (where amino acids attach).

   1. Each tRNA combines with a specific amino acid that has been activated by an enzyme.

   2. One end of the tRNA molecule possesses an **anticodon**, a triplet of nucleotides that recognizes the complementary codon in mRNA. If recognition occurs, the anticodon ensures that the tRNA transfers its activated amino acid molecule in the proper sequence to the growing polypeptide chain.

C. **Ribosomal RNA** associates with many different proteins (including enzymes) to form **ribosomes**.

   1. rRNA associates with mRNA and tRNA during protein synthesis.

   2. rRNA synthesis takes place in the nucleolus and is catalyzed by RNA polymerase I. A single **45S precursor rRNA (pre-rRNA)** is formed and **processed to form ribosomes** as follows (Figure 2.5):

      a. Pre-rRNA associates with ribosomal proteins and is cleaved into the three sizes (28S, 18S, and 5.8S) of rRNAs present in ribosomes.

      b. The **RNP** containing 28S and 5.8S rRNA then combines with 5S rRNA, which is synthesized outside of the nucleolus, to form the **large subunit** of the ribosome.

      c. The RNP containing 18S rRNA forms the **small subunit** of the ribosome.

D. Regulatory RNAs include micro RNA (miRNA), large intergenic noncoding RNA (lincRNA), and small interfering RNAs (siRNAs).

   1. **MicroRNAs (miRNAs)**, first discovered in the roundworm in the 1990s, are very small segments of single-stranded RNA molecules of only 19 to 25 nucleotides in length that function to regulate gene expression. Although miRNAs are transcribed from DNA, they are noncoding and are not translated into proteins. Recent research demonstrated the presence of a diverse population of more than 1,000 human miRNAs that regulate developmental and physiological processes. Some miRNAs methylate specific regions of the DNA, thus preventing transcription from taking place, whereas other miRNAs insert into a matching portion of the mRNA strand, which prevents the translation of the mRNA; thus, the miRNA acts to regulate gene expression. It has been estimated that miRNAs may regulate a third or more of human genes. Because each miRNA can control hundreds of gene targets, they may influence most genetic pathways. In addition to functioning in gene expression, miRNAs also act as "central switchboards" of signaling networks that control stem cell homeostasis as well as various disease processes such as fibrosis, metastasis, and the biology of malignant cells.

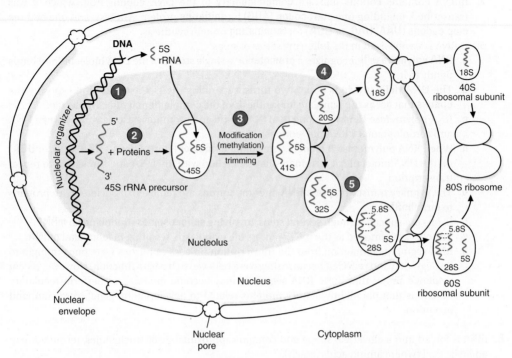

FIGURE 2.5. Formation of ribosomal ribonucleic acid (rRNA) and its processing into ribosomal subunits, which occurs in the nucleolus. (Reprinted with permission from Swanson et al. *BRS Biochemistry, Molecular Biology, and Genetics.* 5th ed. Baltimore, MD: Wolters Kluwer Health/Lippincott Williams & Wilkins; 2009:265.)

2. **Large intergenic noncoding RNAs (lincRNAs)**, more than 200 nucleotides in length, also function in gene regulation. Since each cell of a female possesses two X chromosomes, one of the X chromosomes is transcribed to form lincRNAs that specifically coat that particular X chromosome and prevents the transcription of its genes. Other lincRNAs prevent the transcription of various genes on different chromosomes. Still other lincRNAs compete with certain mRNAs for miRNAs, thereby acting as decoys that protect the mRNAs from the inhibitory actions of miRNAs and facilitating the translation of the mRNA to synthesize a particular protein.

3. **Small interfering RNAs (siRNAs)** are similar to miRNAs; they are 19 to 25 nucleotides in length, but they frequently arise from the genome of RNA viruses that infect a cell (although some siRNAs are transcribed from the cell's own genome). They resemble miRNAs in their mode of action in that they also methylate specific regions of the DNA and thus interfere with the process of transcription.

CLINICAL CONSIDERATIONS **miRNAs** have been shown to repress certain cancer-related genes. Additionally, miRNAs are known to depress angiogenesis, which may become useful in clinically restricting cancer growth. Thus, it is expected that miRNAs may prove useful in the diagnosis and treatment of cancer. Certain other miRNAs appear have been shown to regulate differentiation (i.e., repressing adipocyte formation, an understanding that may lead to a clinical treatment modality for obesity). Still other miRNAs repress certain cancer-related genes, such as lung cancer where human lung cancer cells treated with miRNA had reduced the rate of their proliferation, slowed greatly their capability to migrate, and reduced their invasive abilities. Additionally, the treated cells had a greater rate of apoptosis; thus, it is expected that miRNAs may prove useful in the diagnosis and treatment of cancer.

IX. CELL CYCLE (Figure 2.6)

A. **The cell cycle** varies in length in different types of cells, but is repeated each time a cell divides. It is composed of not only the series of events that prepare the cell to divide into two daughter cells but the process of cell division as well.

1. It is **temporarily suspended** in nondividing resting cells (e.g., peripheral lymphocytes), which are in the **gap outside phase** (**G$_0$ phase**). Such cells may reenter the cycle and begin to divide again.

2. It is **permanently interrupted** in differentiated cells that do not divide (e.g., most cardiac muscle cells and neurons).

B. Two major periods comprise the cell cycle: **interphase** (interval between cell divisions) and **M phase** (**mitosis,** the period of cell division).

1. **Interphase** is considerably longer than the M phase and is the period during which **the cell doubles in size and DNA content**.

a. Interphase is divided into three separate phases (**G$_1$, S**, and **G$_2$**) during which specific cellular functions occur.

(1) **G$_1$ phase (gap one phase)** lasts for hours to several days.

(a) Occurring after mitosis, it is the period during which the cell grows and proteins are synthesized, restoring the daughter cells to normal volume and size.

(b) Certain trigger proteins are synthesized; these proteins enable the cell to reach a threshold (**restriction point**) and proceed to the S phase. Cells that fail to reach the restriction point become resting cells and enter the **G$_0$ phase** (gap outside phase), where they may remain for a few days, months, or years eventually to reenter the cell cycle or remain in the G$_0$ phase permanently (see above).

(2) **S phase (synthetic phase)** lasts 8 to 12 hours in most cells.

(a) DNA is replicated, and histone and non-histone proteins are synthesized, resulting in **duplication of the chromosomes**.

(b) Centrosomes are also duplicated.

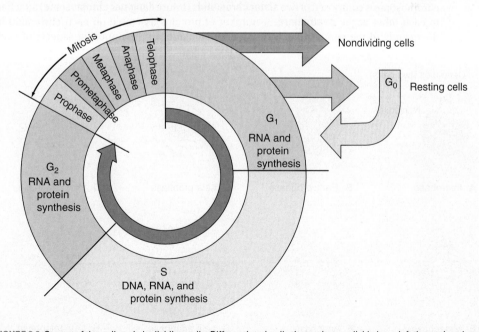

FIGURE 2.6. Stages of the cell cycle in dividing cells. Differentiated cells that no longer divide have left the cycle, whereas resting cells in the G$_0$ state may reenter the cycle and begin dividing again. (Adapted with permission from Widnell CC, Pfenninger KH. *Essential Cell Biology*. Baltimore, MD: Williams & Wilkins; 1990:58.)

    (3) G_2 phase (gap two phase) lasts 2 to 4 hours.

      (a) This phase follows the S phase and extends to mitosis.

      (b) Centrioles duplicate, and each gives rise to a new, daughter centriole; the cell prepares to divide as the energy required for the completion of mitosis is stored; and RNA and proteins necessary for mitosis are synthesized, including tubulin for the spindle apparatus.

  b. Several **control factors** have been identified. These include a category of proteins known as **cyclins** as well as **cyclin-dependent kinases (CDKs)**, which initiate and/or induce progression through the cell cycle.

    (1) During the G_1 phase, **cyclins D and E** bind to their respective CDKs; these complexes enable the cell to enter and advance through the **S phase**. During both the G_1 phase and the S phase, DNA replication is monitored and if errors are detected the cell cycle cannot continue until the errors are corrected. These are known as the **G_1 DNA damage checkpoint** and the **S DNA damage checkpoint**, respectively.

    (2) Cyclin A binds to its CDKs, thus enabling the cell to leave the **S phase** and enter the **G_2 phase** as well as to manufacture **cyclin B**. There are two further DNA checkpoints in the G_2 phase; one is the **unreplicated DNA checkpoint** that cannot be passed unless all of the DNA was replicated in the S phase, and the **G_2 damage checkpoint** that prevents the continuation of the G_2 phase if errors are present in the replicated DNA.

    (3) Cyclin B binds to its CDK, inducing the cell to leave the **G_2 phase** and enter the **M phase**. In the beginning of the M phase, the spindle apparatus is monitored, and if the spindle assembly is faulty the cell cannot leave the M phase. This is referred to as the **spindle assembly checkpoint**. Near the termination of the M phase, the condition of the chromosomes is monitored, and if any of the chromosomes are "sticking" to each other, the cell is not permitted to leave the M phase. This is referred to as the **chromosome segregation checkpoint**.

2. **Mitosis** (Figure 2.7; Table 2.1) lasts 1 to 3 hours. It follows the G_2 phase and completes the cell cycle. It includes segregation of the replicated chromosomes, division of the nucleus (**karyokinesis**), and finally division of the cytoplasm (**cytokinesis**), resulting in the production of two **identical** daughter cells. It consists of five major stages.

  a. **Prophase** begins when the duplicated chromosomes condense and become visible. Each chromosome is composed of two **sister chromatids** (future **daughter chromosome**) attached to each other at the **centromere**. A number of proteins assemble on each chromatid in the vicinity of the centromere, forming a **kinetochore** on the opposing aspects of each

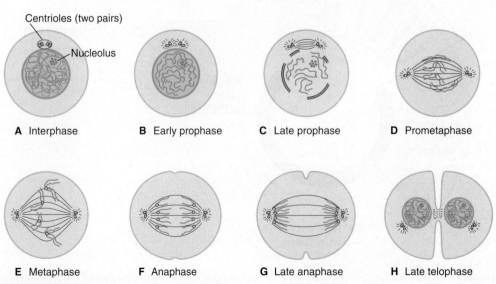

A Interphase   **B** Early prophase   **C** Late prophase   **D** Prometaphase

E Metaphase   **F** Anaphase   **G** Late anaphase   **H** Late telophase

FIGURE 2.7. Events in various phases of mitosis. (Redrawn with permission from Kelly DE, Wood RL, Enders AC. *Bailey's Textbook of Microscopic Anatomy.* 18th ed. Baltimore, MD: Williams & Wilkins; 1984:89.)

t a b l e **2.1** Stages of Mitosis		
Stage	DNA Content	Identifying Characteristics
Prophase (early)	DNA content doubles in the S phase of interphase (4n); also, centrioles replicate	Nuclear envelope and nucleolus begin to disappear. Chromosomes condense; they consist of two sister chromatids attached at centromere.
Prophase (late)		Centrioles migrate to opposite poles and give rise to spindle fibers and astral rays.
Prometaphase	Double complement of DNA (4n)	Nuclear envelope disappears. Kinetochores develop at centromeres, and kinetochore microtubules form.
Metaphase	Double complement of DNA (4n)	Maximally condensed chromosomes align at the equatorial plate of the mitotic spindle.
Anaphase	Double complement of DNA (4n)	Daughter chromatids separate at centromere.
Anaphase (late)		Each chromatid migrates to an opposite pole of the cell along the microtubule (karyokinesis). A cleavage furrow begins to form.
Telophase	Each new daughter cell contains a single complement of DNA (2n)	The furrow (midbody) now deepens between the newly formed daughter cells (cytokinesis). Nuclear envelope reforms, nucleoli reappear, chromosomes disperse forming new interphase nucleus

chromatid. Thus, there will be two kinetochores, one on each chromatid, facing opposite poles of the cell. During prophase, the nucleolus and nuclear envelope begin to dissipate.

(1) The **centrosome** contains **centrioles** and a pericentriolar cloud of material containing γ-**tubulin rings**. It is the principal **microtubule-organizing center (MTOC)** of the cell. As centrosomes migrate to opposite poles of the cell, they set up two MTOCs, one at each pole of the dividing cell, and each MTOC gives rise to three sets of microtubules that will compose the **spindle apparatus** of the cell: **Astral microtubules** arise from the MTOCs in a spoke-like fashion and they ensure that the MTOCs maintain their correct location at the opposite poles of the cell near the cell membrane, and in this fashion astral microtubules facilitate the proper orientation of the spindle apparatus. **Polar microtubules** arise from each MTOC, grow toward each other, and meet near the equator of the cell. They function in ensuring that the two MTOCs are kept apart from each other and maintain their respective locations. **Kinetochore microtubules** emanate from each MTOC and grow toward the chromosomes. Once they reach each chromosome, they attach to the kinetochores of the sister chromatids and, during anaphase, begin the process of dragging sister chromatids to opposing poles of the cell.

b. Prometaphase begins when the nuclear envelope disappears, allowing the chromosomes to disperse apparently randomly in the cytoplasm. Sister chromatids are held together by **cohesisn**, a group of binding proteins, and their compressed condition is maintained by the proteins **condensin**.

c. Metaphase is the phase during which the duplicated condensed chromosomes align at the equatorial plate of the mitotic spindle and become attached to kinetochore microtubules at their kinetochore. If this connection is not stable, **anaphase-promoting complex** interferes with cyclin E, and the cell cannot progress through metaphase.

d. Anaphase begins as sister chromatids separate at the centromere and daughter chromosomes move to the opposite poles of the cell.

(1) The spindle elongates.

(2) In the later stages of anaphase, a **cleavage furrow** begins to form around the cell as the **contractile ring**, a band of actin filaments, contracts.

e. Telophase is characterized by each set of chromosomes reaching the pole, a deepening of the cleavage furrow; the **midbody** (containing overlapping polar microtubules) is now between the newly forming daughter cells.

(1) Microtubules in the midbody are depolymerized, facilitating **cytokinesis** and formation of two identical daughter cells.

(2) The **nuclear envelope** is reestablished around the condensed chromosomes in the daughter cells, and **nucleoli reappear**. Nucleoli arise from the specific **nucleolar organizing regions** (called secondary constriction sites), which are carried on five separate chromosomes in humans (see Section III Nucleolus in this chapter).

(3) The daughter nuclei gradually enlarge, and the condensed chromosomes disperse to form the typical interphase nucleus with heterochromatin and euchromatin.

(4) It appears that at the end of cytokinesis the mother centriole of the duplicated pair moves from the newly forming nuclear pole to the intercellular bridge. This event is necessary to initiate disassembly of the midbody microtubules and complete the separation of the daughter cells. If this event fails, DNA replication is arrested at one of the G_1 checkpoints during the next interphase.

CLINICAL CONSIDERATIONS   **Transformed cells**

1. Transformed cells have lost their ability to respond to regulatory signals controlling the cell cycle, and by this, they may undergo cell division indefinitely, thus becoming cancerous.
2. **Vinca alkaloids** may arrest these cells in mitosis, whereas drugs that block purine and pyrimidine synthesis may arrest these cells in the S phase of the cell cycle.

X. APOPTOSIS (PROGRAMMED CELL DEATH)

Apoptosis is programmed cell death whereby cells are removed from tissues in an orderly fashion as a part of normal maintenance or during development.

A. Cells that undergo programmed cell death have several **morphological features**.
   1. They include chromatin condensation, breaking up of the nucleus, and blebbing of the plasma membrane.
   2. The cell shrinks and is fragmented into membrane-enclosed fragments called **apoptotic bodies**.

B. Apoptotic cells do not pose a threat to surrounding cells, because changes in their plasma membranes make them subject to rapid phagocytosis by macrophages and by neighboring cells. Macrophages that phagocytose apoptotic cells do not release cytokines that initiate the inflammatory response.

   Further, apoptotic cells may be inhibited by several survival factors produced by certain cells, growth factors, hormones, proteins, etc.

C. The signals that induce apoptosis may occur through several mechanisms.
   1. Genes that code for enzymes, called **caspases**, play an important role in the process.
   2. Certain cytokines, such as **tumor necrosis factor**, may also activate caspases that degrade regulatory and structural proteins in the nucleus and cytoplasm, leading to the morphological changes characteristic of apoptosis.

D. Defects in the process of programmed cell death contribute to many major diseases.
   1. Excessive apoptosis causes extensive nerve cell loss in Alzheimer disease and stroke.
   2. Insufficient apoptosis has been linked to cancer and other autoimmune diseases.

XI. MEIOSIS (Figure 2.8)

A. **Meiosis** is a special form of cell division in germ cells (oogonia and spermatozoa) in which the **chromosome number** is reduced from **diploid (2n)** to **haploid (n)**. These events are accomplished via two reduction divisions.
   1. This occurs in developing germ cells in preparation for sexual reproduction. Subsequent fertilization results in **diploid zygotes**.
   2. DNA content of the original diploid cell is doubled (4n) in the S phase preparatory to meiosis.
      a. This phase is followed by two successive cell divisions that give rise to **four haploid cells**.
      b. In addition, **recombination** of maternal and paternal genes occurs by **crossing over** and **random assortment**, yielding the unique haploid genome of the gamete.

B. The **stages of meiosis** are meiosis I (reductional division) and meiosis II (equatorial division).
   1. **Reductional division (meiosis I)** occurs after interphase during the cell cycle, when the DNA content is duplicated, whereas the chromosome number (46) remains unchanged, giving the cell a **4CDNA content** (considered to be the total DNA content of the cell).

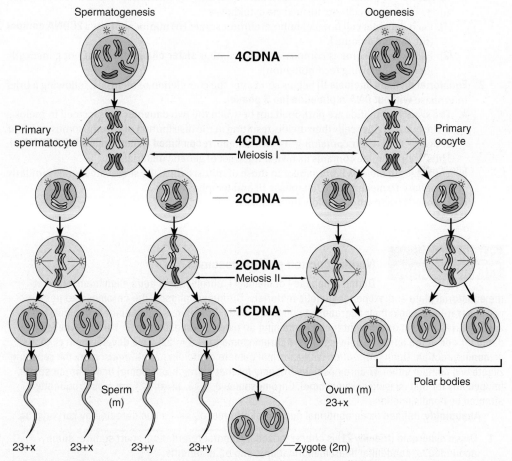

FIGURE 2.8. Meiosis in men and women. Spermatogenesis in the male gives rise to sperm, each containing the haploid number of chromosomes. Oogenesis in the female gives rise to an ovum with the haploid number of chromosomes. Fertilization reconstitutes the diploid number of chromosomes in the resulting zygote. (Adapted with permission from Widnell CC, Pfenninger KH. *Essential Cell Biology.* Baltimore, MD: Williams & Wilkins; 1990:69.)

    a. Prophase I is divided into five stages (leptotene, zygotene, pachytene, diplotene, and diakinesis), which accomplish the following events:

      (1) Chromatin condenses into the visible chromosomes, each containing two chromatids joined at the centromere.

      (2) Homologous maternal and paternal chromosomes pair via the **synaptonemal complex**, forming a **tetrad. Crossing over** (random exchanging of genes between segments of homologous chromosomes) occurs at the **chiasmata**, thus **increasing genetic diversity**.

      (3) The nucleolus and nuclear envelope disappear.

    b. Metaphase I

      (1) Homologous pairs of chromosomes align on the equatorial plate of the spindle in a random arrangement, facilitating genetic mixing.

      (2) Spindle fibers from either pole attach to the **kinetochore** of any one of the chromosome pairs, thus ensuring genetic mixing.

    c. Anaphase I

      (1) This phase is similar to anaphase in mitosis except in mitosis the two chromatids are pulled apart and each is delivered to each pole of the cell, whereas in anaphase I of meiosis the four chromatids are separated in such a fashion that **two chromatids** remain held together as they are being pulled to each pole of the cell.

      (2) Chromosomes migrate to the poles.

    d. Telophase I is similar to telophase in mitosis in that the nuclear envelope is reestablished and two daughter cells are formed via cytokinesis.

      (1) Each daughter cell now contains 23 chromosomes (n) number but has a **2CDNA content** (the diploid amount).

      (2) Each chromosome is composed of **two** similar **sister chromatids** (but not genetically identical following recombination).

  2. Equatorial division (meiosis II) begins soon after the completion of meiosis I, following a brief interphase **without DNA replication (no S phase)**.

    a. The sister chromatids are portioned out between the two daughter cells formed in meiosis I. The two daughter cells then divide, resulting in the distribution of chromosomes into four daughter cells, each containing its own **unique recombined genetic material (1CDNA;n)**. Thus, every gamete contains its own unique set of genetic materials.

    b. The stages of meiosis II are similar to those of mitosis; thus, the stages are named similarly (prophase II, metaphase II, anaphase II, and telophase II).

    c. Meiosis II occurs more rapidly than mitosis.

CLINICAL CONSIDERATIONS   **Nondisjunction of Chromosomes**

    During prophase I of meiosis I, chromosome pairs align themselves at the equatorial plate and exchange genetic materials. During anaphase I, the chromosome pairs will separate and begin their migrations to opposite poles. Sometimes, the members of a pair fail to separate, resulting in one daughter cell containing an extra chromosome (n + 1 = 24), whereas the daughter cell at the opposite pole is minus a chromosome (n − 1 = 22). This development is known as **nondisjunction.** Upon fertilization with a normal gamete containing 23 chromosomes, the resulting zygote will contain either 47 chromosomes (trisomy for that extra chromosome) or 45 chromosomes (monosomy for that missing chromosome). Chromosomes 8, 9, 13, 18, and 21 are most frequently affected by nondisjunction.

    Aneuploidy, defined as an abnormal number of chromosomes, can be detected by karyotyping.

1. **Down syndrome (trisomy 21)** is characterized by mental retardation, short stature, stubby appendages, congenital heart malformations, and other defects.
2. **Klinefelter syndrome (XXY)** is aneuploidy of the sex chromosomes, characterized by infertility, variable degrees of masculinization, and small testes.
3. **Turner syndrome (XO)** is **monosomy** of the sex chromosomes, characterized by short stature, sterility, and various other abnormalities.

Review Test

Directions: Each of the numbered items or incomplete statements in this section is followed by answers or by completions of the statement. Select the ONE lettered answer or completion that is BEST in each case.

1. The nuclear pore complex
   - **(A)** permits free communication between the nucleus and the cytoplasm.
   - **(B)** is bridged by a unit membrane.
   - **(C)** is located only at specific nuclear pore sites.
   - **(D)** permits passage of proteins via receptor-mediated transport.
   - **(E)** has a luminal ring that faces the cytoplasm.

2. Which one of the following nucleotides is present only in RNA?
   - **(A)** Thymine
   - **(B)** Adenine
   - **(C)** Uracil
   - **(D)** Cytosine
   - **(E)** Guanine

3. Anticodons are located in
   - **(A)** mRNA.
   - **(B)** rRNA.
   - **(C)** tRNA.
   - **(D)** snRNP.
   - **(E)** hnRNP.

4. DNA is duplicated in the cell cycle during the
   - **(A)** G_2 phase.
   - **(B)** S phase.
   - **(C)** M phase.
   - **(D)** G_1 phase.
   - **(E)** G_0 phase.

5. A male child at puberty is determined to have Klinefelter syndrome. Although the parents have been informed of the clinical significance, they have asked for an explanation of what happened. Identify the item that should be discussed with the parents.
   - **(A)** Trisomy of chromosome 21
   - **(B)** Loss of an autosome during mitosis
   - **(C)** Loss of the Y chromosome during meiosis
   - **(D)** Nondisjunction of the X chromosome
   - **(E)** Loss of the X chromosome

6. Which one of the following is an inclusion not bounded by a membrane that is observable only during interphase?
   - **(A)** Nuclear pore complex
   - **(B)** Nucleolus
   - **(C)** Heterochromatin
   - **(D)** Outer nuclear membrane
   - **(E)** Euchromatin

7. A structure that is continuous with RER is the
   - **(A)** nuclear pore complex.
   - **(B)** nucleolus.
   - **(C)** heterochromatin.
   - **(D)** outer nuclear membrane.
   - **(E)** euchromatin.

8. Identify the structure that controls movement of proteins in and out of the nucleus.
   - **(A)** Nuclear pore complex
   - **(B)** Nucleolus
   - **(C)** Heterochromatin
   - **(D)** Outer nuclear membrane
   - **(E)** Euchromatin

9. The site of transcriptional activity is the
   - **(A)** nuclear pore complex.
   - **(B)** nucleolus.
   - **(C)** heterochromatin.
   - **(D)** outer nuclear membrane.
   - **(E)** euchromatin.

10. Clumps of nucleoprotein concentrated near the periphery of the nucleus are called
   - **(A)** nuclear pore complex.
   - **(B)** nucleolus.
   - **(C)** heterochromatin.
   - **(D)** outer nuclear membrane.
   - **(E)** euchromatin.

Answers and Explanations

1. **D.** The NPC contains a central aqueous channel that permits passage of small water-soluble molecules. However, movement of proteins in and out of the nucleus is selectively controlled by the NPC via receptor-mediated transport (see Chapter 2 II E).

2. **C.** DNA contains the purines, adenine and guanine, and the pyrimidines, cytosine and thymine. In RNA, uracil, a pyrimidine, replaces thymine (see Chapter 2 VII A, VIII).

3. **C.** Each tRNA possesses a triplet of nucleotides, called an anticodon, which recognizes the complementary codon in mRNA (see Chapter 2 VIII B).

4. **B.** The S (synthesis) phase of the cell cycle is the period during which DNA replication and histone synthesis occur, resulting in duplication of the chromosomes. At the end of the S phase, each chromosome consists of two identical chromatids attached to one another at the centromere (see Chapter 2 IX B).

5. **D.** Klinefelter syndrome occurs only in men. This condition results from nondisjunction of the X chromosome during meiosis, resulting in an extra X chromosome in somatic cells. These cells therefore have a normal complement of autosomal chromosomes (22 pairs), and instead of one pair of sex chromosomes (XY), there is an extra X chromosome. These individuals have an XXY genotype, resulting in 47 total chromosomes rather than the normal complement of 46. This syndrome is an example of trisomy of the sex chromosomes. Down syndrome is an example of an autosomal trisomy, specifically trisomy of chromosome number 21. Both syndromes have profound complications (see Chapter 2 XI B Clinical Considerations).

6. **B.** The nucleolus is an inclusion, not bounded by a membrane, within the nucleus. It is observable during interphase but disappears during mitosis (see Chapter 2 III A).

7. **D.** The outer nuclear membrane is continuous with the RER (see Chapter 2 II A).

8. **A.** The NPC selectively controls movements of water-soluble molecules and proteins in and out of the nucleus (see Chapter 2 II E).

9. **E.** The pale-staining euchromatin is the transcriptionally active chromatin in the nucleus (see Chapter 2 V A).

10. **C.** Heterochromatin is the dark-staining nucleoprotein near the periphery of the nucleus. It is transcriptionally inactive, but may be responsible for proper chromosome segregation during meiosis (see Chapter 2 V A).

3 Cytoplasm and Organelles

I. OVERVIEW—THE CYTOPLASM

The cytoplasm contains three main structural components: **organelles, inclusions**, and the **cytoskeleton**. The fluid component is called the cytosol. The functional interactions among certain organelles result in the uptake and release of material by the cell, protein synthesis, and intracellular digestion.

II. STRUCTURAL COMPONENTS

A. **Organelles** (Figure 3.1) are metabolically active units of cellular matter.

1. The **plasma membrane**, which envelops the cell and forms a boundary between it and adjacent structures, is discussed in Chapter 1.

2. **Ribosomes**

   a. **Structure.** Ribosomes are nonmembranous organelles that are 12 nanometers (nm) wide and 25 nm long and consist of a **small** and a **large subunit**. The two subunits are composed of several types of ribosomal ribonucleic acids (rRNAs) and numerous proteins (Table 3.1; Figure 2.5).

   b. Ribosomes may be free in the cytosol or bound to membranes of the rough endoplasmic reticulum (RER) or the cytoplasmic surface of the outer nuclear membrane. Whether free or bound, the ribosomes constitute a single interchangeable population.

   c. A **polyribosome (polysome)** is a cluster of ribosomes along a single strand of messenger ribonucleic acid (mRNA) where every ribosome is concurrently engaged in protein synthesis.

   d. **Function.** Ribosomes are the sites where **mRNA is translated into protein**. Proteins destined for transport (secretory, membrane, and lysosomal) are synthesized on polyribosomes bound to the RER, whereas proteins not destined for transport are synthesized on polyribosomes in the cytosol. Protein synthesis that forms proteins not destined for transport occurs in the following manner (synthesis of proteins destined to be transported is discussed below in Section III b):

      (1) The **small ribosomal subunit** binds both mRNA and activated transfer ribonucleic acids (tRNAs); the **codons** of the mRNA then **base-pair** with the corresponding **anticodons** of the tRNAs.

      (2) Next, an initiator tRNA recognizes the **start codon (AUG)** on the mRNA.

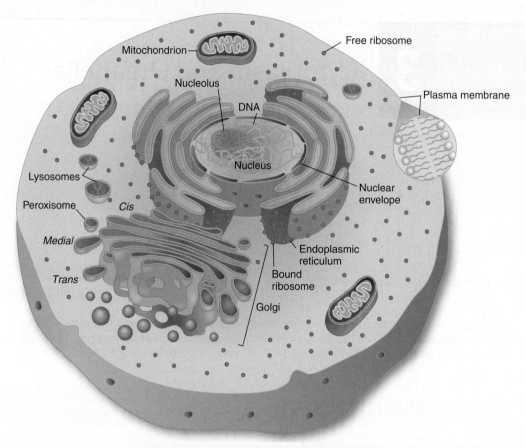

FIGURE 3.1. A eukaryotic cell and its major organelles and inclusions. (Reprinted with permission from Chandar N, Viselli S. *Cell and Molecular Biology.* North American ed. Baltimore, MD: Wolters Kluwer Health/Lippincott Williams & Wilkins; 2010:48.)

  (3) The **large ribosomal subunit** then binds to the complex. The enzyme **peptidyl transferase** located in the large subunit catalyzes peptide bond formation, resulting in addition of amino acids to the growing polypeptide chain.

  (4) A **chain-terminating codon** (**UAA, UAG,** or **UGA**) causes release of the polypeptide from the ribosome, and the ribosomal subunits dissociate from the mRNA.

 3. **Rough endoplasmic reticulum** (Figures 3.1 and 3.2)

  a. **Structure.** RER is a system of membrane-bounded sacs, or cavities. The outer surface of RER is studded with ribosomes, which makes it appear rough. The interior region of RER is called the **cisterna,** or the **lumen.** The outer nuclear membrane is **continuous** with the RER membrane, which brings the perinuclear cisterna into continuity with the cisternae of the RER. The RER membrane also has receptors (**ribophorins**) in its membrane to which the large ribosomal subunit binds.

t a b l e **3.1** Ribosome Composition		
Subunit	rRNA Types	Number of Proteins
Large (60S)	5S	49
	5.8S	
	28S	
Small (40S)	18S	33

rRNA, ribosomal ribonucleic acid.

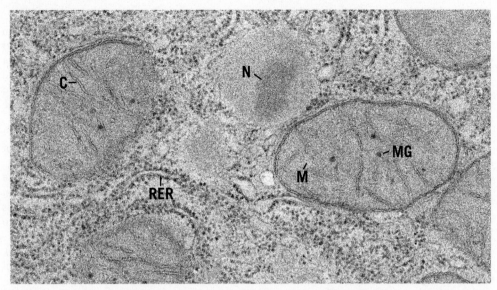

FIGURE 3.2. An electron micrograph showing rough endoplasmic reticulum (RER), portions of several mitochondria and their cristae (C), matrix (M), and matrix granules (MG), and a peroxisome with a nucleoid (N).

    b. RER is abundant in cells synthesizing **secretory proteins**; in such cells, the RER is organized into many parallel arrays.

    c. The RER sac closest to the Golgi apparatus gives rise to buds free of ribosomes that form vesicles known as **transfer vesicles**. This sac is known as a **transitional element** and represents the region of exit from the RER.

    d. Function. The RER is where **membrane-packaged proteins** are synthesized, including secretory, plasma membrane, and lysosomal proteins. In addition, the RER **monitors** the assembly, retention, and even degradation of certain proteins. Proteins that are to be retained in the RER cisternae are marked by the presence of a small peptide composed of a specific sequence of four amino acids at their C terminus; these amino acids form the **KDEL sequence** and are composed of lysine, asparagine, glutamine, and leucine. Proteins that do not sport the KDEL sequence at the C terminus are transported out of the cisternae of the RER.

4. Smooth endoplasmic reticulum (SER)

    a. Structure. SER is an irregular network of membrane-bounded channels that lacks ribosomes on its surface, which makes it appear smooth.

    b. It usually appears as branching, anastomosing **tubules**, or **vesicles**, whose membranes do **not** contain ribophorins.

    c. SER is less common than RER but is prominent in cells synthesizing steroids, triglycerides, and cholesterol.

    d. Function. SER has different functions in different cell types.

        (1) Steroid hormone synthesis occurs in SER-rich cells such as the Leydig cells of the testis, which make testosterone.

        (2) Cells synthesizing fatty acids and phospholipids are rich in SER.

        (3) Drug detoxification occurs in hepatocytes following proliferation of the SER in response to the drug phenobarbital; the oxidases that metabolize this drug are located in the SER.

        (4) Muscle contraction and relaxation involve the release and recapture of Ca^{2+} by the SER in skeletal muscle cells, called the sarcoplasmic reticulum.

5. Annulate lamellae

    a. Structure. Annulate lamellae are parallel stacks of membranes (usually 6–10) that resemble the nuclear envelope, including its pore complexes. They are often arranged with their **annuli** (pores) in register and are frequently **continuous** with the RER.

    b. Function. Annulate lamellae are found in rapidly growing cells (e.g., germ cells, embryonic cells, and tumor cells), but their function and significance remain unknown.

6. **Mitochondria** (Figures 3.1 and 3.2)
    a. **Structure.** Mitochondria are rod-shaped organelles that are 0.2 μm wide and up to 7 μm long. They possess an **outer membrane**, which surrounds the organelle, and an **inner membrane**, which has a high concentration of **cardiolipin**, a phospholipid that does not allow ions to cross the membrane in either direction. The inner membrane invaginates to form **cristae**. Mitochondria are subdivided into an **intermembrane compartment** between the two membranes and an inner **matrix compartment**. Granules within the matrix bind the divalent cations Mg^{2+} and Ca^{2+}.
    b. **Enzymes and genetic apparatus.** Mitochondria contain the following:
        (1) All of the enzymes of the **Krebs (tricarboxylic acid) cycle** are in the matrix, except for succinate dehydrogenase, which is located on the inner mitochondrial membrane.
        (2) **Elementary particles** (visible on negatively stained cristae) represent **adenosine triphosphate (ATP) synthase**, a special enzyme embedded in the inner mitochondrial membrane. It consists of a head portion and a transmembrane H^+ carrier and is involved in **coupling oxidation to phosphorylation** of adenosine diphosphate (ADP) to form ATP (Figure 3.3).
        (3) A **genetic apparatus** in the matrix composed of circular deoxyribonucleic acid (DNA), mRNA, tRNA, and rRNA (with a limited coding capacity), although most mitochondrial proteins are encoded by nuclear DNA.
        (4) Those mitochondrial proteins that are formed in the cytosol are transported into the mitochondria in a very specific fashion. The proteins must possess a terminal amino acid presequence that has a positive charge and the protein has to be accompanied **by cytosolic heat shock protein 70**. These two signals are recognized by a carrier embedded in the outer mitochondrial membrane, known as the **TOM (translocase of the outer mitochondrial membrane complexes)**. The recognition permits the translocation of the protein into the intermembrane compartment via the proteins known as the **ITM (inner mitochondrial membrane complexes)**. Once in the matrix, mitochondrial heat shock protein 70 cleaves the amino acid–positive presequence.

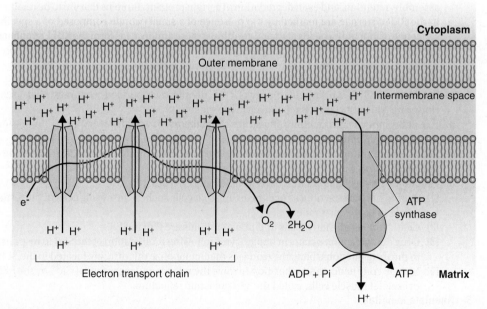

FIGURE 3.3. Chemiosmotic coupling mechanism for generating adenosine triphosphate (ATP) in mitochondria. As electrons move (sequentially) along the enzyme complexes of the electron transport chain, H^+ ions (protons) are pumped from the matrix compartment across the inner mitochondrial membrane into the intermembrane compartment generating a proton gradient. This electrochemical proton gradient drives the production of ATP as protons pass down their electrochemical gradient through ATP synthase and reenter the matrix. As H^+ passes through ATP synthase, this enzyme uses the energy of the proton flow to drive the production of ATP from adenosine diphosphate (ADP) and Pi.

    c. **Origin and proliferation**

       (1) Mitochondria may have **originated as symbionts** (intracellular parasites). According to this theory, anaerobic eukaryotic cells endocytosed aerobic microorganisms that evolved into mitochondria, which function in oxidative processes.

       (2) Mitochondria proliferate by division (fission) of preexisting mitochondria and typically have a 10-day life span. Proteins needed to sustain mitochondria are imported into them from the cytosol.

    d. **Mitochondrial ATP synthesis**

       (1) Mitochondria synthesize ATP via the Krebs cycle, which traps chemical energy and produces ATP by **oxidation** of fatty acids, amino acids, and glucose.

       (2) ATP is also synthesized via a **chemiosmotic coupling mechanism** involving enzyme complexes of the **electron transport chain** (composed of **NADH dehydrogenase complex**, **cytochrome b_1–c complex**, and **cytochrome oxidase complex** through which **energy-rich protons** enter the intermembrane compartment) and **ATP synthase** present in elementary particles of cristae (Figure 3.3). It is through the ATP synthase that the energy-rich protons leave the intermembrane compartment to reenter the matrix compartment where they yield their energy to **ADP + Pi** (where Pi is **inorganic phosphate** derived from the cytosol) to form **ATP**.

       (3) In order to manufacture ATP, the mitochondria require ADP, which is transported into the organelle via **ADP/ATP exchange proteins** located in both the outer and inner mitochondrial membranes. As their name implies, these exchange proteins allow ADP to enter the mitochondrion and ATP to exit the mitochondrion.

    e. **Condensed mitochondria** result from a **conformational change** in the orthodox form (which is the typical morphology). The change occurs in response to an uncoupling of oxidation from phosphorylation.

       (1) In condensed mitochondria, the size of the inner compartment is decreased, and the matrix density is increased. The intermembrane compartment is enlarged.

       (2) Condensed mitochondria are present in **brown fat cells**, which produce **heat**, rather than ATP because they have a special transport protein in their inner membrane that **uncouples** respiration from ATP synthesis (see Chapter 6 IV B 5 b).

       (3) Mitochondria **swell** in response to calcium, phosphate, and thyroxine, which induce an increase in water uptake and an uncoupling of phosphorylation; ATP reverses the swelling.

7. Golgi apparatus (complex) (Figures 3.1, 3.4, and 3.5)

    a. **Structure.** The Golgi apparatus consists of several membrane-bounded **cisternae (saccules)** arranged in a **stack** and positioned and held in place by microtubules. Cisternae are disk-shaped and slightly curved, with flat centers and dilated rims, but their size and shapes vary. A distinct **polarity** exists across the Golgi stack, with many vesicles present on one side (the entry side into the Golgi apparatus) and larger secretory granules (vacuoles) on the other (the exit side of the Golgi apparatus).

    b. **Regions**

       (1) The **cis face** of the Golgi apparatus typically lies deep in the cell toward the nucleus next to the transitional element of the RER. Its outermost cisterna is associated with a network of interconnected tubes and vesicles, called **vesicular–tubular clusters (VTCs)**, which receive **transfer vesicles** from the transitional element of the RER (Figures 3.4 and 3.5). Formerly, the VTC was thought to be a separate, intermediary compartment located between the RER and the Golgi, known as the endoplasmic reticulum–Golgi-intermediate compartment.

       (2) The **medial compartment** of the Golgi apparatus is composed of as many as several cisternae lying between the cis and trans faces.

       (3) The **trans face** of the Golgi apparatus lies at the side of the stack facing the plasma membrane and is associated with vacuoles and secretory granules.

       (4) The *trans*-**Golgi network (TGN)** lies apart from the last cisterna at the *trans* face and is separated from the Golgi stack. It sorts proteins for their final destinations.

    c. **Functions**. The Golgi apparatus processes membrane-packaged proteins synthesized in the RER and also recycles and redistributes membranes.

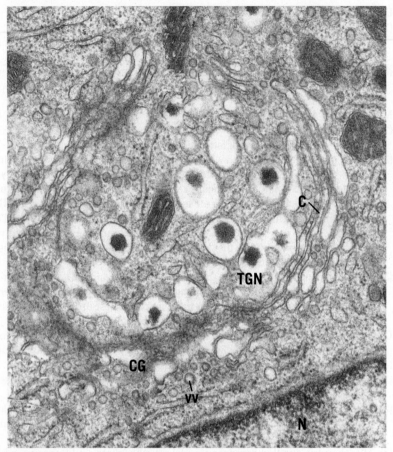

FIGURE 3.4. Electron micrograph of a Golgi apparatus showing a *trans*-Golgi network (TGN) with vacuoles and forming secretory granules, Golgi cisternae (C), and a vesicular–tubular cluster delivering proteins to the *cis*-Golgi (CG) via tiny vesicles (vv). A portion of a nucleus (N) is also evident.

8. **Coated vesicles** are characterized by a visible cytoplasmic surface coat.
   a. **Clathrin-coated vesicles** (Figure 3.6)
      (1) **Structure.** These vesicles are coated with clathrin, which consists of three large and three small polypeptide chains that form a **triskelion** (three-legged structure). Thirty-six clathrin triskelions associate to form a polyhedral cage-like lattice around the vesicle. Proteins called **adaptins** are also part of clathrin-coated vesicles. There are four classes of adaptins, two large ones named α-adaptin and β-adaptin, a medium-sized one known as μ-adaptin, and the smallest one, σ-adaptin. A μ-adaptin, a σ-adaptin, and two of the large adaptins combine to form an **adaptin complex** (also known as an **adaptor**) which assist in the formation of the clathrin coat, capturing cargo receptors containing specific molecules, and they help to establish the vesicle curvature. A guanosine triphosphate (GTP)–binding protein, called **dynamin**, forms a ring around the neck of a budding vesicle or pit and aids in pinching it off the parent membrane to form a free clathrin-coated vesicle (Figure 3.6).
      (2) **Function**
         (a) Clathrin-coated vesicles are formed during **receptor-mediated uptake (endocytosis)** of specific molecules by the cell. After uptake, the vesicles quickly lose their coats, and clathrin and adaptin complexes return to the plasma membrane for recycling (Figure 3.5).

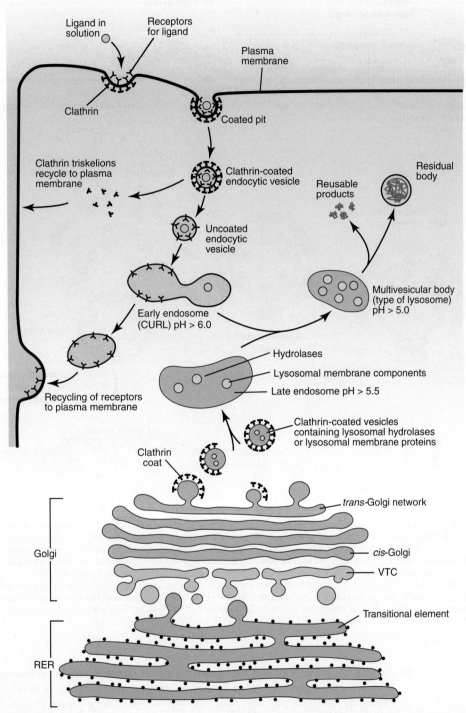

FIGURE 3.5. Receptor-mediated endocytosis of a ligand (e.g., low-density lipoproteins) and the lysosomal degradative pathway. Clathrin triskelions quickly recycle back to the plasma membrane. The receptors and ligands then uncouple in the early endosome (compartment for uncoupling of receptors and ligands [CURL]), which is followed by recycling of receptors back to the plasma membrane. The late endosome is the primary intermediate in the formation of lysosomes (e.g., multivesicular bodies). Material that is phagocytosed or organelles that undergo autophagy do not use the early endosomal pathway. VTC, vesicular–tubular cluster; RER, rough endoplasmic reticulum.

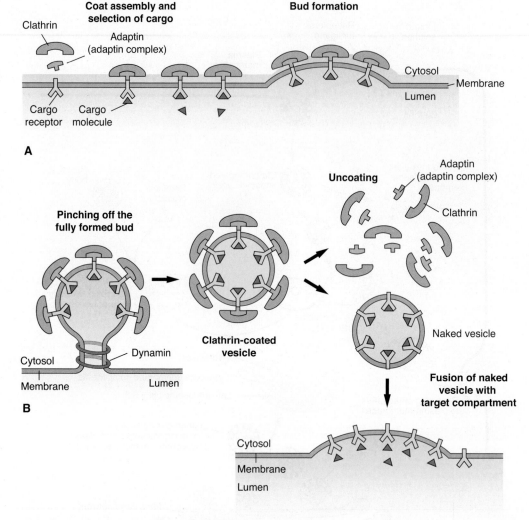

FIGURE 3.6. Formation and disassembly of a clathrin-coated vesicle involved in the transport of selected cargo molecules. **A.** Cargo receptors in the membrane of a donor organelle recognize transport signals on cargo molecules and select specific molecules. Adaptin (adaptin complex) coat proteins recognize and bind the specific cargo receptors that have captured a selected set of cargo molecules, ensuring that only they will be incorporated into the lumen of the new clathrin-coated vesicle. Adaptin also recruits clathrin and binds it to the outer surface of the forming bud. **B.** As the budding vesicle becomes fully formed, dynamin proteins assemble around its neck and constrict it to pinch off the vesicle. The clathrin and adaptin are quickly removed, and the uncoated (naked) vesicle then fuses with the membrane of its target organelle and releases the cargo molecules into its lumen. (Copyright 2002 from *Molecular Biology of the Cell*, 4th ed., by Alberts et al. Adapted with permission from Garland Science/Taylor & Francis LLC.)

(b) Clathrin-coated vesicles also function in the **signal-directed (regulated) transport** of proteins from the TGN either to the secretory granule pathway or to the late endosome–lysosome pathway. After the clathrin-coated vesicle loses its coat, the naked vesicle fuses with a donor membrane compartment, and the clathrin and adaptin molecules are reused within the cell in other transport vesicles (Figure 3.6).

b. Coatomer-coated vesicles

    (1) Structure. These vesicles have coats consisting of coatomer, which does not form a cage-like lattice around vesicles. Coatomer is a large protein complex formed by individual **co**at **p**rotein subunits called **COPs**. Assembly of coatomer depends on the protein **ADP-ribosylation factor (ARF)**, which binds GTP, becomes activated, and recruits coatomer subunits. ARF also helps to select the cargo molecules.

(2) Function

(a) Coatomer-coated vesicles mediate the continuous **constitutive protein transport** (default pathway; bulk flow) within the cell. Specific GTP-binding proteins are present at each step of vesicle budding and fusion, and proteins called **SNAREs** (**SNAP-receptors**) ensure that the vesicle docks and fuses only with its correct target membrane. Coated vesicle SNAREs (v-SNAREs) recognize and bind to complementary target SNAREs (t-SNAREs) to deliver not only cargo molecules but also membrane to the target compartment (Figure 3.7). Once the t-SNAREs and v-SNAREs recognize each other, they enlist the help of two additional cytosolic proteins **NSF (N-ethylmaleimide-sensitive fusion)** protein and **SNAP (soluble NSF attachment protein)**. The four proteins, SNAP, NSF, t-SNARE, and v-SNARE together accomplish the process of fusion between the specific target membrane and the cargo carrying vesicle.

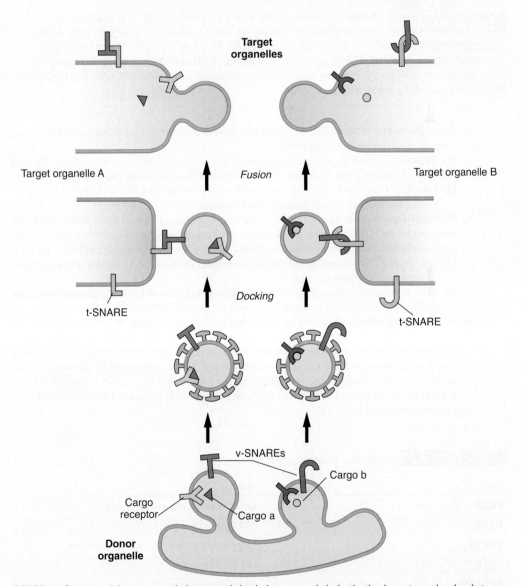

FIGURE 3.7. Coated vesicles are moved along cytoskeletal elements to their destination by motor molecules, but once there, they must recognize and fuse with only the correct target organelle membrane. This is achieved by proteins on the surface of the vesicle, called vesicle SNAREs (v-SNAREs), that recognize and bind to complementary target SNAREs (t-SNAREs) on the membrane of the correct target organelle. First docking of the vesicle and then fusion occurs as the vesicle not only contributes its contents (cargo) but also adds its membrane to that of the organelle. (Copyright 2002 from *Molecular Biology of the Cell*, 4th ed., by Alberts et al. Adapted with permission from Garland Science/Taylor & Francis LLC.)

(b) Coatomer-coated vesicles transport proteins from the RER to the VTC to the Golgi apparatus, from one Golgi cisterna to another, and from the TGN to the plasma membrane.

   1. COP-II transports molecules forward from the RER to the VTC to the *cis*-Golgi **(anterograde transport)**.

   2. COP-I facilitates **retrograde transport** (from the VTC or any Golgi cisternal compartment or from the TGN) to the RER. It is still questionable whether or not COP-I facilitates anterograde transport, but recent findings suggest that they might move forward between Golgi regions (*cis*-Golgi to medial Golgi to *trans*-Golgi) and to the TGN.

CLINICAL CONSIDERATIONS   **Botox.** The interaction of v-SNAREs with t-SNAREs is essential for neurotransmitter release, via exocytosis, at chemical synapses. At the presynaptic nerve terminal, one of the t-SNAREs is SNAP-25, a fusion protein. **Botox** (botulinum neurotoxin A) cleaves SNAP-25 and prevents the synaptic vesicles from anchoring and releasing their neurotransmitter, thus preventing neuromuscular transmission and contraction. This leads to a flaccid paralysis of the postsynaptic muscle.

---

   c. **Caveolin-coated vesicles.** These coated vesicles are less common and less well understood than those of the previous two categories.

   (1) **Structure.** Caveolae are invaginations of the plasma membrane in endothelial and smooth muscle cells. They possess a distinct coat formed by the protein **caveolin**.

   (2) **Function.** Caveolae have been associated with cell signaling and a variety of transport processes, such as transcytosis and endocytosis.

   d. **Retromer-coated vesicles** are present only in the retrieval of cargo from **endosomes** and returned to the TGN. Retromer is composed of four protein subunits, which assemble only on curved endosomal membranes if, and only if, the following two other conditions are met:

   (1) the cytoplasmic component of the cargo receptor protein is available for binding to one of the retromer subunits. and

   (2) if the membrane possesses a particular **inositol phospholipid**, known as **phosphoinositide (PIP)** that is recognized by another one of the retromer subunits.

   e. **Inositol phospholipids.** It should be noted that inositol phospholipids form only one-tenth of all membrane phospholipids, yet they have essential functions in membrane transport. Because their hydroxyl groups are easily phosphorylated and dephosphorylated and they may have as many as three phosphate groups, they can be recognized by the various coat proteins that form coated vesicles. Therefore, the presence of the various types of PIPs and their ability to be altered to different forms act as signaling molecules for the various coat proteins (see Table 3.2).

t a b l e **3.2** Membrane Locations of PIPs	
PIP	Location
PI(3)P	Early endosomes; phagosome membrane
PI(4)P	TGN; lateral cell membrane
PI(4,5)P$_2$	Golgi; lateral cell membrane; apical cell membrane
PI(3,5)P$_2$	Late endosomes
PI(3,4,5)P$_3$	Apical cell membrane

PI(3)P indicates that there is only one phosphate group, and it is located at the 3' position; PI(3,5)P$_2$ indicates that there are two phosphate groups, where one is at the 3' and the other at the 5' position; PI(3,4,5)P$_3$ indicates that there are three phosphate groups, one at the 3', one at the 4', and the third one at the 5' position.
PIP, phosphoinositide; TGN, *trans*-Golgi network.

t a b l e **3.3** Locations of Selected Rab-GTPs on Intracellular Membranes	
Membrane	**Rab-GTPs (Rab Protein)**
Cell membrane	Rab5A
Clathrin-coated vesicles	Rab5A
Synaptic vesicles	Rab3A
Secretory granules	Rab3A and SEC4
RER	Rab1, Rab18
cis-Golgi	Rab1 and Rab2
Medial Golgi	Rab6
trans-Golgi	Rab6
Recycling endosomes	Rab4 and Rab11
TGN	Rab9
Early endosomes	Rab5C and Rab8
Late endosomes	Rab7 and Rab9
Lipid droplets	Rab18

RER, rough endoplasmic reticulum; TGN, *trans*-Golgi network.

    f. Rab proteins. Another large family of monomeric GTPases, known as **Rab proteins (Rab-GTPs)**, is also involved in the molecular mechanism of membrane transport. There are more than 70 types of Rab proteins (Table 3.3), and they are considered to be peripheral, rather than integral, proteins that are attached to vesicle and/or target membranes via prenyl groups. The target membranes also possess **Rab effector proteins** (**tethering proteins**) that recognize specific Rab-GTPs, bind to them, and in this fashion direct the vesicle to the target membrane, where v-SNAREs are able to contact t-SNAREs, thus facilitating membrane fusion. If the Rab-GTP is not recognized, then the vesicle cannot dock, assuring that the particular vesicle can fuse only with its intended target membrane. Subsequent to the fusion of the vesicle with its target membrane, the Rab protein is recycled to its membrane of origin.

9. Lysosomes

    a. Structure. Lysosomes are dense membrane-bound organelles of diverse shape and size that function to degrade material. They may be identified in sections of tissue by cytochemical staining for **acid phosphatase**. Lysosomes possess special membrane proteins whose luminal aspects possess a substantial layer of sugar molecules that shield them from the 50 or so types of acid hydrolases housed in this organelle. Moreover, lysosomal membranes are also rich in cholesterol and **lysobiphosphatidic acid**, where the latter is believed to prevent the hydrolytic enzymes from digesting the lysosomal membrane. Furthermore, ATP-powered proton pumps in the lysosome membrane maintain an **acid pH** (<5).

    b. Formation. Lysosomes are formed when sequestered material fuses with a **late endosome**, and enzymatic degradation begins. Formation of a lysosome via one lysosomal pathway (Figure 3.5) involves the following intermediates:

    (1) Early endosomes

      (a) These irregular vesicles near the cell periphery form part of the pathway for receptor-mediated endocytosis and contain receptor–ligand complexes.

      (b) They are also known as the **compartment for uncoupling of receptors and ligands** (**CURL**).

      (c) Their acidic interiors (pH < 6) are maintained by ATP-driven proton pumps. The acidity aids in the uncoupling of receptors and ligands; receptors return to the plasma membrane, and ligands move to a late endosome.

    (2) Late endosomes

      (a) Late endosomes play a **key role** in various lysosomal pathways and are therefore sometimes known as the intermediate compartment.

      (b) These irregular vesicles (pH < 5.5) deep within the cell receive ligands via microtubular transport of vesicles from early endosomes.

    (c) Late endosomes contain **both lysosomal proenzymes (inactive acid hydrolases) and lysosomal membrane proteins**; these are formed in the RER as proenzymes, transported to the Golgi complex for processing, and delivered in separate vesicles to late endosomes.[1]

    (d) These lysosomal proteins and proenzymes are folded in such a fashion within the RER that they display a **signal region** that becomes modified in the Golgi apparatus to accept **mannose-6-phosphate (M-6-P)**, which is inserted into the signal region within the TGN. The presence of M-6-P ensures that they will be packaged specifically into those vesicles that are destined for early and late endosomes, organelles whose membranes possess **M-6-P receptors**.

    (e) Once late endosomes have received a full complement of lysosomal enzymes, they begin to degrade their ligands and are classified as **lysosomes**.

  c. Types of lysosomes (Figure 3.8). Lysosomes are named after the content of recognizable material; otherwise, the general term **lysosome** is used.

    (1) Multivesicular bodies are formed by fusion of an early endosome containing endocytic vesicles with a late endosome.

    (2) Phagolysosomes are formed by fusion of a **phagocytic vacuole** with a late endosome or a lysosome.

    (3) Autophagolysosomes are formed by fusion of an **autophagic vacuole** (Figure 3.9) with a late endosome or lysosome. Autophagic vacuoles are formed when cell components

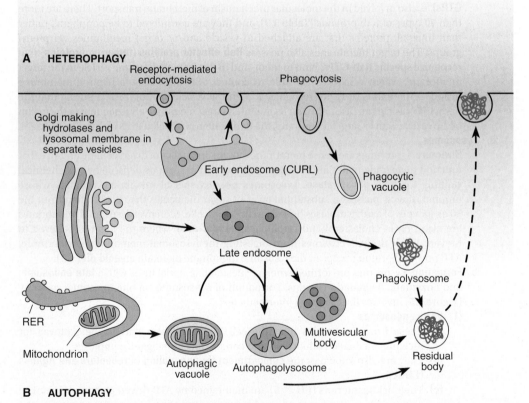

FIGURE 3.8. Heterophagy refers to the intracellular digestion of material taken into the cell from outside (*top of illustration*), whereas autophagy is the digestion of parts of the cell itself (*bottom*). The different pathways and the types of lysosomes involved in each pathway are shown. RER, rough endoplasmic reticulum.

---

[1]The terms primary and virgin lysosomes, formerly used for tiny vesicles believed to be lysosomes that have not yet engaged in digestive activity, are no longer used.

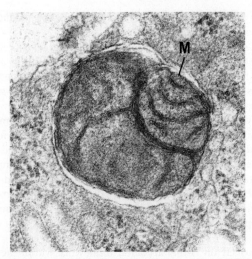

FIGURE 3.9. Electron micrograph of an autophagic vacuole containing mitochondria (M). Once an autophagic vacuole fuses with a late endosome or lysosome (to form an auto-phagolysosome) further digestion occurs, making the organelles inside unrecognizable and resulting in a structure identified simply as a lysosome.

targeted for destruction become enveloped by smooth areas of membranes derived from the RER.

(4) **Residual bodies** are lysosomes of any type that have expended their capacity to degrade material. They contain **undegraded material** (e.g., lipofuscin and hemosiderin) and eventually may be excreted from the cell.

10. **Peroxisomes** (Figure 3.2)
    a. **Structure.** Peroxisomes (also known as **microbodies**) are membrane-bound, spherical, or ovoid organelles that may be identified in cells by a cytochemical reaction for the enzyme **catalase**. In stained preparations, they appear as small organelles (0.15–0.25 μm in diameter); they may be larger in hepatocytes. Peroxisomes may contain a **nucleoid**, a crystalline core consisting of urate oxidase (uricase); the human peroxisome lacks a nucleoid.
    b. They originate from preexisting peroxisomes, which grow by importing specific cytosolic proteins that are recognized by a family of receptor proteins (called **peroxins**) in the peroxisomal membrane. Then the peroxisome divides by fission; it has a life span of approximately 5 to 6 days.
    c. **Function.** Peroxisomes contain various **enzymes** whose functions vary from the oxidation of long-chain fatty acids to the synthesis of cholesterol to the detoxification of substances such as ethanol and in the process form H_2O_2, a molecule exceptionally harmful to cells. However, the enzyme catalase, composed of four **apocatalase** molecules each of which binds a **heme**, catalyzes the breakdown of H_2O_2 into water. Other peroxisomal enzymes initiate the synthesis of **plasmalogen**, the major phospholipid component of myelin.

CLINICAL CONSIDERATIONS — Peroxisomal diseases

1. **Zellweger syndrome** is a genetic disease in which normal peroxisomes are absent. Infants with this syndrome have profound neurological disorders and liver and kidney problems, and usually die within a few months. Electron micrographs of biopsies from these patients reveal empty peroxisomes, lacking enzymes. Although peroxisomal enzymes may be synthesized, they become dislocated in the cytosol.
2. **Adrenoleukodystrophy** is caused by the inability of peroxisomes to metabolize fatty acids. Therefore, lipids accumulate in the nervous system and adrenal glands, impairing their function.
3. **Plasmalogen deficiency** has been suggested as a possible contributing factor to the incidence of Trisomy-21 and Alzheimer disease as well as in syndromes involving malformed myelin sheaths.

B. **Inclusions.** Inclusions are accumulations of material that is **not metabolically active**. They are usually present in the cytosol only **temporarily**.

1. **Glycogen** appears as small clusters (or in hepatocytes as larger aggregates, known as **rosettes**) of electron-dense 20- to 30-nm β-particles, which are similar in appearance to but larger than ribosomes. Glycogen is not bound by a membrane but frequently lies close to the SER. Glycogen serves as a **stored energy source** that can be degraded to glucose, which enters the bloodstream to elevate blood sugar levels.

2. **Lipid droplets** vary markedly in size and appearance depending on the method of fixation, and they are not bound by a membrane. Lipid droplets are storage forms of **triglycerides** (an energy source) and **cholesterol** (used in the synthesis of steroids and membranes).

3. **Lipofuscin** appears as membrane-bound, electron-dense granular material varying greatly in size and often containing lipid droplets. Lipofuscin represents a residue of undigested material present in residual bodies. Because the amount of this material increases with age, it is called **age pigment**. It is most common in nondividing cells (e.g., cardiac muscle cells, neurons), but is also found in hepatocytes.

C. **Cytoskeleton.** The cytoskeleton is the structural framework within the cytosol. It functions in maintaining cell shape, stabilizing cell attachments, facilitating endocytosis and exocytosis, and promoting cell movement. It includes the following major components:

1. **Microtubules**
   a. **Structure.** Microtubules are straight, hollow tubules 25 nm in diameter and made of **tubulin**. They have a rigid wall composed of 13 protofilaments, each of which consists of a linear arrangement of tubulin dimers; each dimer consists of nonidentical α- and β-**tubulin subunits** that are linked end to end, so that an α-tubulin subunit of one dimer is linked to the β-tubulin subunit of the next dimer.
   b. Microtubules are **polar**, in that they have a **plus end** (β-tubulin end) and a **minus end** (α-tubulin). Polymerization (assembly) and depolymerization (disassembly) occur preferentially at the plus end, but only when **GTP**, in the presence of magnesium ions, is bound to tubulin dimers. The minus end of a microtubule is usually not free, but is affixed to the microtubule-organizing center (discussed below C.2.).
   c. **Microtubules have microtubule-associated proteins** (MAPs, such as MAP1, MAP2, MAP3, MAP4, and MAP tau), which stabilize them, control their lengthening, and bind them to other cytoskeletal components and organelles. Other MAPs, such as Lis 1, facilitate neuronal migration, which permits the development of gyri and sulci in the brain.

CLINICAL CONSIDERATIONS   Individuals who do not possess the Lis 1 MAPs are born with smooth cerebral hemispheres, a condition known as **lissencephaly**. Children with this condition rarely survive past 15 years of age and display various grades of mental retardation. Those most severely affected die during the first few months of life.

   d. Microtubules are also associated with **kinesin** and **cytoplasmic dynein**, two force-generating proteins (**motor proteins**), which serve as motors for vesicle or organelle movement. Kinesin moves cargo toward the plus end of the microtubule (outward, toward the cell periphery), whereas cytoplasmic dynein moves it toward the minus end (inward, toward the center of the cell).
   e. **Function.** Microtubules maintain cell shape; aid in the transport of macromolecules, vesicles, and organelles within the cytosol; assemble into the mitotic spindle during mitosis and ensure the correct distribution of chromosomes to daughter cells; and assist in the formation of cell appendages called cilia and flagella, which beat rhythmically and precisely.

2. **Centrosome (Microtubule Organizing Center, MTOC) and Centrioles** (see Figures 2.7 and 3.10)
   a. **Structure.** The **centrosome** is located near the nucleus. It contains two **centrioles** and a cloud of **pericentriolar material**. The centrioles exist as a pair of cylindrical rods (each 0.2 μm wide and 0.5 μm long) at right angles to one another. Each member of the pair is

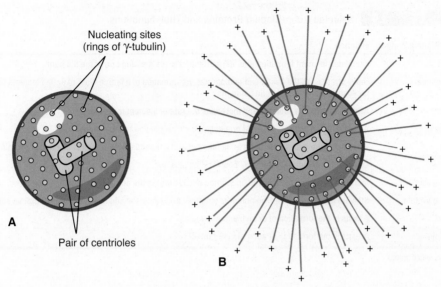

FIGURE 3.10. Polymerization of tubulin at a centrosome. **A.** A centrosome consists of an amorphous cloud of material containing γ-tubulin rings that initiate microtubule polymerization. Within the cloud is a pair of centrioles. **B.** A centrosome with attached microtubules. The minus end of each microtubule is embedded in the centrosome, having grown from a nucleating ring, whereas the plus end of each microtubule is free in the cytoplasm. (Copyright 2004 from *Essential Cell Biology*, 2nd ed., by Alberts et al. Adapted with permission from Garland Science/Taylor & Francis LLC.)

composed of nine triplets of microtubules (9 + 0 axoneme pattern) arranged radially in the shape of a pinwheel and sport a narrow ring of unknown material surrounding their distal ends (the ends away from the nucleus), known as the **distal ring**. The two centrioles of the pair differ from each other because one is older, the **mature centriole**, since it was formed in an earlier predecessor of the present cell. The younger centriole is referred to as the **immature centriole**. The mature centriole possesses structures of unknown function known as **appendages** that are associated with the distal ring and **satellites** projecting from the centriole's distal aspect. The proximal ends of both mature and immature centrioles are connected to the nuclear envelope by some proteinaceous material.

   b. The centrioles **self-duplicate** in the S phase of the cell cycle, as each parent centriole forms a **procentriole** at right angles to itself.

   c. Centrioles also form **basal bodies**, which appear identical to unpaired centrioles and which give rise to the axonemes of cilia and flagella.

   d. Function

     (1) The centrosome is the major microtubule-organizing center in the cell.

     (2) The **pericentriolar cloud** of material contains hundreds of ring-shaped structures composed of γ-**tubulin**, and each ring serves as a starting point for the polymerization of one microtubule.

     (3) Centrioles play no role in nucleating microtubules, but they help to maintain the organization of the centrosome.

     (4) The centrosome itself is also duplicated during interphase (S phase), and then separates to form the poles of the mitotic spindle, where microtubules originate and converge.

3. Actin filaments (microfilaments)

   a. Structure. Actin filaments measure 7 nm in diameter and are composed of globular actin monomers (**G actin**) linked into a **double helix** (F actin). They are thin, flexible, and abundant in cells.

   b. Actin filaments display **polarity** similar to that of microtubules; that is, their polymerization and depolymerization occur preferentially and more rapidly at the **plus end** (**barbed end**) than at the **minus end** (**pointed end**). Free G actin subunits possess ATP bound to them, and when they bind to the growing actin filament, the subunit acts as an enzyme and hydrolyses the ATP, releasing energy, and the resultant ADP becomes buried deep in the groove of the

t a b l e **3.4**	Selected Actin-Binding Proteins and Their Functions
Actin-Binding Protein	**Function**
Formin	Facilitates filament formation and stays attached to the growing end of the filament
ARP complex	Stays attached to the minus end and permits the formation of a lattice work of actin filaments by facilitating branching of actin filaments
Profilin	Attaches to G actin subunits and increases the rate of filament formation
Thymosin	Attaches to G actin subunits and prevents them from binding to the actin filament
Cofilin	Attaches to the minus end of the actin filament and enhances the process of filament shortening
Gelsolin	Cleaves the filament and remains bound to the plus end
Tropomyosin	Increases filament stability and, in striated muscle masks the active binding site to myosin
Capping protein	Stabilizes the filament and maintains its length by preventing the addition or deletion of G actin subunits
Fimbrin	Assists in the formation of actin filament bundles
α-Actinin	Assists in the formation of actin filament bundles

ARP, actin-related protein.

filament and the filament is lengthened. During the lengthening of the actin filament, the speed of ATP dephosphorylation becomes faster. When G actin monomers are removed from the minus end, they have ADP attached to them, and in the cytosol the nucleotide becomes phosphorylated to ATP.

c. Many **actin-binding proteins** associate with G actin and F actin and in that fashion accelerate or decelerate the lengthening or shortening of the actin filament as well as permit branching of the filament (Table 3.4). During filament formation, actin monomers are added to the plus end and may be deleted from the minus end. In certain conditions, known as **treadmilling**, the same number of G actin monomers is added to the plus end as is removed from the minus end.

d. Actin filaments are abundant at the periphery of the cell, where they are anchored to the plasma membrane via one or more intermediary proteins (e.g., α-actinin, vinculin, and talin).

e. **Function.** Actin filaments play a role in many **cellular processes**, such as establishing focal contacts between the cell and the extracellular matrix, locomotion of non-muscle cells, formation of the contractile ring (in dividing cells), formation of a rigid core of microvilli, and the folding of epithelia into tubes during development.

4. **Intermediate filaments** are 8 to 10 nm in diameter. They constitute a population of heterogeneous filaments that are the products of at least 70 different genes. In spite of their diversity, intermediate filaments have numerous common characteristics, namely that their basic unit is a **monomer**, composed of a rod-shaped protein whose longest region is an alpha helical structure, the **central domain**, with a globular N terminal (**head**) and a globular C terminal (**tail**). Two of these monomers coiled around each other to form a dimer. Two dimers assemble head to tail, in an antiparallel, staggered **tetramer formation**. Eight tetramers assemble side by side and are compressed into **unit length filaments** (**ULFs**) that form 10-nm subunits. Many ULFs assemble end to end to form the mature intermediate filaments. Although it was believed that intermediate filaments are rigid in nature, they have been demonstrated to move, change their shapes, and stretch to a certain extent without breaking. There are four types of intermediate filaments in the cytoplasm and one type located in the nucleus as well as a special type located only in the cytoplasm of the cells of the lens of the eye (see Table 3.5). In general, intermediate filaments **provide mechanical strength** to cells; they lack polarity and do not require GTP or ATP for assembly, which occurs along the entire length of the filament.

5. **Plectin** is a 500-kDa protein that has a ubiquitous presence in most cells. It acts to attach microfilaments, intermediate filaments, and microtubules to each other and in that fashion provides a very stable configuration to the cytoskeleton. Plectin is also present in striated muscles and assists desmin in maintaining the regular arrangement of myofibrils. Additionally, plectin has been shown in reinforcing the cell–cell junctions by binding some of the structural molecules to the cytoskeleton.

table 3.5	Major Types of Intermediate Filaments		
Type	Protein	Location	Function
I	Acidic keratins	Various types of epithelial cells	They are the tonofilaments associated with desmosomes and hemidesmosomes; in nails and hair they are known as trichocytic (hard) keratins
II	Basic keratins		
III	Vimentin*	Endothelial cells, leukocytes, fibroblasts	Architectural support for plasma membranes; fix organelles in position.
	Desmin†	Muscle cells	Links myofibrils to each other at Z disks
	GFAP†	Glia and astrocytes	Provides structural support
	Peripherin	Axons of PNS	Assists in elongation of axons?
	Synemin	Muscle cells	Binds to α-actinin and desmin
IV	NF-L (70 kDa)‡	Axons of neurons	NF-L, NF-M, and NF-H all function to provide support for axons and establishes the axon diameter
	NF-M (140 kDa)‡	Axons of neurons	
	NF-H (210 kDa)‡	Axons of neurons	
	Nestin	Developing neurons and glia	Provides support for embryonic cells and is not present in mature cells
	α-Internexin	Axons of neurons	Copolymerizes with the other neurofilaments
	Syncoilin	Muscle	Binds to desmin
V	Nuclear lamins A, B, and C	Nuclei of all human cells	Forms a two-dimensional meshwork, the nuclear lamina, deep to the inner nuclear membrane to organize the peripheral nuclear chromatin; also form the framework of the nucleoplasm.
VI	Phakinin and filensin**	Lens fiber cells of the eye	These beaded filaments of the lens fibers of the eye maintain lens transparency.

GFAP, glial fibrillary acidic protein.
*Vimentin is the most common intermediate filament with a wide distribution.
†Desmin and GFAP may copolymerize with vimentin; they are sometimes categorized as vimentin-like filaments. Vimentin is the most commonly found intermediate filament in a variety of cells.
‡NF-L (Neurofilaments light), NF-M (Neurofilaments medium), and NF-H (Neurofilaments heavy). NF-L copolymerizes to form neurofilaments with either NF-M or NF-H.
**Phakinin and filensin copolymerize to form beaded filaments. They are found only in the lens fiber cells of the eye.

CLINICAL CONSIDERATIONS **Tumor diagnosis** is often based on immunocytochemical identification of the intermediate filaments in the tumor cells because the type of intermediate filament present identifies the tissue from where the metastatic cancer cells originated. For example, an undifferentiated tumor that has metastasized to the bladder can be identified as a carcinoma (of epithelial origin) if it stains immunocytochemically in a histological section after applying a cytokeratin antibody.

III. INTERACTIONS AMONG ORGANELLES

Organelles are involved in important cellular processes, such as the uptake and release of material by cells, protein synthesis, and intracellular digestion. These various interactions provide the basis for a functional approach to examine some dynamics of cell biology.

A. **Uptake and release of material by cells**
1. **Endocytosis** is the **uptake (internalization) of material by cells.** Endocytosis includes pinocytosis, receptor-mediated endocytosis, and phagocytosis.
   a. **Pinocytosis ("cell drinking") is the nonspecific (random) uptake** of extracellular fluid and material in solution into pinocytic vesicles.

b. Receptor-mediated endocytosis is the **specific uptake** of a substance (**ligand**), such as low-density lipoproteins (LDLs) and protein hormones, by a cell that has a plasma membrane receptor for that ligand. It involves the following sequence of events (Figure 3.5):

(1) A ligand **binds specifically** to its receptors on the cell surface.

(2) Ligand–receptor complexes cluster into a **clathrin-coated** pit, which invaginates and gives rise to a clathrin-coated vesicle containing the ligand.

(3) The cytoplasmic clathrin coat is rapidly **lost**, leaving an **uncoated endocytic vesicle** containing the ligand.

CLINICAL CONSIDERATIONS **Familial hypercholesterolemia** is associated with a decreased ability of cells to take in cholesterol, which normally is ingested by receptor-mediated endocytosis of LDLs.

1. This disease is caused by an inherited genetic defect that results in an inability to synthesize LDL receptors or in the synthesis of defective receptors unable to bind either to LDLs or to clathrin-coated pits.

2. It is characterized by an elevated level of cholesterol in the bloodstream. This facilitates early development of **atherosclerosis,** which may be fatal.

---

c. Phagocytosis ("cell eating") is the uptake of microorganisms, other cells, and particulate matter (frequently of foreign origin) by a cell. Phagocytosis usually involves cell surface receptors. It is characteristic of cells—particularly **macrophages** and **neutrophils**—that degrade proteins and cellular debris, and involves the following sequence of events:

(1) A macrophage binds via its **Fc receptors** to a bacterium coated with the antibody immunoglobulin G (IgG) or via its C3b receptors to a complement-coated bacterium.

(2) Binding progresses until the plasma membrane completely envelops the bacterium, forming a phagocytic vacuole.

2. Exocytosis is the **release of material** from the cell via fusion of a secretory granule membrane and the plasma membrane. **It requires interaction of receptors in both the secretory granule membrane and the plasma membrane** as well as the **coalescence** (adherence and joining) of the two phospholipid membrane bilayers. Exocytosis takes place in both regulated and constitutive secretion.

a. Regulated (signal-directed) **secretion** is the release, in response to an **extracellular signal,** of enzymes, neurosecretions, and other materials **stored** in the cell.

b. Constitutive secretion (default pathway) is the more or less **continuous** release of material (e.g., collagen and plasma proteins) without any intermediate storage step. An extracellular signal is **not** required for constitutive secretion.

3. Membrane recycling maintains a relatively constant plasma membrane surface area following exocytosis. In this process, the secretory granule membrane added to the plasma membrane surface during exocytosis is **retrieved** through endocytosis via clathrin-coated vesicles. This membrane is returned to the TGN via early endosomes for further recycling. Figure 3.11 illustrates endocytic pathways used by cells. More specific information concerning the mechanisms of membrane recycling and transference was presented in earlier sections of this chapter (see Section 8, Coated vesicles).

B. Protein synthesis

1. Synthesis of membrane-packaged proteins involves translation of mRNAs encoding the protein on polyribosomes at the surface of the RER, transport of the growing polypeptide chain across the RER membrane and **into the cisterna (lumen)**, and the processing of the polypeptide/protein within the RER. These water-soluble proteins will bud from the RER and be transported in vesicles either for transfer into the **lumen** (or interior) **of another organelle** or for **secretion** from the cell.

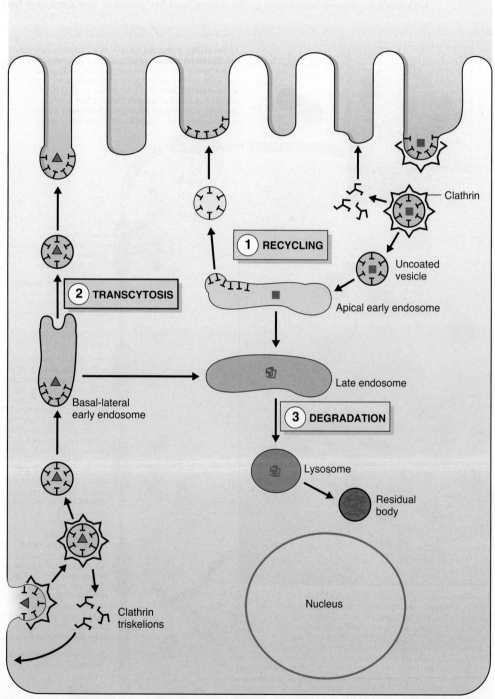

FIGURE 3.11. Pathways used by receptors and ligands following endocytosis. (1) Recycling of receptors to the same plasma membrane surface. (2) Transcytosis from one surface (e.g., basal–lateral) to another (e.g., apical). Transcytosis can occur in either direction, but separate early endosome compartments near the domain of vesicle entry are used. (3) Degradation: If not retrieved from either early endosome compartment, the ligands move to a common late endosome, which subsequently becomes a lysosome, where degradation is completed.

a. A three-step process translates mRNA as follows:

(1) mRNA binds to the small subunit of a ribosome that has three additional binding sites (A, P, and E) for tRNA molecules (Figure 3.12). The tRNA anticodon sites base-pair with complementary codon sites in the mRNA, and because only **one particular type**

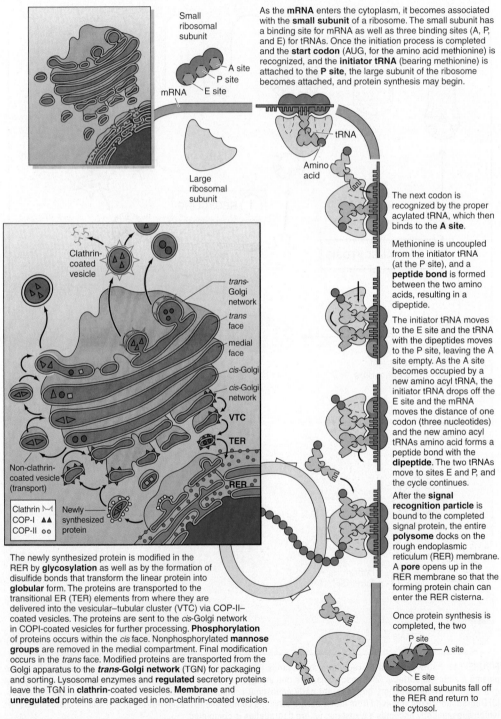

Small ribosomal subunit

A site
P site
E site

mRNA

Large ribosomal subunit

tRNA

Amino acid

As the **mRNA** enters the cytoplasm, it becomes associated with the **small subunit** of a ribosome. The small subunit has a binding site for mRNA as well as three binding sites (A, P, and E) for tRNAs. Once the initiation process is completed and the **start codon** (AUG, for the amino acid methionine) is recognized, and the **initiator tRNA** (bearing methionine) is attached to the **P site**, the large subunit of the ribosome becomes attached, and protein synthesis may begin.

The next codon is recognized by the proper acylated tRNA, which then binds to the **A site**.

Methionine is uncoupled from the initiator tRNA (at the P site), and a **peptide bond** is formed between the two amino acids, resulting in a dipeptide.

The initiator tRNA moves to the E site and the tRNA with the dipeptides moves to the P site, leaving the A site empty. As the A site becomes occupied by a new amino acyl tRNA, the initiator tRNA drops off the E site and the mRNA moves the distance of one codon (three nucleotides) and the new amino acyl tRNAs amino acid forms a peptide bond with the **dipeptide**. The two tRNAs move to sites E and P, and the cycle continues.

After the **signal recognition particle** is bound to the completed signal protein, the entire **polysome** docks on the rough endoplasmic reticulum (RER) membrane. A **pore** opens up in the RER membrane so that the forming protein chain can enter the RER cisterna.

Once protein synthesis is completed, the two

Clathrin-coated vesicle

*trans-*Golgi network

trans face

medial face

cis-Golgi

cis-Golgi network

VTC

TER

Non-clathrin-coated vesicle (transport)

RER

Clathrin	⋈	Newly synthesized protein
COP-I	▲▲	
COP-II	∘∘	

The newly synthesized protein is modified in the RER by **glycosylation** as well as by the formation of disulfide bonds that transform the linear protein into **globular** form. The proteins are transported to the transitional ER (TER) elements from where they are delivered into the vesicular–tubular cluster (VTC) via COP-II–coated vesicles. The proteins are sent to the *cis*-Golgi network in COPI-coated vesicles for further processing. **Phosphorylation** of proteins occurs within the *cis* face. Nonphosphorylated **mannose groups** are removed in the medial compartment. Final modification occurs in the *trans* face. Modified proteins are transported from the Golgi apparatus to the ***trans*-Golgi network** (TGN) for packaging and sorting. Lysosomal enzymes and **regulated** secretory proteins leave the TGN in **clathrin**-coated vesicles. **Membrane** and **unregulated** proteins are packaged in non-clathrin-coated vesicles.

P site
A site
E site

ribosomal subunits fall off the RER and return to the cytosol.

FIGURE 3.12. A diagram illustrating protein synthesis (From Gartner LP, Hiatt JL. *Color Atlas of Histology.* 5th ed. Baltimore, MD: Lippincott William & Wilkins; 2009:8.)

of many tRNAs in a cell can base-pair with each codon, it is the **codon** that determines which amino acid will be added to the peptide chain.

(2) Once the start codon (AUG for methionine) is recognized and the initiator tRNA (bearing methionine) is attached to the P site, a **large ribosome subunit** combines with the small subunit, and protein synthesis begins.

(3) The next codon is recognized by an aminoacyl tRNA bearing the proper amino acid, which then binds to the A site (first step). Methionine at the P site forms the first peptide bond with the incoming amino acid forming a dipeptide (second step).

(4) The mRNA moves a distance of one codon (three nucleotides) through the small subunit, and the "spent" initiator tRNA moves to the E site and is ejected, leaving the A site empty so that a new aminoacyl tRNA can bind (third step).

(5) The A site then becomes occupied by an aminoacyl tRNA bearing the next amino acid to be added, which forms a peptide bond with the growing chain at the P site, and the initiator tRNA is ejected from the E site and the process repeats over and over until the stop codon is reached and protein synthesis ceases.

The ribosome moves along the mRNA in the 5′ to 3′ direction using acylated tRNAs as adapters to add each amino acid to the end of the growing peptide chain, which is always located at the P site of the large subunit of the ribosome.

b. Transport of the newly formed peptide into the RER cisterna occurs by a mechanism described by the **signal hypothesis** as follows (Figure 3.13):

(1) mRNAs for secretory, membrane, and lysosomal proteins contain codons that encode a short polypeptide known as the **leading signal sequence**.

(2) When the signal sequence is formed on the ribosome, a ribonucleated protein (a complex of RNA and protein) known as the **signal recognition particle (SRP)** in the cytosol binds to it.

(3) Synthesis of the growing chain stops until the SRP facilitates the relocation of the polysome to **SRP receptors** in the RER membrane.

(4) The large subunits of the ribosomes interact with ribosome receptor proteins, which bind them to the RER membrane. The SRP detaches, and multisubunit **protein**

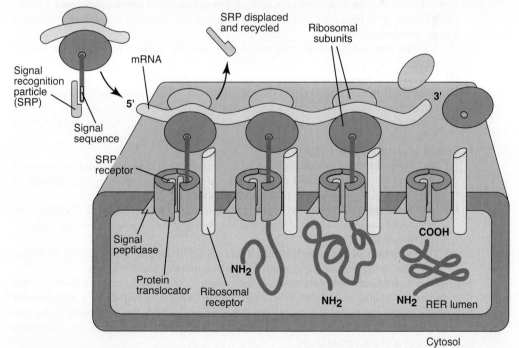

FIGURE 3.13. The signal hypothesis. The signal sequence of a newly formed secretory polypeptide binds to a signal recognition particle (SRP) that delivers the ribosome–peptide–SRP complex to a receptor on the rough endoplasmic reticulum (RER). The SRP is recycled, and the polypeptide is translocated into the cisterna of the RER, where a signal peptidase cleaves off the signal sequence.

translocators form a pore across the RER membrane. Synthesis resumes, and the newly formed polypeptide is threaded through the pore and into the RER cisterna (lumen).

   c. Posttranslational modification in the RER

   (1) After the newly formed polypeptide enters the cisterna, a **signal peptidase** cleaves the signal sequence from it.

   (2) The polypeptide is glycosylated.

   (3) Disulfide bonds form, converting the linear polypeptide into a globular form.

   d. Protein transport from the RER to the cis-Golgi (Figure 3.14)

   (1) Transitional elements of the RER give rise to **COP-II coatomer–coated vesicles** containing newly synthesized protein.

   (2) These vesicles move to the **VTCs**, where they fuse with the membranes to deliver the protein.

   (3) The **VTC** appears to be the first way station for the segregation of anterograde versus retrograde transport in the secretory pathway. Either proteins move forward toward the **cis-Golgi**, or if they are RER-resident proteins that escaped from the RER, they are captured by a specific membrane receptor protein and returned in **COP-I coatomer– coated vesicles** to the RER along a microtubule-guided pathway.

   e. Anterograde transport from the VTC to the *cis*-Golgi is via COP-II coatomer–coated vesicles.

   f. Movement of material anterograde among the Golgi subcompartments may occur by cisternal maturation and/or by vesicular transport, as follows:

   (1) Cisternae-containing proteins may change in biochemical composition as they move intact across the stack.

   (2) Vesicles (COP-II-coated, according to some investigators) may bud off one cisterna and fuse with the dilated rim of another cisterna.

   (3) Although both mechanisms have been observed, the precise way that anterograde transport occurs across the Golgi stack of cisternae is unresolved.

   (4) **Retrograde** vesicular transport occurs between Golgi cisternae and between the Golgi and the VTC or RER via COP-I-coated vesicles.

   g. Protein processing in the Golgi complex (Figure 3.14) occurs as proteins move from the cis to the trans face of the Golgi complex through **distinct cisternal subcompartments**. Protein processing may include the following events, each of which occurs in a different cisternal subcompartment:

   (1) Proteins targeted for lysosomes are tagged with mannose 6-phosphate in the cis cisterna.

   (2) Mannose residues are removed in cis and medial cisternae.

   (3) Some proteins undergo terminal glycosylation with sialic acid residues and galactose.

   (4) Sulfation and phosphorylation of amino acid residues take place.

   (5) A membrane similar in composition and thickness to the plasma membrane is acquired.

   h. Sorting of proteins in TGN (Figure 3.14)

   (1) **Regulated secretory proteins** are sorted from membrane and lysosomal proteins and delivered via clathrin-coated vesicles to condensing vacuoles, in which removal of water via ionic exchanges yields **secretory granules**.

   (2) **Lysosomal proteins** are sorted into clathrin-coated regions of the TGN that have receptors for mannose 6-phosphate and are delivered to late endosomes via clathrin-coated vesicles.

   (3) **Plasma membrane proteins** are sorted into coatomer-coated regions of the TGN and delivered to the plasma membrane in COP-II coatomer–coated vesicles.

2. Synthesis of transmembrane proteins also takes place on polyribosomes at the surface of the RER, but rather than entering the lumen, the transfer process is **halted** (by a **stop-transfer sequence**), and the transmembrane protein becomes anchored in the RER membrane. The ultimate destination of this protein will be the RER membrane, the membrane of another organelle, or the plasma membrane.

3. Synthesis of cytosolic proteins takes place on polyribosomes lying **free** in the cytosol and is directed by mRNAs that **lack** signal codons. Such proteins (e.g., protein kinase and hemoglobin) are released directly into the cytosol.

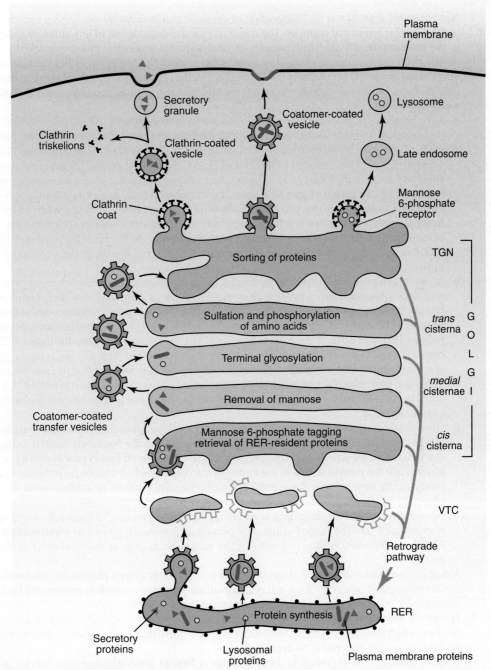

FIGURE 3.14. The pathways of secretory proteins in separate compartments of the Golgi complex. Proteins synthesized in the rough endoplasmic reticulum (RER) include secretory (▲), membrane (/), and lysosomal (o) proteins. These proteins bud off the transitional element of the RER via COP-coated vesicles and enter the vesicular–tubular cluster (VTC). From here they are transported to the *cis*-Golgi via COP-coated vesicles. Anterograde passage through the Golgi cisternae is either via COP-coated vesicles or by cisternal maturation. Cisternal maturation coupled with retrograde vesicular transport of Golgi enzymes is currently a favored view. Only COP-I vesicles are thought to function in retrograde transport (from Golgi to VTC or RER), but both COP-II and COP-I may function in anterograde transport. Not all proteins undergo all of the chemical modifications (e.g., only lysosomal proteins undergo tagging with mannose 6-phosphate). Final sorting occurs in the *trans*-Golgi network (TGN).

C. Intracellular digestion

1. **Nonlysosomal digestion** is the degradation of cytosolic constituents by mechanisms outside of the vacuolar lysosomal pathway. The major site for the degradation of unwanted proteins is the **proteasome**, a cylindrical complex of nonlysosomal proteases. Proteins marked for destruction are enzymatically tagged with **ubiquitin**, a relatively small protein 76 amino acids long that is commonly occurring in the cytoplasm and the nucleus. It is the ubiquitination that delivers them to the proteasome, where they are broken down to small peptides, seven to eight amino acids long.

   a. Each proteasome is a 26S nonmembranous, cylindrical organelle with a hollow center; it is composed of three subunits, a 20S **core particle** and two **regulatory particles**, 19S each, capping each end (entry face [top] and exit face [bottom]) of the proteasome. The core particle is 15 nm tall with a diameter of 11 to 12 nm whose central lumen may be as small as 1.3 nm in diameter or as large as 5.3 nm. Viewed from the side, the core particle is seen to be composed of four ring-shaped units, named α, β, β, and α, counting from entry face to exit face. The two α subunits bind the regulatory particles, whereas the luminal aspects of the two β subunits function as proteolytic enzymes. The regulatory subunit at the entry face acts as a lid that controls access to the lumen of the proteasome, whereas the regulatory subunit on the exit face permits the release of the products of proteolysis.

   b. In order for a protein to be permitted entry into the lumen of the proteasome, the protein has to be ubiquitinated, a process that requires a set of three enzymes that attach a ubiquitin molecule to the targeted protein. The first enzyme, **ubiquitin-activating enzyme (E1)**, activates ubiquitin so that the second enzyme, **ubiquitin-conjugating enzyme (E2)**, can bind to the targeted protein. The third enzyme, **ubiquitin-ligase (E3)** can now transfer the ubiquitin molecule to the targeted protein. This process is repeated several times, so that a number of ubiquitin molecules may be attached to each other, forming a **polyubiquitin chain** bound to the targeted protein. E1, E2, and especially E3, come in many forms, indicating that recognition of a specific targeted protein is probably enzyme specific.

   c. Once the targeted protein is polyubiquitinated (at least four ubiquitin molecules must be bound to the protein) it may bind, in the presence of ATP, to the regulatory particle at the entry face. The regulatory particle unhinges and, similar to a lid that is attached to a pot, lifts to allow the protein access to the lumen of the core particle. However, in order for the protein to be able to enter the narrow lumen of the core particle, two things must take place: (1) the target protein must be deubiquitinated and (2) the targeted protein must be unfolded, where the unfolding is an energy-requiring process. The unfolded protein is introduced into the lumen of the core particle, a procedure known as **translocation**. The targeted protein is then degraded by the enzymatic activity of the β subunits of the proteasome.

   Although most proteins must be ubiquitinated before they may enter a proteasome, there are certain exceptions, especially if the cell is under stressful conditions such as exposure to high temperature, infectious agents, or higher than normal oxygen levels.

2. **Lysosomal digestion** (Figure 3.8) is the degradation of material within various types of lysosomes by lysosomal enzymes. Different lysosomal compartments are involved, depending on the origin of the material to be degraded.

   a. **Heterophagy** is the ingestion and degradation of **foreign material** taken into the cell by receptor-mediated endocytosis or phagocytosis.

      (1) Digestion of **endocytosed** ligands occurs in **multivesicular bodies** (Figure 3.8).

      (2) Digestion of **phagocytosed** microorganisms and foreign particles begins and may be completed in **phagolysosomes**.

   b. **Autophagy** is the segregation of an organelle or other cell constituents within membranes from the RER to form an **autophagic vacuole** (Figure 3.9), which is subsequently digested in an **autophagolysosome**.

   c. **Crinophagy** is the fusion of **hormone secretory granules** and lysosomes and their subsequent digestion. Crinophagy is used to remove **excess numbers** of secretory granules from the cell.

CLINICAL CONSIDERATIONS **Lysosomal storage diseases** are hereditary disorders caused by a deficiency in specific lysosomal acid hydrolases. Therefore, **lysosomes** are unable to degrade certain compounds, which accumulate and interfere with cell function.

1. **Tay-Sachs disease** is characterized by glycolipids (namely, G_{M2} gangliosides) accumulating in the lysosomes of neurons as a result of a deficiency of the enzyme hexosaminidase A. The disease is most common in children of central European Jewish descent. The large buildup of gangliosides in neurons of the brain results in marked degenerative changes in the central nervous system, and death usually occurs before the age of 4 years.

2. A hallmark of **Hurler syndrome** is that glycosaminoglycans (GAGs) and proteoglycans accumulate in the heart, brain, liver, and other organs. This rare inherited disease is caused by a deficiency in any 1 of 10 lysosomal enzymes involved in the sequential degradation of GAGs. Clinical features of Hurler syndrome include skeletal deformities, enlarged organs, progressive mental deterioration, deafness, and death before the age of 10 years.

3. **Glycogen storage diseases** are caused by a hereditary defect in an enzyme involved in either the synthesis or the degradation of glycogen. As a result, glycogen accumulates most often in the liver, skeletal muscle, and the heart, but the major organ involvement depends on the particular enzymatic defect. There are at least 10 distinct glycogen storage diseases.

Review Test

Directions: Each of the numbered items or incomplete statements in this section is followed by answers or by completions of the statement. Select the ONE lettered answer or completion that is BEST in each case.

1. Which of the following organelles divides by fission?

(A) Golgi complex
(B) RER
(C) Peroxisome
(D) SER
(E) Centriole

2. A 30-year-old man with very high blood cholesterol levels (290 mg/dL) has been diagnosed with premature atherosclerosis. His father died of a heart attack at age 45, and his mother, aged 44, has coronary artery disease. Which of the following is the most likely explanation of his condition?

(A) He has a lysosomal storage disease and cannot digest cholesterol.
(B) He has a peroxisomal disorder and produces low levels of hydrogen peroxide.
(C) The SER in his hepatocytes has proliferated and produced excessive amounts of cholesterol.
(D) He has a genetic disorder and synthesizes defective LDL receptors.
(E) He is unable to manufacture endosomes.

3. Movement of protein from the RER to the VTC takes place in which of the following cell components?

(A) A caveolin-coated vesicle
(B) A clathrin-coated vesicle
(C) A coatomer I–coated vesicle
(D) A coatomer II–coated vesicle
(E) An early endosome

4. The retrieval of secretion granule membrane immediately after exocytosis occurs in which of the following cell components?

(A) A caveolin-coated vesicle
(B) A clathrin-coated vesicle
(C) A coatomer I–coated vesicle
(D) A coatomer II–coated vesicle
(E) An early endosome

5. Movement of protein from trans to *cis*-Golgi cisternae occurs in which of the following cell components?

(A) A caveolin-coated vesicle
(B) A clathrin-coated vesicle
(C) A coatomer I–coated vesicle
(D) A coatomer II–coated vesicle
(E) An early endosome

6. Uncoupling of endocytosed ligands from receptors takes place in which of the following cell components?

(A) A caveolin-coated vesicle
(B) A clathrin-coated vesicle
(C) A coatomer I–coated vesicle
(D) A coatomer II–coated vesicle
(E) An early endosome

7. Movement of acid hydrolases from the TGN to a late endosome takes place in which of the following cell components?

(A) A caveolin-coated vesicle
(B) A clathrin-coated vesicle
(C) A coatomer I–coated vesicle
(D) A coatomer II–coated vesicle
(E) An early endosome

8. Which of the following cytoskeletal components is associated with kinesin?

(A) Keratin
(B) Lamin A
(C) Microfilament
(D) Microtubule
(E) Neurofilament

9. Which of the following consists of globular actin monomers linked into a double helix?

(A) Keratin
(B) Lamin A
(C) Microfilament
(D) Microtubule
(E) Neurofilament

10. Which of the following has a rigid wall composed of 13 protofilament strands?

(A) Keratin
(B) Lamin A
(C) Microfilament
(D) Microtubule
(E) Neurofilament

11. Which of the following provides structural support to astrocytes?

(A) Keratin
(B) Lamin A
(C) Microfilament
(D) Microtubule
(E) Neurofilament

12. This tissue section from a tumor has been immunochemically stained for the intermediate filament protein glial fibrillary acidic protein (GFAP). Based on the reddish-brown staining observed (*arrow*), the tumor has originated from which of the following?

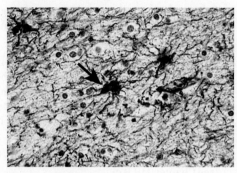

(A) Oligodendrocytes
(B) Chondrocytes
(C) Neurons
(D) Endothelial cells
(E) Fibroblasts

Answers and Explanations

1. **C.** A peroxisome originates from preexisting peroxisomes. It imports specific cytosolic proteins and then undergoes fission. The other organelle that divides by fission is the mitochondrion (see receptor-mediated Chapter 3 II A 10).

2. **D.** Cells import cholesterol by the receptor-mediated uptake of LDLs in coated vesicles. Certain individuals inherit defective genes and cannot make LDL receptors, or they make defective receptors that cannot bind to clathrin-coated pits. The result is an inability to internalize LDLs, which leads to high levels of LDLs in the bloodstream. High LDL levels predispose a person to premature atherosclerosis and increase the risk of heart attacks (see Chapter 3 III A 1 Clinical Considerations).

3. **D.** Transport of protein from the RER to the VTC occurs via (COP-II) coatomer-coated vesicles (see Chapter 3 III B c).

4. **B.** Membrane recycling after exocytosis of the contents of a secretion granule occurs via clathrin-coated vesicles (see Chapter 3 III A 3).

5. **C.** Transfer of material among the cisternae of the Golgi complex in a retrograde direction takes place via (COP-I) coatomer-coated vesicles (see Chapter 3 III B e).

6. **E.** The uncoupling of ligands and receptors internalized by receptor-mediated endocytosis occurs in the early endosome (see Chapter 3 II A 9 b).

7. **B.** Proteins targeted for lysosomes (via late endosomes) leave the TGN in clathrin-coated vesicles (see Chapter 3 II A 8 a).

8. **D.** Kinesin is a force-generating protein associated with microtubules. It serves as a molecular motor for the transport of organelles and vesicles outward, away from the centrosome (see Chapter 3 II C 1).

9. **C.** Globular actin monomers (G actin) polymerize into a double helix of filamentous actin (F actin), also called a microfilament, in response to the regulatory influence of a number of actin-binding proteins (see Chapter 3 II C 2).

10. **D.** A microtubule consists of α- and β-tubulin dimers polymerized into a spiral around a hollow lumen to form a fairly rigid tubule. When cross-sectioned, the microtubule reveals 13 protofilament strands, which represent the tubulin dimers present in one complete turn of the spiral (see Chapter 3 II C 1).

11. **E.** Glial filaments are a type of intermediate filament composed of GFAP and present in fibrous astrocytes. These filaments are supportive, but they may play additional roles in both normal and pathologic processes in the central nervous system (see Chapter 3 II C 3).

12. **A.** The intermediate filament protein GFAP is present in glial cells, including microglia, oligodendrocytes, fibrous astrocytes, and Schwann cells. Vimentin is found in cells of connective tissue origin, which include fibroblasts, chondrocytes, and endothelial cells. Neurons contain intermediate neurofilaments, which would not stain for either GFAP or vimentin (Chapter 3 II C 3 Clinical Considerations).

chapter 4

Extracellular Matrix

I. OVERVIEW—THE EXTRACELLULAR MATRIX

A. Structure. The extracellular matrix (ECM) is an **organized meshwork of macromolecules** surrounding and underlying cells. Although it varies in composition, in general it consists of an amorphous **ground substance** (containing primarily glycosaminoglycans [GAGs], proteoglycans, and glycoproteins [multiadhesive glycoproteins]) and **fibers** (Figure 4.1).

B. Functions. The ECM, along with water and other small molecules (e.g., nutrients, ions), constitutes the **extracellular environment**. By affecting the metabolic activities of cells in contact with it, the ECM may alter the cells and influence their shape, migration, cell–cell interactions, cell division, and their differentiation. Additionally, the ECM provides physical support against compressive as well as tensile forces.

II. GROUND SUBSTANCE

A. Glycosaminoglycans (GAGs), are long, unbranched polysaccharides composed of **repeating identical disaccharide units**.
   1. An **amino sugar**, either *N*-acetylglucosamine or *N*-acetylgalactosamine, is always one of the repeating disaccharides.
   2. Because GAGs are commonly **sulfated** and usually possess a **uronic acid sugar**, which has a carboxyl group in the repeating disaccharide unit, they have a strong **negative charge**.
   3. GAGs are generally linked to a **core protein**.
   4. The attraction of osmotically active cations (e.g., Na^+) to GAGs results in a heavily hydrated matrix that strongly **resists compression**.
   5. Their extended random coils occupy large volumes of space because they do not fold compactly.
   6. GAGs may be classified into four main groups on the basis of their chemical structure (Table 4.1).
      a. Hyaluronic acid (hyaluronan) is a very large unsulfated molecule up to 20 μm in length and as much as 10,000 kDa in weight; but it is not attached to a core protein.
      b. The other three GAG groups are **chondroitin sulfate** and **dermatan sulfate, heparin** and **heparan sulfate**, and **keratan sulfate**.

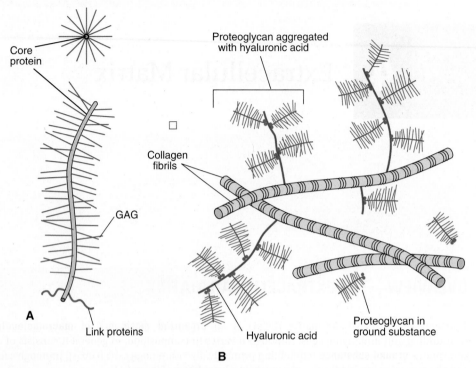

FIGURE 4.1. Components of the extracellular matrix (ECM). **A.** Proteoglycan molecule, two views. **B.** Relationships among various ECM molecules. GAG, glycosaminoglycan. (Adapted with permission from Henrikson RC, Kaye GI, Mazurkiewicz JE. *NMS Histology.* Baltimore, MD: Lippincott Williams & Wilkins; 1997:104.)

CLINICAL CONSIDERATIONS Taking the popular dietary supplement **chondroitin sulfate** and/or **glucosamine** has been reported to reduce the risk of osteoarthritis, joint degeneration, and cartilage deterioration, but the findings are equivocal. In a recent large-scale study, patients with knee osteoarthritis experienced significantly less pain and increased function while taking these compounds when compared with patients on placebo, but radiographic evidence from examining knee joint degeneration was complicated by the fact that the placebo group had a smaller loss of cartilage than had been anticipated on the basis of prior research results, so no definite conclusions could be reached.

table **4.1** Classification of Glycosaminoglycans

Group	Glycosaminoglycans	Linked to Core Protein	Sulfated	Major Locations in Body
I	Hyaluronic acid	No	No	Synovial fluid, vitreous humor, cartilage, skin, most connective tissues
II	Chondroitin sulfate	Yes	Yes	Cornea, cartilage, bone, adventitia of arteries
	Dermatan sulfate	Yes	Yes	Skin, blood vessels, heart valves
III	Heparin	Yes	Yes	Lung, skin, liver, mast cells
	Heparan sulfate	Yes	Yes	Basal laminae, lung, arteries, cell surfaces
IV	Keratan sulfate	Yes	Yes	Cornea, cartilage, nucleus pulposus of intervertebral disks

B. **Proteoglycans** consist of a **core protein from which many GAGs extend**. These large molecules are shaped like a bottlebrush (Figure 4.1A).
   1. Proteoglycans may attach to hyaluronic acid via their core proteins to form large complex aggregates.
   2. Their core proteins, their molecular size, and the number and types of GAGs they contain show marked heterogeneity.
   3. **Function.** Proteoglycans act as binding sites for **growth factors** (e.g., fibroblast growth factor) and **other signaling molecules**. They confer unique attributes on the ECM in certain locations (e.g., **selective permeability** in the filtration barrier of the glomerulus).

C. **Glycoproteins (multiadhesive glycoproteins)** are multifunctional molecules whose domains bind to components of the ECM and to receptors on the cell surface, thereby promoting adhesion between the cell and the matrix (Table 4.2).
   1. **Fibronectin**
      a. **Types and location**
         (1) Matrix fibronectin forms fibrils in the ECM.
         (2) Cell-surface fibronectin is a protein that transiently attaches to the surface of cells.
         (3) Plasma fibronectin is a circulating plasma protein that functions in blood clotting, wound healing, and phagocytosis.
      b. **Function.** Fibronectin is a **multifunctional** molecule.
         (1) Fibronectin has domains for **binding collagen, heparin**, various **cell-surface receptors**, and **cell adhesion molecules (CAMs)**.
         (2) It **mediates cell adhesion** to the ECM by binding to fibronectin receptors on the cell surface.

CLINICAL CONSIDERATIONS **Wound healing** in adults involves the formation of **fibronectin tracks** along which cells migrate to their destinations.

1. In **connective tissue**, wound healing is often characterized by migration of fibroblasts across blood clots, where they adhere to fibronectin.
2. In **epithelia**, wound healing involves reepithelialization, which depends on the **basal lamina serving as a scaffold** for cell migration to cover the denuded area; epithelial cell proliferation and replacement then occur.

table 4.2 Major Glycoproteins of the Extracellular Matrix

Glycoprotein	Location	Function
Fibronectin	Most connective tissues	Binds collagen, heparan sulfate, various cell-surface receptors, and CAMs, thus mediating cell adhesion to the ECM.
Laminin	Basal laminae of epithelial cells and external laminae of muscle cells and Schwann cells	Anchors cells to their basal laminae (and external lamina), thus assisting in adhering epithelial cells to the underlying connective tissue.
Entactin	Basal laminae of epithelial cells and external laminae of muscle cells and Schwann cells	Links laminin to type IV collagen of the basal laminae (and external laminae).
Tenascin	Embryonic connective tissue	Facilitates cell–matrix adhesion, thus assisting in cell migration.
Chondronectin	Cartilage	Assists cartilage cells in adhering to their matrix.
Osteonectin	Bone	Assists bone cells in adhering to their matrix. Influences calcification of the bone matrix.

CAMs, cell adhesion molecules;

2. Laminin is located in basal laminae, where it is synthesized by adjacent epithelial cells, and in external laminae surrounding muscle cells and Schwann cells.

    a. The arms of this large **cross-shaped glycoprotein** have binding sites for cell-surface receptors (integrins), heparan sulfate, type IV collagen, and entactin.

    b. Function. Laminin mediates interaction between epithelial cells and the ECM by anchoring the cell surface to the basal lamina.

3. Entactin is a component of all basal (and external) laminae.

    a. This sulfated adhesive glycoprotein **binds laminin**.

    b. Function. Entactin links laminin with type IV collagen in the lamina densa.

4. Tenascin is an adhesive glycoprotein most abundant in embryonic tissues.

    a. Tenascin is secreted by glial cells in the developing nervous system.

    b. Function. Tenascin promotes cell–matrix adhesion and thus plays a role in cell migration.

5. Chondronectin, a glycoprotein in cartilage, attaches chondrocytes to type II collagen.

    a. This **multifunctional** molecule has binding sites for collagen proteoglycans and cell-surface receptors.

    b. Function. By influencing the composition of its ECM, chondronectin plays a role in the development and maintenance of cartilage.

6. Osteonectin

    a. This ECM calcium-binding glycoprotein found in bone is synthesized by osteoblasts.

    b. It has binding sites for type I collagen and for integrins of osteoblasts and osteocytes.

    c. Function. Osteonectin plays a role in bone formation and remodeling and in maintaining bone mass by influencing calcification.

D. Fibronectin receptors, which belong to the **integrin family of receptors,** are transmembrane proteins consisting of two polypeptide chains.

    1. Because they enable cells to adhere to the ECM, they are known as **CAMs**.

    2. They bind to fibronectin via a specific tripeptide sequence (Arg-Gly-Asp; RGD sequence); other extracellular adhesive proteins also contain this sequence.

    3. Function. They link fibronectin outside the cell to cytoskeletal components (e.g., to actin) inside the cell (Figure 4.2) and may activate cell-signaling pathways that determine the cell's behavior; conversely, the cell can enhance or inhibit its ability to bind to the ECM.

III. FIBERS

A. Collagen is the most abundant structural protein of the ECM. It exists in at least 25 molecular types, which vary in the amino acid sequence of their three α-chains (Table 4.3). There are four major categories of collagens into which the 25 or so different molecular types of collagens may be classed. They are fibril-forming, fibril-associated, network-forming, and transmembrane collagens. Before the discussion of the members of these major categories, fibril-forming collagen synthesis and network-forming collagens have to be described.

    1. Collagen synthesis and assembly into **fibrils** occur via a series of **intracellular** and **extracellular** events (Figure 4.3).

        a. Intracellular events in collagen synthesis occur in the following sequence:

            (1) Preprocollagen synthesis occurs at the rough endoplasmic reticulum (RER) and is directed by messenger ribonucleic acid (mRNA) that encodes the different types of α-chains to be synthesized.

            (2) Hydroxylation of specific proline and lysine residues of the forming polypeptide chain occurs within the RER. The reaction is catalyzed by specific **hydroxylases** that require vitamin C as a cofactor.

            (3) Attachment of sugars (glycosylation) to specific hydroxylysine residues also occurs within the RER.

            (4) Procollagen triple-helix formation takes place in the RER and is precisely regulated by **propeptides** (extra nonhelical amino acid sequences) at both ends of each α-chain. The three α-chains align and coil into a triple helix.

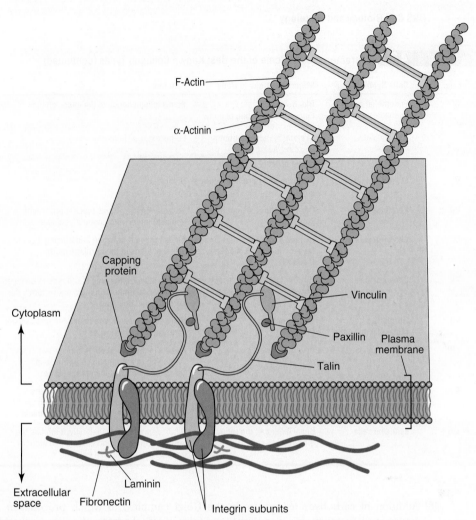

FIGURE 4.2. Integrin receptors such as the fibronectin receptor link molecules outside the cell with components inside the cell. This is common at focal contacts (adhesion plaques), where the integrins serve as transmembrane linkers that mediate reciprocal interactions between the cytoskeleton and the extracellular matrix. (Adapted from Gartner LP, Hiatt JL. *Color Textbook of Histology.* 2nd ed. New York, NY: Saunders; 2001:46.)

table 4.3	Characteristics of Some of the Best Known Collagen Types		
Molecular Type	**Cells Synthesizing**	**Major Locations in Body**	**Function**
I	Fibroblasts	Dermis of skin, tendons, ligaments, fibrocartilage, capsules of some organs	Resists tension
	Osteoblasts	Bone matrix	The arrangement of collagen fibers in compact bone reduces the presence of cleavage planes
	Odontoblasts	Dentin matrix	Structural support and provides a degree of elasticity to dentin
II	Chondroblasts	Hyaline and elastic cartilages	Resists intermittent pressure
III	Fibroblasts	Dermis of skin and capsules of some organs	Forms structural framework
	Reticular cells	Lymph nodes, spleen	
	Smooth muscle cells	Smooth muscle	Forms external lamina
	Schwann cells	Nerve fibers	
	Hepatocyte	Liver	Forms reticular fibers

(continued)

| t a b l e **4.3** Characteristics of Some of the Best Known Collagen Types (continued) |

Molecular Type	Cells Synthesizing	Major Locations in Body	Function
IV	Endothelial cells Epithelial cells	Blood vessels Epidermis and lining of body cavities	Forms lamina densa of the basal lamina
	Muscle cells	Skeletal muscles, smooth muscles, heart	Forms external lamina
	Schwann cells	Nerve fibers	
V	Mesenchymal cells	Placenta and dermal-epidermal junction	Unknown
VII	Keratinocytes	Dermal-epidermal junction	Forms anchoring fibrils that secure lamina densa to underlying connective tissue
IX	Chondrocytes	Hyaline and elastic cartilages (associated with collagen types II and XI)	Binds to type II collagen and affixing it to the proteoglycans of the cartilage matrix
XI	Chondrocytes	Hyaline and elastic cartilages as well as type I collagen	Acts to stabilize the type II and type IX collagen substructure of the cartilage matrix; forms the core of type I collagen
XII	Fibroblasts Mesenchymal cells	Dermis of skin Placenta	Binds to surface of type I collagen and assist it in resisting tensile forces
XIII	Various cell types	In various tissues	Assists in the formation of focal adhesions by binding to fibronectin, integrins, and components of the lamina reticularis
XVII	Epidermis of the skin	Hemidesmosomes	It has domains that are embedded in the epidermal cell membrane binding both to keratins as well as to integrins and laminin
XVIII	Epithelial cells	Basal lamina of the retina of the eye	When degraded enzymatically, it inhibits the formation of new blood vessels and induces apoptosis of endothelial cells

(5) Addition of carbohydrates occurs in the Golgi complex, to which procollagen is transported via transfer vesicles. With the addition of carbohydrates, the oligosaccharide side chains are completed.

(6) Secretion of procollagen occurs by exocytosis after secretory vesicles from the *trans*-Golgi network are guided to the cell surface along microtubules.

CLINICAL CONSIDERATIONS   **Scurvy** is associated with a **deficiency of vitamin C.**

1. Scurvy is caused by the synthesis of poorly hydroxylated tropocollagen, which is unable to form either a stable triple helix or collagen fibrils.
2. **Symptoms** include bleeding gums and eventual tooth loss.
3. Administration of vitamin C reverses the disease.

---

   b. **Extracellular events in collagen synthesis** occur in the following sequence:
      (1) Cleavage of procollagen is catalyzed by the enzymes **procollagen peptidases**, which are located on the extracellular aspect of the cell membrane and remove most of the propeptide sequences at the ends of each α-chain, yielding **tropocollagen** molecules.
      (2) Self-assembly of tropocollagen occurs as insoluble tropocollagen molecules that aggregate near the cell surface. The cell establishes longitudinal furrows in its membrane, and the procollagen molecules are discharged into these furrows and are converted into tropocollagen molecules (as just described).
         (a) **Fibrils** characteristic of types I, II, III, V, and VII collagen are produced.
         (b) These fibrils have a transverse banding periodicity of 67 nm in types I, II, and III collagen (Figures 4.4 and 4.5); the periodicity varies in other types of collagen.

INTRACELLULAR EVENTS

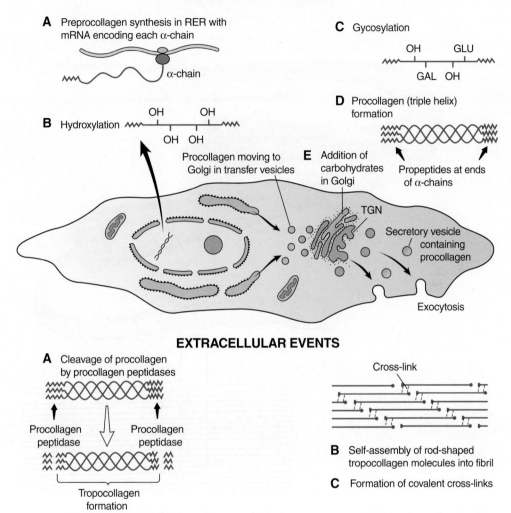

A Preprocollagen synthesis in RER with mRNA encoding each α-chain

α-chain

B Hydroxylation OH OH / OH OH

C Gycosylation OH GLU / GAL OH

D Procollagen (triple helix) formation

Procollagen moving to Golgi in transfer vesicles

E Addition of carbohydrates in Golgi

Propeptides at ends of α-chains

TGN

Secretory vesicle containing procollagen

Exocytosis

EXTRACELLULAR EVENTS

A Cleavage of procollagen by procollagen peptidases

Procollagen peptidase   Procollagen peptidase

Tropocollagen formation

Cross-link

B Self-assembly of rod-shaped tropocollagen molecules into fibril

C Formation of covalent cross-links

FIGURE 4.3. The intracellular and extracellular steps involved in the synthesis of a collagen fibril. RER, rough endoplasmic reticulum; mRNA, messenger ribonucleic acid; TGN, *trans*-Golgi network. (Adapted with permission from Junqueira LC, Carneiro J, Kelley RO. *Basic Histology.* 9th ed. Norwalk, CT: Appleton & Lange; 1998:101.)

(c) The formation of type I collagen requires a core of type XI collagen as well as the inclusion of type III and type V, and type XII collagens.

(d) The formation of type II collagen fibers requires the addition of chondroitin sulfate–enriched type IX collagen fibers.

(3) Covalent bond formation (cross-linking) occurs between adjacent tropocollagen molecules and involves formation of lysine- and hydroxylysine-derived aldehydes. This cross-linking imparts great tensile strength to collagen fibrils.

CLINICAL CONSIDERATIONS   **Ehlers-Danlos type IV syndrome**

1. This syndrome results from a genetic defect in transcription of deoxyribonucleic acid (DNA) or translation of mRNA encoding **type III collagen**, the major component of **reticular fibers.**
2. Clinical findings include skin that is thin, translucent, fragile, easily bruised, and sometimes stretchy (elastic) and joints that are abnormally flexible and that may be easily dislocated.
3. Patients often present with a rupture of the bowel and/or large arteries, where reticular fibers normally ensheath smooth muscle cells.

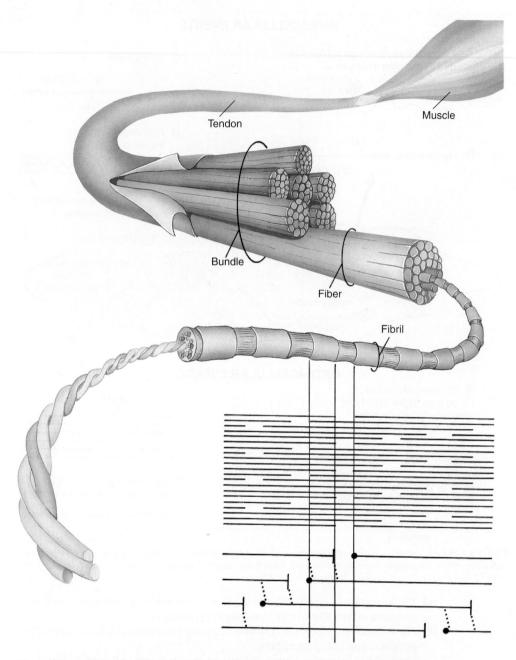

Each collagen fiber bundle is composed of smaller fibrils, which in turn consist of aggregates of **tropocollagen molecules**. Tropocollagen molecules self-assemble in the extracellular environment in such a fashion that there is a gap between the tail of the one and the head of the succeeding molecule of a single row. As fibrils are formed, tails of tropocollagen molecules overlap the heads of tropocollagen molecules in adjacent rows. Additionally, the **gaps** and **overlaps** are arranged so that they are in register with those of neighboring (but not adjacent) rows of tropocollagen molecules. When stained with a heavy metal, such as osmium, the stain preferentially precipitates in the gap regions, resulting in the repeating **light** and **dark** banding of collagen.

FIGURE 4.4. The levels of organization in collagen fibers. As seen by light microscopy, collagen fibers consist of collagen fibrils, which typically reveal a 67-nm cross-banding when observed by electron microscopy. The periodicity along the collagen fibril is due to the precise arrangement of tropocollagen molecules, which overlap each other, producing gap regions where electron-dense stains penetrate and produce a transverse banding across the fibril. (Reprinted with permission from Gartner LP, Hiatt JL. *Color Atlas and Text of Histology.* 6th ed. Baltimore, MD: Wolters Kluwer Health/Lippincott Williams & Wilkins; 2013:66.)

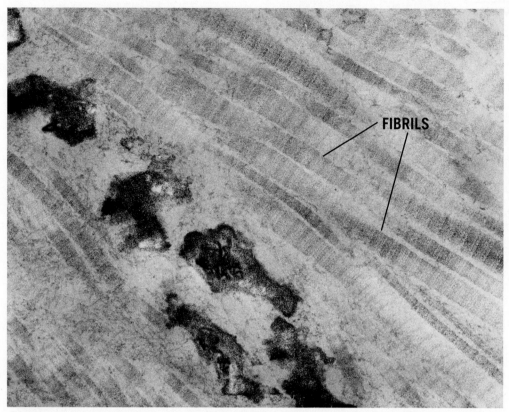

FIBRILS

FIGURE 4.5. Electron micrograph showing a number of collagen fibrils with their characteristic 67-nm cross-banding. The large black structures represent calcium phosphate deposits.

2. Synthesis of network-forming collagens, specifically **type IV collagen**, is unique in that it assembles into a meshwork rather than fibrils.
   a. Type IV collagen constitutes most of the **lamina densa** of basal laminae and external laminae.
   b. It differs from other collagen types as follows:
      (1) The propeptide sequences are not removed from the ends of its procollagen molecules.
      (2) Its triple-stranded helical structure is interrupted in many regions.
      (3) It forms head-to-head dimers that interact to form lateral associations, creating a sheet-like meshwork.

CLINICAL CONSIDERATIONS **Alport syndrome** is the result of genetic defects in the genes that are responsible for the formation of collagen types III, IV, and V, which result in the abnormal type IV collagen assembly. Since the lamina densa of the basal lamina is formed mostly by type IV collagen, individuals afflicted by Alport syndrome present with glomerulonephritis that results in end-stage kidney disease. These individuals also have hearing disorders and an anomaly of the lens of their eyes known as lenticonus, a bulge that occurs in the lens during development; the consequence of the bulge may be a herniated lens. Since the gene that codes for type IV collagen is located on the X chromosome, Alport syndrome occurs much more frequently in males than in females.

3. **Classes of Collagens**
   a. **Fibril-forming collagens** (types I, II, III, V, and XI) are the most common of the collagens; their subunits are the tropocollagen molecules that assemble to form long, flexible fiber bundles whose tensile strength is greater than that of stainless steel of the same diameter. This class of collagen, because of their staggered arrays of tropocollagen molecules,

display a **67-nm cross-banding**. Each tropocollagen molecule, as mentioned above, is composed of three α-chains wrapped around each other, where each α-chain is about 1,000 amino acids long. Because every third amino acid in each α-chain is a **glycine**, the smallest of the amino acids, the three chains can form a very tight helix by bending around these amino acids. Moreover, **hydroxyproline** and **hydroxylysine** molecules also abound in all three α-chains; the hydroxyprolines of each α-chain form tight bonds with each other, assisting in the maintenance of the tight helix. The hydroxylysines bind to each other across neighboring tropocollagen molecules, thus assisting in the formation of collagen fiber bundles.

b. **Fibril-associated collagens** (types IX and XII) are bound to the surfaces of fibril-forming collagens and thereby they stabilize the collagen framework of the tissues in which they reside by adhering not only to the collagen fibers but also to the molecules of the ground substance. **Type IX collagens** are associated with type II collagens of cartilage, and **type XII collagens** are localized on the surface of type I collagens of the dermis and placenta.

c. **Network-forming collagens** (types IV and VII), unlike the other types of collagen, have procollagen as their subunits. As described above, procollagen possesses the propeptide sequences at both ends of the molecule, which, in fibril-forming collagens, are removed by procollagen peptidase in the extracellular environment. Procollagen molecules are unable to assemble in the style of tropocollagen molecules; hence, they do not form fibers. Instead, the procollagen molecules form head-to-head dimers that interact forming lateral associations, creating a **sheet-like meshwork. Type IV collagen** forms the lamina densa of the basal lamina, and **type VII** collagens form the anchoring fibrils that secure the lamina densa to the lamina reticularis of the underlying connective tissue.

d. **Transmembrane collagens** (types XIII, XVII, and XVIII) are associated with focal adhesions, hemidesmosomes, and the basal laminae, respectively.

CLINICAL CONSIDERATIONS **Knobloch syndrome (type I)** is an inherited disease resulting from the malformation of type XVIII collagen. The symptoms include encephalocele, the formation of large brain vesicles that jut out through a defect of the bony skull due to incomplete fusion of the neural tube during embryonic development, as well as sporadic detachment of the retina, and nearsightedness that may become evident by the time the child is a year old.

B. **Elastic fibers**
1. **Components**
    a. **Elastin**, an amorphous structural protein, imparts remarkable elasticity to the ECM; 90% of elastic fibers or elastic sheets are composed of elastin.
        (1) Elastin is unusual in that its lysine molecules form unique linkages with one another.
        (2) Lysine residues of four different chains form covalent bonds called **desmosine cross-links** to create an extensive elastic network.
        (3) Like a rubber band, after being stretched, the elastin returns to its original shape once the tensile force is released.
    b. **Fibrillin-1**, a glycoprotein, organizes elastin into fibers and is the main component of the **peripheral microfibrils** of elastic fibers.
        (1) The amino terminus of one fibrillin-1 interacts with the carboxyl terminus of another fibrilin-1 molecule to form pencil-like head-to-tail assembly of fibrilin-1 molecules to form microfibrils.
        (2) Fibrillin-1 possesses binding sites for tropoelastin, which form cross-links with each other.
        (3) Heparin competes with tropoelastin for binding sites on fibrilin-1, which probably has a regulatory effect on elastic fiber formation.

   c. **Fibulin-5**, a protein, forms bonds with integrin molecules of cells such as vascular smooth muscle cells and endothelial cells of blood vessels, and also facilitates the formation of elastic fibers.

     (1) Fibulin-5 also binds to microfibrils and tropoelastin.

     (2) It has been shown that during wound healing fibulin-5 is present in an increased concentration than in undamaged blood vessels.

   d. **Type VIII collagen** is often associated with elastic fibers, most probably to limit the extent of elastic fiber stretching, protecting the elastic fibers from being damaged by overstretching.

2. **Synthesis of elastic fibers** is carried out by **fibroblasts** in elastic ligaments, **smooth muscle cells** in large arteries, and **chondrocytes** and **chondroblasts** in elastic cartilage.

   a. Synthesis begins with the elaboration of **fibrillin microfibril templates** that are arranged in a parallel array near regions of the cell surface.

   b. These cells manufacture and exocytose a soluble form of elastin, known as **tropoelastin**, and fibulin-5 which bind not only to each other but also to fibrillin-1.

   c. Tropoelastin molecules cross-link with each other to form insoluble, mature elastin.

   d. Additional factors, such as heparan sulfate, microfibril-associated glycoproteins, and fibrillin-2, have been implicated in the assembly of elastic fibers.

CLINICAL CONSIDERATIONS

Marfan syndrome results from mutations in the genes encoding **fibrillin**, a critical component of elastic fibers.

1. Patients with this condition have unusually long, slender limbs and long fingers.

2. The lens of the eye often dislocates; cardiovascular problems are common; and the aorta may rupture, causing death.

3. Treatment includes drugs that decrease blood pressure, and in severe cases surgery replacing the aorta.

Review Test

Directions: Each of the numbered items or incomplete statements in this section is followed by answers or by completions of the statement. Select the ONE lettered answer or completion that is BEST in each case.

1. Which one of the following statements about the fibronectin receptor is true?

(A) It is located exclusively in the basal lamina.

(B) It is a cross-shaped glycoprotein.

(C) It mediates the linkage of molecules outside the cell with cytoskeletal elements inside the cell.

(D) It belongs to the entactin family of receptors.

(E) Its absence is associated with scurvy.

2. Which one of the following events in collagen synthesis occurs outside of the cell?

(A) Synthesis of preprocollagen

(B) Hydroxylation of lysine residues

(C) Triple-helix formation

(D) Carbohydrate addition to procollagen

(E) Cleavage of procollagen by procollagen peptidases

3. A medical student goes to the emergency department and is diagnosed with a ruptured bowel, the result of a genetic condition called Ehlers-Danlos type IV syndrome. Which one of the following statements about this patient's condition is true?

(A) He has a defect in the synthesis of mRNA encoding type I collagen.

(B) He has a defect in the genes encoding type IV collagen.

(C) He has defective type II collagen.

(D) He has an increased risk of breaking his bones.

(E) He has a defect in the translation of mRNA for type III collagen.

4. Which one of the following statements about hyaluronic acid is true?

(A) It is a component of elastic fibers.

(B) It is a glycosaminoglycan.

(C) It is a proteoglycan with a shape resembling a bottlebrush.

(D) It is sulfated.

(E) It is a small molecule.

5. Which one of the following statements about osteonectin is true?

(A) It is present in the lacunae of bone.

(B) It is a proteoglycan.

(C) It binds to type II collagen.

(D) It influences calcification of bone.

(E) It is synthesized by osteoclasts.

6. Which of the following statements about scurvy is true?

(A) One of its symptoms is bowlegs.

(B) It is caused by excessive glycosylation of tropocollagen.

(C) It is caused by a deficiency of vitamin A.

(D) It is associated with structurally defective elastic fibers.

(E) It is alleviated by eating citrus fruits.

7. Which one of the following is a glycoprotein across which fibroblasts migrate during wound healing?

(A) Fibrillin

(B) Fibronectin

(C) Elastin

(D) Entactin

(E) Laminin

8. Which of the following is an adhesive glyco-protein that links type IV collagen with laminin in the lamina densa?

(A) Fibrillin
(B) Fibronectin
(C) Elastin
(D) Entactin
(E) Tenascin

9. Which one of the following is a main component of peripheral microfibrils in an elastic fiber?

(A) Fibrillin
(B) Fibronectin
(C) Elastin
(D) Entactin
(E) Laminin

10. Which one of the following is present in the basement membrane and is manufactured by connective tissue cells?

(A) Fibrillin
(B) Fibronectin
(C) Elastin
(D) Entactin
(E) Laminin

Answers and Explanations

1. **C.** The fibronectin receptor is a transmembrane protein that enables cells to adhere to the ECM. Laminin is a cross-shaped glycoprotein in the basal lamina, where entactin is also present (see Chapter 4 II D).

2. **E.** In the extracellular space, peptidases cleave off end sequences of procollagen to yield tropocollagen, which self-assembles to form collagen fibrils (see Chapter 4 III A 1).

3. **E.** Ehlers-Danlos type IV syndrome is associated with a defect in the synthesis and translation of mRNA for type III reticular collagen (see Chapter 4 III A 1 Clinical Considerations).

4. **B.** Hyaluronic acid is a glycosaminoglycan, not a proteoglycan. The core protein of proteoglycans can attach to hyaluronic acid forming large aggregates (see Chapter 4 II A).

5. **D.** Osteonectin synthesized by osteoblasts influences the calcification of bone and binds to type I collagen in the bone matrix. Type II collagen is found in cartilage (see Chapter 4 II C).

6. **E.** Scurvy is caused by a deficiency of vitamin C, a necessary cofactor in the hydroxylation of preprocollagen. Citrus fruits are rich in vitamin C (see Chapter 4 III A 1 Clinical Considerations).

7. **B.** Fibronectin forms tracks along which cells migrate. During wound healing in connective tissue, fibroblasts adhere to fibronectin in blood clots, facilitating the healing process (see Chapter 4 II C 1 Clinical Considerations).

8. **D.** Entactin is a sulfated adhesive glycoprotein in basal and external laminae that binds both type IV collagen and laminin (see Chapter 4 II C).

9. **A.** Fibrillin is the major component of the peripheral microfibrils of elastic fibers (see Chapter 4 III B).

10. **B.** Fibronectin is synthesized by cells of the connective tissue, usually fibroblasts, and is located in the lamina reticularis near the lamina densa (see Chapter 4 II C 1).

chapter 5

Epithelia and Glands

I. OVERVIEW—EPITHELIA

A. **Structure.** Epithelia are **specialized layers of tissue** arising from all three embryonic germ layers, namely, the ectoderm, mesoderm, and endoderm, that line the internal and cover the external surfaces of the body except in certain areas such as tooth surfaces and articular cartilages. An epithelium consists of a **sheet of cells** lying close together with little extracellular space. These cells have distinct biochemical, functional, and structural domains that confer **polarity**, or sidedness; thus, these cells are said to have **apical, lateral**, and **basal epithelial domains** (or as some authors prefer: **basolateral domain**).

1. **A basement membrane**, composed of a basal lamina and a lamina reticularis, separates the epithelium from underlying connective tissue and blood vessels.

2. Epithelia are **avascular** and receive nourishment by diffusion of molecules through the **basal lamina to which they are attached**.

B. **Classification** (Table 5.1). Epithelia are classified into various types based on the **number** of cell layers (one cell layer is **simple**; more than one is **stratified**) and the **shape of the superficial cells**

t a b l e   5.1 Classification of Epithelia

Type	Shape of Superficial Cell Layer	Typical Locations
One cell layer		
Simple squamous	Flattened	Endothelium (lining of blood vessels), mesothelium (lining of peritoneum and pleura)
Simple cuboidal	Cuboidal	Lining of distal tubule in kidney and ducts in some glands, surface of ovary
Simple columnar	Columnar	Lining of intestine, stomach, and excretory ducts in some glands
Pseudostratified	All cells rest on basal lamina, but not all reach the lumen; thus the epithelium appears falsely stratified	Lining of trachea, primary bronchi, nasal cavity, and excretory ducts in parotid gland
More than one cell layer		
Stratified squamous (not keratinized)	Flattened (nucleated)	Lining of esophagus, vagina, mouth, and true vocal cords
Stratified squamous (keratinized)	Flattened (without nuclei)	Epidermis of skin
Stratified cuboidal	Cuboidal	Lining of ducts in sweat glands
Stratified columnar	Columnar	Lining of large excretory ducts in some glands and cavernous urethra
Transitional	Dome-shaped (when relaxed), flattened (when stretched)	Lining of urinary passages from renal calyces to the urethra

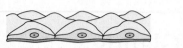

A   Simple squamous

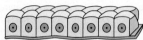

B   Simple cuboidal

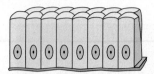

C   Simple columnar

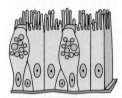

D   Pseudostratified
ciliated columnar
with goblet cells

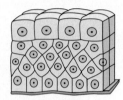

E   Transitional

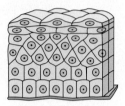

F   Stratified squamous
nonkeratinized

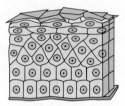

G   Stratified squamous
keratinized

FIGURE 5.1. Classifications of epithelia.

(Figure 5.1). Therefore, all cells composing a simple epithelium contact the basal lamina, whereas in stratified epithelia only the deepest cell layer contacts the basal lamina. **Pseudostratified** epithelia give the appearance of having multiple cell layers, but they are composed of a single cell layer only, as evidenced by the fact that all cells that compose this type of epithelium are in contact with the basal lamina (Figure 5.2).

C. **Function**
   1. **Transcellular transport** of molecules from one epithelial surface to another occurs by various processes, including the following:
      a. **Diffusion** of oxygen and carbon dioxide across the epithelial cells of lung alveoli and capillaries
      b. **Carrier protein–mediated** transport of amino acids and glucose across intestinal epithelia
      c. **Vesicle-mediated** transport of immunoglobulin A (IgA) and other molecules
   2. **Absorption** occurs via **endocytosis** or **pinocytosis** (see Chapter 3 III A) in various organs (e.g., the proximal convoluted tubule of the kidney; see Chapter 18 II).
   3. **Secretion** of various molecules (e.g., hormones, mucinogen, proteins) occurs by **exocytosis**.

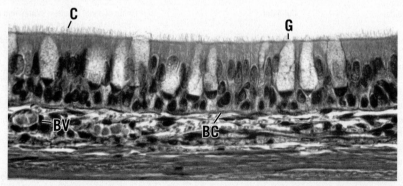

FIGURE 5.2. A light micrograph of pseudostratified ciliated (C) columnar epithelium with goblet cells (G) lining the trachea. All of the cells in this epithelium rest on the basal lamina (note the basal cell [BC]), but not all of them extend to the lumen, giving a falsely stratified appearance. Blood vessels (BV) containing red blood cells are seen in the underlying connective tissue.

4. **Selective permeability** results from the presence of **tight junctions** between epithelial cells and permits fluids with different compositions and concentrations to exist on separate sides of an epithelial layer (e.g., intestinal epithelium).
5. **Protection** from abrasion and injury is provided by the **epidermis,** the epithelial layer of the skin.

CLINICAL CONSIDERATIONS **First-degree burns** are lesions caused by heat, friction, or other agents.

1. Damage is limited to the superficial layers of the **epithelium** (usually the epidermis of the skin).
2. Redness and edema occur, but blisters do not form.
   a. Mitotically active cells remain viable in the deeper layers of the epidermis.
   b. They divide and replace the damaged or destroyed cells.

II. LATERAL EPITHELIAL SURFACES (Figure 5.3)

These surfaces contain specialized molecules that form **junctions** that permit cells to adhere to each other and restrict movement of materials between adjacent cells (paracellular route) into and out of the lumen lined by the epithelium.

A. **The junctional complex** is an intricate arrangement of membrane-associated **cell adhesion molecules** that function in cell-to-cell attachment of columnar epithelial cells. It corresponds to the terminal bar observed in epithelia by light microscopy and consists of three distinct components that are visible by electron microscopy.

1. The **tight junction** (**zonula occludens**; plural: zonulae occludentes) is a zone that surrounds the entire apical perimeter of adjacent cells and is formed by **fusion of the outer leaflets** of the cells' plasma membranes (Figure 5.3).
   a. In freeze-fracture preparations of this zone, the tight junction is visible as a branching anastomosing network of intramembrane **strands (ridges)** on the plasma membrane inner leaflet next to the cytoplasm (P-face) and **grooves** on the corresponding external E-face, the inner aspect of the outer leaflet (Figure 5.3). The strands consist of transmembrane **proteins** of each cell **attached directly to one another**, thus sealing off the extracellular space.
   b. The intramembrane strands that close off the paracellular route possess four groups of transmembrane proteins: claudins, occludins, nectins, and junctional adhesive molecules (JAMs).
      (1) **Claudins** are believed to bear the greatest responsibility in closing off the paracellular route by creating a physical barrier that prevents the movement of material between the cells. However, claudins do form small aqueous pores that allow water and small ions to penetrate this barrier.
      (2) **Occludins** are also present in most, but not all, epithelial cell tight junctions. Their role is not understood as yet.
      (3) **Nectins** are also present in the zonula occludens, and their extracellular domains form a part of the physical barrier.
      (4) **JAMs** are similar to nectins in that their extracellular domains probably impede the movement of molecules in the extracellular space of the tight junction.
         These four proteins have to be reinforced so that they maintain their proper position, and this reinforcement is due to the presence of **actin filaments (F-actin)** of the cytoskeleton. However, there are intermediary proteins that are capable of binding both to F-actin as well as to the four proteins just described. These are the three **zonula occludens proteins, ZO-1, ZO-2,** and **ZO-3,** as well as a fourth protein, known as **afadin**. These four intermediary proteins are located on the cytoplasmic aspect of the region of the cell membrane involved in the formation of the tight junction and, in that fashion, are interposed between the F-actin and the claudins, occludins, nectins, and JAMs, forming a strong bond that maintains the integrity of the tight junction.

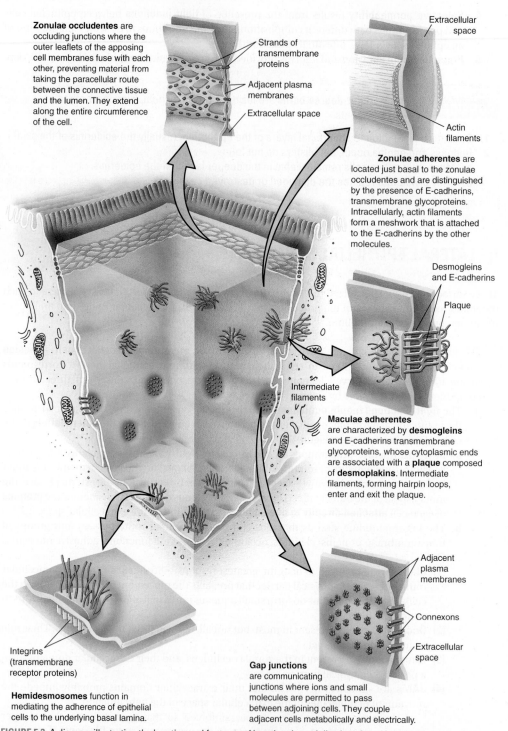

Zonulae occludentes are occluding junctions where the outer leaflets of the apposing cell membranes fuse with each other, preventing material from taking the paracellular route between the connective tissue and the lumen. They extend along the entire circumference of the cell.

Strands of transmembrane proteins

Adjacent plasma membranes

Extracellular space

Extracellular space

Actin filaments

Zonulae adherentes are located just basal to the zonulae occludentes and are distinguished by the presence of E-cadherins, transmembrane glycoproteins. Intracellularly, actin filaments form a meshwork that is attached to the E-cadherins by the other molecules.

Desmogleins and E-cadherins

Plaque

Intermediate filaments

Maculae adherentes are characterized by **desmogleins** and E-cadherins transmembrane glycoproteins, whose cytoplasmic ends are associated with a **plaque** composed of **desmoplakins**. Intermediate filaments, forming hairpin loops, enter and exit the plaque.

Adjacent plasma membranes

Connexons

Extracellular space

Integrins (transmembrane receptor proteins)

Hemidesmosomes function in mediating the adherence of epithelial cells to the underlying basal lamina.

Gap junctions are communicating junctions where ions and small molecules are permitted to pass between adjoining cells. They couple adjacent cells metabolically and electrically.

FIGURE 5.3. A diagram illustrating the location and features of junctional specializations found in epithelial cells: the junctional complex, the desmosome, the gap junction, and the hemidesmosome. (From Gartner LP, Hiatt, JL. *Color Atlas of Histology.* 5th ed. Baltimore, MD: Lippincott, William & Wilkins; 2009:33.)

    c. The tight junction **prevents** not only the movement of substances into the **extracellular space** from the lumen but also intermingling of the transmembrane proteins of the apical with those of the lateral domains. This ability (its tightness) is directly related to the number and complexity of the intramembrane strands and to the function of the epithelia housing the particular tight junction.

    d. The **fascia occludens**, a ribbon-like area of fusion between transmembrane proteins on adjacent **endothelial cells** lining capillaries, is analogous to the zonula occludens but does not encircle the perimeter of the entire cell.

2. Anchoring junctions of epithelial cells consist of four types, two on the cell's lateral domain, **zonula adherens** (plural: zonulae adherentes) and **desmosome** (**macula adherens**; plural: maculae adherentes) and two, discussed in the section below, on the cell's basal domain, namely **hemidesmosomes** and **focal adhesions**.

    a. The adhering junction, **zonula adherens**, surrounds the entire perimeter of epithelial cell, and is located just basal to and reinforcing the zonula occludens (Figure 5.3).

        (1) It is characterized by a 10-to 20-nm separation between the adjoining cell membranes where the extracellular portions of the transmembrane glycoprotein **E-cadherin** molecules occupy the intercellular space.

        (2) A mat of **actin filaments** is located on each of the cytoplasmic surfaces of the zonulae adherentes. The actin filaments are linked to each other via the actin-binding proteins α-**actinin**, and are linked, via another actin-binding protein **vinculin**, to the protein **catenin**, which also binds to the intracellular portion of the **E-cadherin** molecules. It is in this fashion that the E-cadherin molecules are reinforced by the α-actinin filaments of the cytoskeleton. The extracellular moieties of E-cadherins of adjacent cells face each other in the extracellular space and, in the presence of Ca^{2+} ions, bind to each other, promoting **adhesion** of adjacent cells to each other.

        (3) **Fasciae adherentes**, ribbon-like adhesion zones in the **intercalated disks** of cardiac muscle, are analogous to zonulae adherentes, but they do not surround the entire perimeter of the cardiac muscle cells.

    b. **Desmosomes (maculae adherentes)** are small, discrete, disk-shaped **adhesive sites**. Desmosomes are commonly found at sites other than the junctional complex, where they join epithelial cells to each other.

        (1) Desmosomes are characterized by having five regions, two intracellular regions in each cell, namely the **outer dense plaque** and **inner dense plaque,** and an extracellular region, known as the **extracellular core,** in the space between the two cells.

        (2) The extracellular moieties of the transmembrane glycoproteins, **desmogleins** and **desmocollins**, members of the E-cadherin superfamily, of one cell contact desmogleins and desmocollins of the other cell in the extracellular space. In order for these glycoproteins to form strong adhesive bonds with their counterparts, Ca^{2+} ions must be present. These extracellular moieties of desmogleins and desmocollins of each cell form the extracellular core and hold the two cells to each other.

        (3) The intracellular moieties of desmogleins and desmocollins form bonds with the desmosomal plaque proteins **plakoglobins** and **plakophilins**. Additional large proteins, known as **desmoplakins**, contact both plakoglobins and plakophilins, and together they form the **outer dense plaque** that presses against the cytoplasmic aspect of each cell membrane.

        (4) The desmoplakins are large molecules, and their tails extend farther into the cytoplasm where they contact and form bonds with the **keratin intermediate filaments** of the epithelial cell. This region of bonding between the desmoplakins and the intermediate filaments forms the **inner dense plaque**, and it is here that the cytoskeleton is affixed to the site of adhesion.

B. Gap junctions (communicating junctions; nexus) are not part of the junctional complex and are frequent components of certain tissues other than epithelia (e.g., central nervous system, cardiac muscle, and smooth muscle).

    1. Gap junctions are small aqueous pores that are inserted into the plasma membranes that **couple adjacent cells** metabolically and electrically (see Figure 5.3).

2. A gap junction is composed of subunits, called **connexons** (**hemichannels**), which extend beyond the cell surface into the **gap** (a 2-nm-wide intercellular space) (Figure 5.3). Two connexons, one in the plasma membrane of each adjacent cell contacting each other in the intercellular space, form a single gap junction.

    a. **Connexons** consist of six subunits (composed of proteins called **connexins**), which are arranged radially around a central channel with a diameter of 1.5 nm (see Figure 5.3).

    b. Precise **alignment** of connexons on adjacent cells produces a junction where they form **cell-to-cell channels** permitting the passage of ions and small molecules with a molecular weight of less than 1 kDa (kilodaltons) but preventing these molecules from escaping into the extracellular space.

    c. Since there are different connexons, depending on the amino acid sequence of their connexins, gap junctions may be homotypic or heterotypic.

    d. Connexins may alter their conformation to shut off communication between cells, especially if one of the cells is dying.

    e. Usually, a large number of gap junction channels are clustered together to form a **gap junction plaque** where exchange of ions and small second messenger molecules may occur.

    f. Connexons are in abundant supply where intercellular communication and coordination is essential such as in smooth and cardiac muscles, nerves, and certain epithelia.

CLINICAL CONSIDERATIONS

Deafness

Mutations of certain connexins genes, which are abundant in the cochlea, are responsible for deafness.

Bone development and mineralization

Certain genes code for connexins located in gap junctions between osteoblasts and osteocytes in developing bone. When a particular gene (Cx43) is deleted, skeletal defects develop and bone mineralization is delayed.

    Darier disease (also known as **keratosis follicularis**) is recognizable due to the pus-filled, dry, dark regions on the skin (although the pus may be absent). It is an inherited, autosomal dominant, noncontagious condition. Histologically, the keratinocytes of the skin (especially those of the stratum spinosum and stratum granulosum) are rounded, and because the desmosomal contacts are compromised, the intercellular connections are weakened and ineffective, leading to acantholysis. The distinguishing characteristics of the disease are a specific scent of the affected skin and the fragility of the fingernails. On the average, 1 in 100,000 people is afflicted by Darier disease worldwide. The condition appears to be due to a problem of **intracellular trafficking** of **desmoplakin** to the lateral cell membrane during desmosomal assembly.

C. Lateral interdigitations (plicae) are irregular fingerlike projections that **interlock** adjacent epithelial cells. These lateral interdigitations are most frequently present in cells that function in fluid and/ or electrolyte transport (e.g., epithelial lining of the intestines, proximal tubules of the kidney).

III. BASAL EPITHELIAL SURFACES (Figures 5.3 and 5.4)

A. The basement membrane is a narrow, flexible, PAS-positive (i.e., it stains purplish with periodic acid–Schiff reagent) acellular supportive structure that is consistently interposed between the epithelium and the underlying connective tissue. The thickness of the basement membrane depends on its location, so that it is much thicker in thick skin than in the lining of the trachea, but on the average it is usually 0.3 μm wide. When viewed with the electron microscope, the basement membrane is resolved to be composed of two layers, the **basal lamina**, approximately 100 nm in thickness, and the **lamina reticularis**, which is at least 200 nm in thickness (Figure 5.4).

    1. The basal lamina is manufactured by the **epithelial layer** and is composed of two regions, the electron-lucent **lamina lucida**, which is in direct contact with the basal plasma membrane of

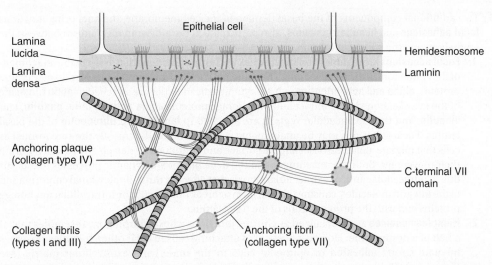

FIGURE 5.4. Basal specializations beneath an epithelium. (Adapted with permission from Keene DR, Sakai LY, Lunstrum GP, et al. Type VII collagen forms an extended network of anchoring fibrils. *J Cell Biol.* 1987;104:611.)

the epithelial cells, and the electron-dense **lamina densa**, which is located between the lamina lucida and the lamina reticularis. Although some authors now believe the lamina lucida to be a fixation artifact and suggest that the lamina densa constitutes the entirety of the basal lamina, the research results are inconclusive enough that in this textbook both the components are detailed.

a. Lamina lucida, the electron-lucent component of the basal lamina, is approximately 50 nm wide and is composed of the extracellular regions of the laminin receptors, **integrin** and **dystroglycan molecules** of the basal plasma membrane. The proteoglycans, **laminin** and **entactin** are also components of the lamina lucida although they coat the surface of the adjacent lamina densa. Therefore, the integrins and dystroglycans form bonds with the laminin in the lamina lucida, and their intracytoplasmic regions form bonds with components of the cytoskeleton, specifically with **talins** and α-**actinins**. In this fashion, the basal plasma membrane becomes affixed to the lamina lucida.

b. The **lamina densa** is a 50-nm-thick dense, flexible feltwork of type IV collagen that is interposed between the lamina lucida and the lamina reticularis. On the lamina lucida side, the lamina densa is coated not only with laminin and entactin but also by **perlacan**, a proteoglycans that is richly endowed with the glycosaminoglycans heparan sulfate. Laminin binds not only to the integrins and dystroglycans but also to heparan sulfate of perlacan and to type IV collagen of the lamina densa. Moreover, entactin also binds to both laminin and type IV collagen, and in this fashion a strong adhesion is formed between the lamina lucida and the lamina densa, and the sheath of epithelial cells is firmly attached to the basal lamina. The surface of the lamina densa that faces the lamina reticularis is also coated by **perlacan** as well as another proteoglycans, **fibronectin** that is synthesized by fibroblasts of the connective tissue. (There is another type of fibronectin, manufactured by cells of the liver; see Chapter 10, Blood and Hemopoiesis.)

c. The **lamina reticularis** is usually 200 nm or more in thickness, and it is composed of **type III collagen**, **type VII collagen** (**anchoring fibrils**), **type XVIII collagen**, and some **type I collagen** fibers as well as **microfibrils** (composed of **fibrillin**). Fibronectin binds to the various types of collagen fibers as well as to the heparan sulfate moieties of perlacan. Additionally, type VII collagen fibrils and microfibrils bind to various components of the lamina reticularis, thereby further securing the lamina densa to the lamina reticularis. Type I and type III collagen fibers loop up from the connective tissue, tethering the lamina reticularis to the superficial surface of the connective tissue. All of these bonds and interactions firmly attach the epithelium to the connective tissue via the various macromolecular components of these structures.

B. Two additional components of the basal domain of the cell membrane, the anchoring junctions **focal adhesions** and **hemidesmosomes**, also participate in the adhesion mechanism between the epithelium and the connective tissue.

    1. Focal adhesions are regions of relatively weak anchoring junctions that assist in the attachment of the epithelium to the basal lamina. The principal components are clusters of transmembrane proteins, **alpha and beta integrins**, whose cytoplasmic moieties are attached to **actin filaments** of the cytoskeleton via the intracellular anchorage proteins **alpha actinin, talin, paxillin**, and **vinculin**, and their extracellular regions are attached to **laminin** and **fibronectin** of the basal lamina. Focal adhesions may be attachments of long duration, but mostly they are formed as cells that migrate along the basal lamina surface and continuously detach and reattach during their movement. Both the attachment and the detachment are dynamic processes that occur due to intracellular and/or extracellular signals that alter the three-dimensional conformation of the integrin molecules, causing them to form or break bonds with the intracellular anchorage proteins and with the proteoglycans of the basal lamina.

    2. Hemidesmosomes are specialized anchoring junctions whose morphology resembles that of a half of a desmosome. However, instead of attaching cells to each other, hemidesmosomes mediate strong **adhesion** of epithelial cells to the underlying extracellular matrix (see Figure 5.3). Unlike focal adhesions, hemidesmosomes are mostly of longer duration and provide a firmer attachment of the cell to the basal lamina. Moreover, instead of binding to actin filaments of the cytoskeleton, they are bound to the more robust intermediate filaments.

        a. There are two types of hemidesmosomes: the **classical type** (**type I**) located in the stratum basale of skin, in the lining of the esophagus, in the masticatory and lining mucosae of the oral cavity, as well as in the cells of pseudostratified epithelia of structures such as the trachea, and **type II hemidesmosomes** are present mostly in the simple columnar epithelia of the intestinal lining. Type I hemidesmosomes are more complex, whereas type II hemidesmosomes have much fewer components.

            (1) Type I hemidesmosomes have several components, namely the dense cluster of transmembrane proteins α6β4 **integrin**, whose intracytoplasmic moieties bind to the protein **erbin** and the **plakin** proteins **plectin** and **bullous pemphigoid antigen 230** (**BP230**). It is these two plakin proteins that connect α6β4 integrins to the intermediate filaments (**keratin-5** and **keratin-14**, also known as **tonofilaments**). Erbin assists in the binding of the integrin molecule to BP230. Two additional proteins are associated with the α6 component of the integrin, namely **bullous pemphigoid antigen 180** (**BP 180**, also known as **type XVII collagen**) and **cluster of differentiation protein 151** (**CD151**). BP 180 binds intracellularly to both the α6 component of the integrin and to plectin, and extracellularly to the α6 component of the integrin and to laminin of the basal lamina. The extracellular moieties of α6β4 integrins also bind to the **laminins** and **type IV collagens** of the basal lamina. **CD151** functions to ensure that enough integrin molecules are recruited to the area so that hemidesmosome formation can occur. The intracytoplasmic components of the hemidesmosome form an electron-dense, plaque-like structure that resembles but is different from the outer dense plaque of a desmosome.

            (2) Type II hemidesmosomes are much simpler than the classical hemidesmosomes, in that they are composed only of the dense cluster of transmembrane proteins α6β4 **integrin** whose intracytoplasmic moieties bind to the **plakin** protein **plectin**, which in turn binds to the intermediate filaments **keratin-8** and **keratin-18** (**tonofilaments**). As in type I hemidesmosomes, the intracytoplasmic components form an electron-dense, plaque-like structure that resembles but is different from the outer dense plaque of a desmosome.

        b. Because of the large number of α6β4 integrins and their connection to the tougher intermediate filaments rather than to the less sturdy actin filaments, hemidesmosomes form much stronger anchoring junctions than focal adhesions. However, similar to focal adhesions, the presence of Ca^{2+} ions are necessary for the formation and maintenance of these anchoring junctions, and the cell is able to form and disassemble hemidesmosomes as required. Both the formation and disassembly are regulated by a series of intracellular and extracellular signaling events, many of which act during the formation of new cells that either become anchored to the basal lamina or are moving toward the free surface of the epithelium.

c. Keratin filaments (tonofilaments) in the cell terminate in the hemidesmosome plaque, allowing these junctions to **link** the cytoskeleton with the components of the extracellular matrix.

CLINICAL CONSIDERATIONS   **Bullous pemphigoid** is an **autoimmune disease** in which antibodies against hemidesmosomes are produced.

1. This disease is characterized by chronic generalized blisters in the skin.
2. These blisters cause the epithelium to separate from the underlying substratum.

C. **Basal plasma membrane infoldings** are common in **ion-transporting epithelia** (e.g., distal convoluted tubule of the kidney, striated ducts in salivary glands).
1. They form deep invaginations that compartmentalize mitochondria.
2. **Function.** They increase the surface area and bring ion pumps (Na^+-K^+ adenosine triphosphatase [ATPase]) in the plasma membrane close to their energy supply (ATP produced in mitochondria).

IV. APICAL EPITHELIAL SURFACES

These surfaces may possess specialized structures such as microvilli, stereocilia, and cilia. Flagella, modified cilia that are present only in spermatozoa, are discussed in Chapter 20, The Male Reproductive System.

A. **Microvilli** are fingerlike projections of epithelia approximately 1 μm long that **extend into a lumen** and increase the cell's surface area.
1. A **glycocalyx** (sugar coat) is present on their surfaces (see Chapter 1 II C).
2. A bundle of approximately 25 to 30 **actin filaments** runs longitudinally through the core of each microvillus, extending from the tip of the microvillus into the **terminal web**, a zone of intersecting filaments in the apical cytoplasm.
   a. The actin filaments within the microvillus are bound to each other by the actin-binding proteins **villin, fimbrin, espin**, and **fascin**, and the actin filaments at the perimeter of the actin bundle are affixed to the plasmalemma of the microvillus by **calmodulin** and **myosin I**.
   b. The actin filaments are arranged in a specific orientation within the microvillus, so that their **plus ends (barbed ends)** extend to the tip of the microvillus, where they are embedded in an amorphous material known as **villin**. The **minus ends (pointed ends)** of the bundle of actin filaments extend into the terminal web of the epithelial cell, where they are affixed to the spectrin and actin filaments of the terminal web.
3. The **myosin II** and **tropomyosin** molecules located at the terminal web can interact to contract the apical region of the cell, thereby causing the microvilli to diverge from each other, increasing the intermicrovillar spaces. These enlarged intermicrovillar spaces facilitate the increased transport of materials into the cell.
4. Microvilli constitute the **brush border** of kidney proximal tubule cells and the **striated border** of intestinal absorptive cells.

B. **Stereocilia** are very **long** (15–20 μm in length) **microvilli** (*they are not cilia*) in the hair cells of the inner ear, in the epididymis, and in the vas deferens of the male reproductive tract. The core of the stereocilia is composed of actin filaments that are attached to each other by **fimbrin** and to the plasmalemma of the stereocilia by **villin-2** and **ezrin** (but not in the hair cells of the inner ear). As in microvilli, the barbed ends of the actin filament bundle extend to the tip of the stereocilia, where villin is absent, and their pointed ends reach and are anchored in the cell web.

C. **Cilia** are of two types, motile and nonmotile (primary) cilia.
  1. The **actively motile cilia** are processes of the cell that are 7 to 10 μm long extending from certain epithelia (e.g., tracheobronchial and oviduct epithelium) that propel substances along their surfaces. They contain a **core** of longitudinally arranged **microtubules** (the **axoneme**), which arises from a basal body during ciliogenesis.
     a. The **axoneme** (Figure 5.5A) consists of 9 doublet microtubules uniformly spaced around 2 central microtubules (**9 + 2 configuration**), where each doublet microtubule is composed of a complete microtubule, referred to as **microtubule A** that consists of the normal 13 protofilaments, and an incomplete microtubule, known as **microtubule B** consisting of only 10 protofilaments. Microtubule A shares three of its protofilaments with microtubule B so that microtubule B has a completely closed structure. Each central microtubule consists of 13 protofilaments. Cilia have the following additional components:
        (1) Inner and outer ciliary dynein arms, which extend unidirectionally from one member of each doublet microtubule and interact with adjacent doublets, so that they slide past one another. These arms consist of **ciliary dynein**, with a head, that is, an **ATPase** that splits ATP to liberate the energy necessary for active movement of a cilium.
        (2) Radial spokes that extend from each of the nine outer doublets toward the central sheath.
        (3) Central sheath, which surrounds the two central microtubules; this sheath and the radial spokes regulate the ciliary beat.
        (4) Nexin, an elastic protein that connects adjacent doublet microtubules to each other and helps to maintain the shape of the cilium.
        (5) Tektin, proteins that resemble intermediate filaments and form a physical support to the axoneme by forming linear backbones that attach at the outer aspects (away from the central sheet) of the junction of each microtubule A with its microtubule B.
     b. The **basal body** (Figure 5.5B) is a cylindrical structure at the **base of each cilium** that consists of nine triplet microtubules arranged radially in the shape of a pinwheel

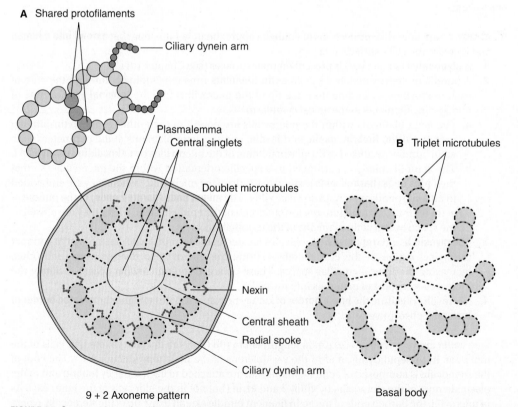

FIGURE 5.5. Cross-sections of a cilium and basal body. (Part A adapted with permission from Junqueira LC, Carneiro J, Kelley RO. *Basic Histology.* 9th ed. Norwalk, CT: Appleton & Lange; 1998:45. Part B adapted with permission from West JB. *Best and Taylor Physiological Basis of Medical Practice.* 12th ed. Baltimore, MD: Williams & Wilkins; 1991:12).

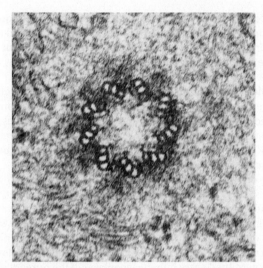

FIGURE 5.6. Electron micrograph of a cross-sectioned centriole. Notice the nine triplet microtubules arranged radially in the shape of a pinwheel. This is known as the 9 + 0 configuration (compare with the cilium), and little central organization is observed.

(**9 + 0 configuration**). It resembles a centriole (see Figure 5.6) but has a less complex central organization. The inner two triplets of the basal body give rise to the doublet microtubules of the cilium axoneme. The outermost, third microtubule, referred to as **microtubule C**, of the triplet is also incomplete. It is composed of only 10 protofilaments and shares 3 of microtubule B's protofilaments so that microtubule C is also a completely closed structure. The region where the basal body and the axoneme merge with each other is frequently referred to as the **transition zone**. It is the basal body and structures coupled with it that not only secure the cilium to the cell but also function in ensuring that all cilia of the cell beat in the same direction. Structures that are associated with the basal body are the alar sheet, basal feet, and striated rootlets.

(1) A funnel-shaped fibrous membrane, known as the **alar sheet**, attaches to the microtubules C of the basal body at the transition zone and sweeps upward to merge with the cell membrane at the origin of the cilium. The alar sheet not only ensures a strong attachment of the basal body to the plasmalemma but also functions as a semipermeable membrane that limits access to the ciliary cytoplasm.

(2) Attached to the basal body is a structure known as the **basal foot** that is believed to ensure that all cilia of the same cell are facing in the same direction, thereby controlling the synchronous, unidirectional bending of all cilia of the same cell.

(3) Extending from the basal body, and securing it into the cytoplasm, are the protofilaments, known as the **striated rootlet**, which affixes the cilium relatively deeply into the apical cytoplasm.

c. Ciliary movement occurs as the dynein arms of a doublet grasp and "climb" along the "back" of the adjacent doublet, thereby bending the cilia in a preferred direction. This is an energy-requiring process and is fueled by the ATPase activity of the dynein arms. As the cilium bends, the elastic proteins of the axoneme become stretched. Once the cilium is bent sufficiently, the dynein arms relax their grasp on the adjacent doublet, and the cilium snaps back to its original position propelling materials located at its tip, thus moving material, such as mucus in the tracheal lumen, along the epithelial surface. The process of "snapping back" does not require energy because it is fueled by the stretched elastic proteins returning to their resting positions.

d. Transport of material occurs within the motile cilia, primary cilia, and flagella, referred to as **axonemal transport**. Within cilia it is known as **intraciliary transport**, and within flagella it is known as **intraflagellar transport**. The transport of tubulin dimers and other molecules required by the cilia occurs via carrier proteins, known as **raft proteins** that pick up cargo, such as tubulin dimers. The raft proteins then become attached to **kinesin** or to

dynein, motor proteins that ferry cargo along microtubules in an anterograde or retrograde direction, respectively. **Anterograde** is from the basal body toward the tip of the cilium, and **retrograde** is in the opposite direction, from the tip of the cilium toward the basal body. Defects in the intraciliary transport result in various anomalies, some with even lethal consequences.

2. A single **nonmotile cilium (primary cilium)** is present on nearly every human cell that is in the G_0 stage of the cell cycle. These structures were believed to be nonfunctional evolutionary remnants, but recently it has been demonstrated that they have essential functions in the organization of signaling pathways not only during embryonic development but also in the adult organism. It has been amply demonstrated that impaired primary cilia are responsible for various anomalous conditions, known as **ciliopathies**.

   a. The axoneme of primary cilia differs from those of motile cilia in that they possess no central singlets; thus, they have a **9 + 0 configuration**; moreover, the central sheet, outer and inner dynein arms, and most radial spokes are absent.

   b. A set of proteins, known as **BBSome** (named after Bardet–Biedl syndrome), is located at the distal end of the basal body and is responsible for the formation as well as the proper functioning of the primary cilium. It is the BBSome protein complex that determines which molecules are permitted entry into the cytoplasm of the primary cilium. Disruption of the BBSome is responsible for a number of ciliopathies, including Bardet–Biedl syndrome.

   c. If a cell leaves the G_0 stage of the cell cycle and enters the G_1 phase, the primary cilium becomes resorbed, and the **basal body** returns to its previous function as a centriole.

   d. Primary cilia of a particular region, such as the kidney tubule or fibroblasts, are oriented in the same direction, and this precise alignment is dictated by the **basal foot**. This precise alignment permits the primary cilia to perform their functions, whether in the monitoring of the flow of the ultrafiltrate in the kidney tubule or in the migration of fibroblasts in the proper direction during wound healing.

   e. It has been demonstrated that a number of ion channels and select receptors are present only in the membranes of primary cilia. The specific reason for this exclusivity has not been elucidated, but it is believed that it may have some association with the **intraciliary transport mechanism**, and disturbances of this particular cellular event are responsible for the various **ciliopathies**.

CLINICAL CONSIDERATIONS

1. **Immotile cilia syndrome** results from a genetic defect that causes an abnormal ciliary beat or the absence of a beat.
   a. In this syndrome, cilia have axonemes that lack ciliary dynein arms and have other abnormalities.
   b. The syndrome is associated with recurrent lower respiratory tract infections, reduced fertility in women, and sterility in men.

2. **Polycystic kidney disease (PKD)**, a genetic disorder, is an autosomal dominant disease occurring in about two per thousand births. There are three mutations responsible for this anomaly, namely PKD-1, PKD-2, and PKHD-1, but most cases are due to mutations in gene PKD-1 located on chromosome 16. For an unknown reason, individuals with these mutations develop abnormal primary centrioles, resulting in abnormal cell cycles as well as defective calcium transport within the cell. During embryonic development, cysts begin forming on the kidneys and increase in size and number. As these cysts continue to gain fluid and become larger, they apply pressure on the uriniferous tubules and prevent them from performing their function. In most patients, the symptoms, such as pain in the back and sides as well as headaches, become evident by the 40th year of life, and eventually the kidney function of the patients is reduced until they have to be placed on renal dialysis and become eligible for kidney transplant.

3. **Bardet–Biedl syndrome** is a disorder due to disruptions in the normal functioning of BBSome located at the base of the basal body of the primary cilium. The manifestations of this syndrome are varied and include night blindness, speech disorder, malformations of the rods and cones of the retina with a subsequent loss of vision, presence of extra digits on the hands and feet, kidney failure, urogenital defects, and obesity. Many patients succumb to kidney failure.

V. GLANDS

They originate from an epithelium that penetrates the connective tissue and forms secretory units.

A. **Structure.** A gland consists of a functional portion (**parenchyma**) of secretory and ductal epithelial cells, which is separated by a basal lamina from supporting connective tissue elements (**stroma**).

B. **Classification.** Glands are classified into three types based on the site of secretion. **Exocrine glands** secrete into a duct or onto a surface. **Endocrine glands** secrete into the bloodstream. **Paracrine glands** secrete into the local extracellular space.
   1. **Exocrine glands**
      a. **Unicellular glands** are composed of a single cell (e.g., goblet cells in tracheal epithelium).
      b. **Multicellular glands** (Figure 5.7)
         (1) Classification is based on two criteria.
            (a) Multicellular glands are classified according to **duct branching** as **simple glands** (duct does not branch) or **compound glands** (duct branches).
            (b) They are further classified according to the **shape of the secretory unit** as **acinar** or **alveolar** (saclike or flasklike) or **tubular** (straight, coiled, or branched).

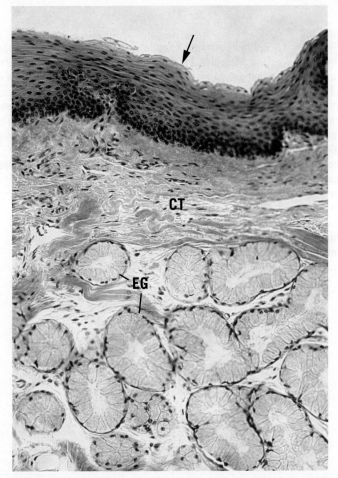

FIGURE 5.7. Light micrograph showing stratified squamous nonkeratinized epithelium (*arrow*) lining the lumen of the esophagus. This epithelium is thick, and cells in its upper layers are flattened or squamous, whereas the basal cells that undergo mitosis and give rise to cells of the upper layer are cuboidal. Esophageal cardiac glands (EG) are present in the connective tissue (CT) layer (lamina propria) deep to the epithelium. These glands are located in the vicinity of the esophageocardiac junction, and they are lined by simple columnar epithelial cells that secrete mucus.

   (2) A connective tissue capsule may surround the gland, or septa of connective tissue may divide the gland into **lobes** and smaller **lobules.**
   (3) Glands may have **ducts** between lobes (**interlobar**), within lobes (**intralobar**), between lobules (**interlobular**), or within lobules (**intralobular**), such as striated and intercalated ducts.
   (4) Multicellular glands secrete various substances.
      (a) *Mucus* is a viscous material that usually protects or lubricates cell surfaces.
      (b) *Serous* secretions are watery and often rich in enzymes.
      (c) *Mixed* secretions contain both mucous and serous components.
   (5) Mechanisms of secretion vary.
      (a) In **merocrine** glands (e.g., parotid gland), the secretory cells release their contents by exocytosis.
      (b) In **apocrine** glands (e.g., lactating mammary gland), part of the apical cytoplasm of the secretory cell is released along with the contents.
      (c) In **holocrine** glands (e.g., sebaceous gland), the entire secretory cell along with its contents is released.
 2. **Endocrine glands** may be **unicellular** (e.g., individual endocrine cells in gastrointestinal and respiratory epithelia) or **multicellular** (e.g., adrenal gland), and they **lack a duct system**. In multicellular glands, secretory material is released into fenestrated capillaries, which are abundant just outside the basal lamina of the glandular epithelium.

CLINICAL CONSIDERATIONS

   1. Epithelia sometimes undergo **metaplasia** in response to persistent injury. Metaplasia is the conversion of one type of differentiated epithelium into another. Most commonly, a glandular epithelium is transformed into a squamous epithelium. However, in cases of chronic acid reflux from the stomach into the lower esophagus, the stratified squamous nonkeratinized epithelium is replaced by a glandular mucus-secreting epithelium (**Barrett epithelium**) similar to that found lining the cardia of the stomach. This helps to protect the esophagus against the injurious effects of the acid and pepsin, but is also a well-known precursor of esophageal adenocarcinoma.
   2. **Epithelial cell tumors** occur when cells fail to respond to normal growth regulatory mechanisms.
      a. These tumors are **benign** when they remain **local**.
      b. They are **malignant** when they **invade neighboring tissues**. Then they may (or may not) **metastasize** to other parts of the body.
         i. **Carcinomas** are malignant tumors that arise from **surface epithelia**.
         ii. **Adenocarcinomas** are malignant tumors that arise from **glands**.

Review Test

Directions: Each of the numbered items or incomplete statements in this section is followed by answers or by completions of the statement. Select the ONE lettered answer or completion that is BEST in each case.

1. Which one of the following statements about the desmosome is true?

(A) It is sometimes called a nexus.
(B) It permits the passage of large proteins from one cell to an adjacent cell.
(C) It has a plaque made up of many connexons.
(D) It facilitates metabolic coupling between adjacent cells.
(E) It is a disk-shaped adhesion site between epithelial cells.

2. A medical student who has chronic lower respiratory infections seeks the advice of an ear, nose, and throat specialist. A biopsy of the student's respiratory epithelium reveals alterations in certain epithelial structures. This patient is most likely to have abnormal

(A) microvilli.
(B) desmosomes.
(C) cilia.
(D) hemidesmosomes.
(E) basal plasmalemma infoldings.

3. Which one of the following statements about the gap junction is true?

(A) It extends as a zone around the apical perimeter of adjacent cells.
(B) It possesses dense plaques composed in part of desmoplakins.
(C) It permits the passage of ions from one cell to an adjacent cell.
(D) Its adhesion is dependent upon calcium ions.
(E) It possesses transmembrane linker glycoproteins.

4. Which one of the following statements about glands is true?

(A) Exocrine glands lack ducts.
(B) Simple glands have ducts that branch.
(C) Endocrine glands secrete into ducts.
(D) Serous secretions are watery.
(E) Holocrine glands release their contents by exocytosis.

5. Which one of the following statements about epithelia is true?

(A) They are polarized.
(B) They are vascular.
(C) They are completely surrounded by a basal lamina.
(D) They contain wide intercellular spaces.
(E) They are not part of the wall of blood vessels.

6. Which one of the following statements about cilia is true?

(A) They possess a 9 + 0 configuration of microtubules.
(B) They do not contain an axoneme.
(C) They contain ciliary dynein arms.
(D) They are nearly identical to centrioles.
(E) They play a major function in absorption.

7. Which one of the following statements about stratified squamous epithelium is true?

(A) The surface layer of cells is always keratinized.
(B) The cells in its most superficial layer are flattened.
(C) Its basal cells rest on an elastic lamina.
(D) Its cells lack desmosomes.
(E) It lines the ducts of sweat glands.

8. Which one of the following is an autoimmune disease?

(A) Adenocarcinoma
(B) Bullous pemphigoid
(C) Carcinoma
(D) First-degree burn
(E) Immotile cilia syndrome

9. Which one of the following is a hereditary disease that may be associated with infertility?

(A) Adenocarcinoma
(B) Bullous pemphigoid
(C) Carcinoma
(D) Edema
(E) Immotile cilia syndrome

10. Which one of the following is a tumor arising from glandular epithelium?

(A) Adenocarcinoma
(B) Bullous pemphigoid
(C) Carcinoma
(D) Edema
(E) Immotile cilia syndrome

11. Which of the following is a condition affecting the epidermis of the skin in which blisters do not form?

(A) Adenocarcinoma
(B) Bullous pemphigoid
(C) Carcinoma
(D) First-degree burn
(E) Immotile cilia syndrome

Answers and Explanations

1. **E.** Desmosomes are sites of adhesion characterized by dense cytoplasmic plaques and associated keratin filaments. Only gap junctions permit cell-to-cell communication of small molecules via their connexon channels (see Chapter 5 II A).

2. **C.** Individuals with abnormal respiratory cilia commonly have recurrent respiratory infections if the cilia are unable to clear the respiratory epithelium of microorganisms, debris, and so forth. The student may have immotile cilia syndrome, which is caused by a genetic defect, resulting in cilia with axonemes that lack ciliary dynein arms and thus are unable to beat (see Chapter 5 IV C 2 Clinical Considerations).

3. **C.** The gap junction channel regulates the passage of ions and small molecules from cell to cell, excluding those having a molecular weight greater than 1200 Da. The tight junction is the zone of adhesion around the apical perimeter of adjacent cells. The other statements are characteristics of desmosomes (see Chapter 5 II B).

4. **D.** Serous secretions produced by glands are often rich in enzymes and watery in consistency. Exocrine glands secrete into ducts, and endocrine glands lack ducts. Merocrine glands use exocytosis to release their products (see Chapter 5 V B).

5. **A.** Epithelia are polarized, meaning they show sidedness and have apical and basolateral surfaces with specific functions (see Chapter 5 I A).

6. **C.** Cilia contain an axoneme with ciliary dynein arms extending unidirectionally from one member of each doublet. Ciliary dynein has ATPase activity, and when it splits ATP, the adjacent doublets slide past one another and the cilium moves. Microvilli, not cilia, function in absorption (see Chapter 5 IV C).

7. **B.** Stratified squamous epithelium is characterized by flattened cells with or without nuclei in its superficial layer. It may or may not be keratinized, and it rests on a basal lamina produced by the epithelium. Stratified cuboidal epithelium lines the ducts in sweat glands (see Chapter 5 I B).

8. **B.** Bullous pemphigoid is an autoimmune disease. Affected individuals form antibodies against their own hemidesmosomes (see Chapter 5 III B Clinical Considerations).

9. **E.** Immotile cilia syndrome results from a genetic defect that prevents synthesis of ciliary dynein ATPase, resulting in cilia that cannot actively move. Men are sterile because their sperm are not motile (the flagella in their tails lack this enzyme). Women may be infertile because cilia along their oviducts may fail to move oocytes toward the uterus (see Chapter 5 IV C 2 Clinical Considerations).

10. **A.** Adenocarcinomas are epithelial tumors that originate in glandular epithelia. Carcinomas originate from surface epithelia (see Chapter 5 V B 2 Clinical Considerations).

11. **D.** First-degree burns damage the upper layers of the epidermis only, and blisters do not form in the skin (see Chapter 5 I C Clinical Considerations).

chapter 6

Connective Tissue

I. OVERVIEW—CONNECTIVE TISSUE

A. **Structure**. Connective tissue is formed primarily of **extracellular matrix (ECM)**, consisting of **ground substance** and **fibers**, in which various connective tissue **cells** are embedded.

B. **Function**. Connective tissue **supports** organs and cells, acts as a **medium for exchange** of nutrients and wastes between the blood and tissues, **protects** against microorganisms, **repairs** damaged tissues, and **stores fat**.

II. EXTRACELLULAR MATRIX

The ECM provides a medium for the transfer of nutrients and waste materials between connective tissue cells and the bloodstream.

A. **Ground substance** is a colorless, transparent, gel-like material in which the cells and fibers of connective tissue are embedded.
   1. It is a complex mixture of **glycosaminoglycans, proteoglycans**, and **glycoproteins** (see Chapter 4).
   2. Ground substance serves as a lubricant, helps to prevent invasion of tissues by foreign agents, and resists forces of compression.

B. **Fibers** (collagen, reticular, and elastic) are long, slender protein polymers present in different proportions in different types of connective tissue.
   1. **Collagen fibers.** Although there are at least 25 different types of collagen, the most common collagen types in connective tissue proper are **types I** and **III collagen** (see Chapter 4, Table 4.3), both consisting of many closely packed **tropocollagen** fibrils. The diameter of individual type I collagen fibrils varies greatly (10–300 nm). These fibrils may aggregate and form cable-like structures up to several centimeters in length and display 67-nm periodicity (see Chapter 4 and Figure 4.4).
      a. Collagen fibers are produced in a two-stage process, involving both intracellular and extracellular events (see Chapter 4 and Figure 4.3).
      b. Collagen fibers have great tensile strength, which imparts both flexibility and strength to tissues containing them.

c. Bone, skin, cartilage, tendon, and many other structures of the body contain collagen fibers.

2. **Reticular fibers** are extremely **thin** (0.5–2.0 μm) in diameter and are composed primarily of **type III collagen**; they have higher carbohydrate content than other collagen fibers.
   a. Type III collagen fibers constitute the architectural framework of certain organs and glands.
   b. Because of their high carbohydrate content, they stain black with silver salts.

3. **Elastic fibers** are coiled branching fibers 0.2 to 1.0 μm in diameter that sometimes form loose networks.
   a. These fibers may be stretched up to 150% of their resting length.
   b. They consist of a central amorphous substance known as **elastin** that is surrounded by thin **microfibrils**. The latter are composed of **fibrillin-1**, which is bound to elastin by the protein **fibulin-5** (see Chapter 4 III B).
   c. Elastic fibers require special staining to be observed by light microscopy.

III. CONNECTIVE TISSUE CELLS

Connective tissue cells include many types with different functions. Some originate locally and remain in the connective tissue (**fixed cells**), whereas others originate elsewhere and remain only temporarily in connective tissue (**transient cells**) (Figure 6.1). **Fixed connective tissue cells** include fibroblasts, pericytes, adipose cells, mast cells, and fixed macrophages. **Transient connective tissue cells** include certain macrophages, lymphocytes, plasma cells, neutrophils, eosinophils, and basophils.

A. **Fixed cells of connective tissue**
1. **Fibroblasts** arise from mesenchymal cells and are the predominant cells in connective tissue proper (Figure 6.2). They often possess an oval nucleus with two or more nucleoli. Fibroblasts seldom undergo mitosis except in wound healing. They may differentiate into other cell types under certain conditions (see Clinical Considerations).

   Active fibroblasts are spindle shaped (fusiform) and contain well-developed rough endoplasmic reticulum (RER) and many Golgi complexes. Myosin is located throughout the cytoplasm, and actin and α-actinin are located at the cell periphery. **Synthetically active**, they produce procollagen, collagen, and elastic fibers and most of the ground substance as well as other components of the ECM.

CLINICAL CONSIDERATIONS **Fibroblasts** undergo mitosis only during wound healing. However, under certain conditions, fibroblasts may differentiate into adipose cells, or during fibrocartilage formation, they may differentiate into chondrocytes. In addition, under pathological conditions, fibroblasts may differentiate into osteoblasts.

2. **Pericytes (adventitial cells; perivascular cells)** are derived from embryonic mesenchymal cells and may retain a **pluripotential role**.
   a. They possess characteristics of endothelial cells as well as smooth muscle cells because they contain actin, myosin, and tropomyosin, suggesting that they may function in contraction where they assist to modify blood flow through capillaries.
   b. They are smaller than fibroblasts, are located mostly along capillaries, and are completely enveloped by their own basal lamina, which is continuous with the basal lamina of the capillary endothelium.
   c. During blood vessel formation and repair, they may differentiate into fibroblasts, smooth muscle cells, as well as endothelial cells of blood vessel walls.

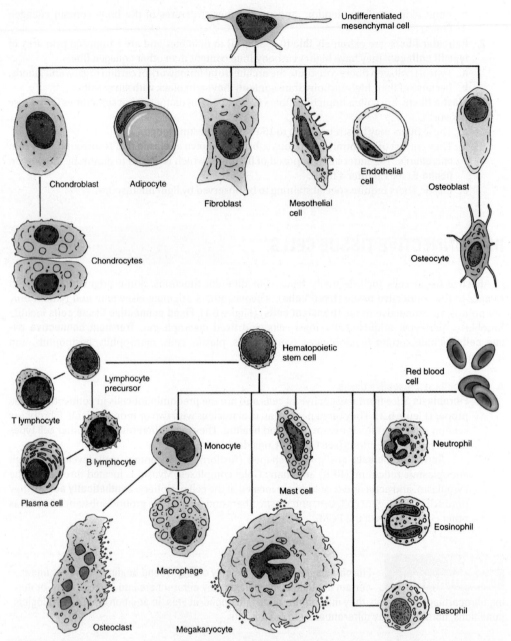

FIGURE 6.1. Origin of connective tissue cells. Cells arising from undifferentiated mesenchymal cells are formed in connective tissue and remain there. Cells arising from hematopoietic stem cells are formed in the bone marrow and reside transiently in connective tissue. (Reprinted with permission from Gartner LP, Hiatt JL. *Color Textbook of Histology.* 3rd ed. Philadelphia, PA: Saunders (Elsevier); 2007:112.)

3. **Adipose cells (adipocytes)** (Figures 6.1 and 6.3) arise from mesenchymal cells and perhaps from fibroblasts. Adipogenesis occurs pre- and postnatally, and its rate is reduced in aging. Adipocytes do not normally undergo cell division because they are fully differentiated cells. However, they do increase in number in early neonatal life. There is debate about normal proliferation of adipocytes beyond 2 years after birth, although in obese individuals the cells not only become enlarged but also form new fat cells. They are surrounded by a basal lamina

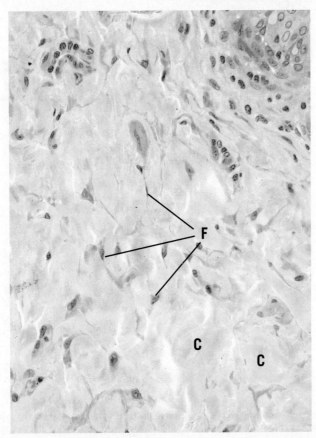

FIGURE 6.2. Light micrograph of monkey bladder (×270) illustrating fibroblasts (F) and collagen bundles (C) within the connective tissue.

and are responsible for the **synthesis, storage**, and **release of fat**. There are two types of fat cells, unilocular and multilocular.

   a. **Unilocular adipose cells** contain a single large fat droplet. To accommodate the large fat droplet, the cytoplasm and nucleus are squeezed into a thin rim around the cell's periphery.

   (1) These cells have plasmalemma **receptors** for insulin, growth hormone, norepinephrine, and glucocorticoids to **control the uptake and release of free fatty acids and triglycerides.**

   (2) They are surrounded by a basal lamina and are responsible for the **synthesis, storage**, and **release of fat.**

   b. **Multilocular adipose cells** are smaller than unilocular adipose cells, and the fat is stored as many small fat droplets, and thus the spherical nucleus is centrally located.

4. **Mast cells** (Figure 6.1) arise from myeloid stem cells in bone marrow and usually reside near small blood vessels. Although they share many structural and functional characteristics with basophils, they develop from different precursors and are not related.

   a. These cells are one of the largest cells of connective tissue proper. They possess a central spherical nucleus; their cytoplasm is filled with coarse, deeply stained metachromatic granules; their contents (known as **primary mediators**) are listed in Table 6.1.

   b. Their surfaces are folded, and in electron micrographs they have a well-developed Golgi complex, scant RER, and many dense lamellated granules. Two populations of mast cells exist. **Connective tissue mast cells** possess secretory granules containing heparin.

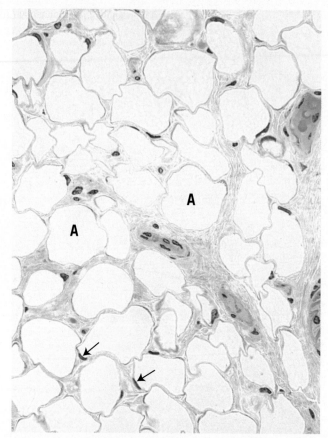

FIGURE 6.3. Light micrograph of monkey skin (×270). Observe the fat cells (adipocytes) (A) and their nuclei (*arrows*) that have been displaced to the periphery of the cell. Note that the fat was extracted during processing.

t a b l e **6.1**	Major Mediators Released by Mast Cells	
Substance	Intracellular Source	Action
Primary mediators		
Histamine	Granules	Vasodilator; increases vascular permeability; causes contraction of bronchial smooth muscle; increases mucus production
Heparin	Granules	Anticoagulant; inactivates histamine
Eosinophil chemotactic factor	Granules	Attractant for eosinophils to site of inflammation
Neutrophil chemotactic factor	Granules	Attractant for neutrophils to site of inflammation
Aryl sulfate	Granules	Inactivates leukotriene C_4, limiting inflammatory response
Chondroitin sulfate	Granules	Binds and inactivates histamine
Neutral proteases	Granules	Protein cleavage to activate complement; increases inflammatory response
Secondary mediators		
Prostaglandin D_2	Membrane lipid	Causes contraction of bronchial smooth muscle; increases mucus secretion; vasoconstriction
Leukotrienes C_4, D_4, E_4	Membrane lipid	Vasodilators; increases vascular permeability; contraction of bronchial smooth muscle
Bradykinins	Membrane lipid	Causes vascular permeability; responsible for pain sensation
Thromboxane A_2	Membrane lipid	Causes platelet aggregation; vasoconstriction
Platelet-activating factor	Activated by phospholipase A_2	Attracts neutrophils and eosinophils; causes vascular permeability; contraction of bronchial smooth muscle

The other population, the smaller **mucosal mast cells** whose secretory granules contain chondroitin sulfate, is located in the mucosa of the alimentary canal and of the respiratory tract. Interestingly, there are no mast cells in the central nervous system presumably to prevent the possibility of an inflammatory response.

c. When mast cells become activated during a type I hypersensitivity reaction (see next item), phospholipids of their cell membranes can be converted into arachidonic acid by the enzyme phospholipase A_2. Arachidonic acid is, in turn, converted into **secondary mediators** (e.g., leukotrienes and prostaglandins; see Table 6.1).

d. Mast cells mediate **immediate (type I) hypersensitivity** reactions (**anaphylactic reactions**) as follows:

(1) After the first exposure to an allergen, plasma cells manufacture immunoglobulin E (IgE) antibodies, which bind to **Fc receptors** (**FcεRI receptors**) on the surface of mast cells and basophils, causing these cells to become **sensitized**. Common antigens that may evoke this response include plant **pollens, insect venoms**, certain **drugs**, and **foreign serum**.

(2) During the second exposure to the same allergen, the membrane-bound IgE binds the allergen. Subsequent cross-linking and clustering of the allergen–IgE complexes trigger degranulation of mast cells and the release of primary and secondary mediators (Figure 6.4 and Table 6.1; see Chapter 12).

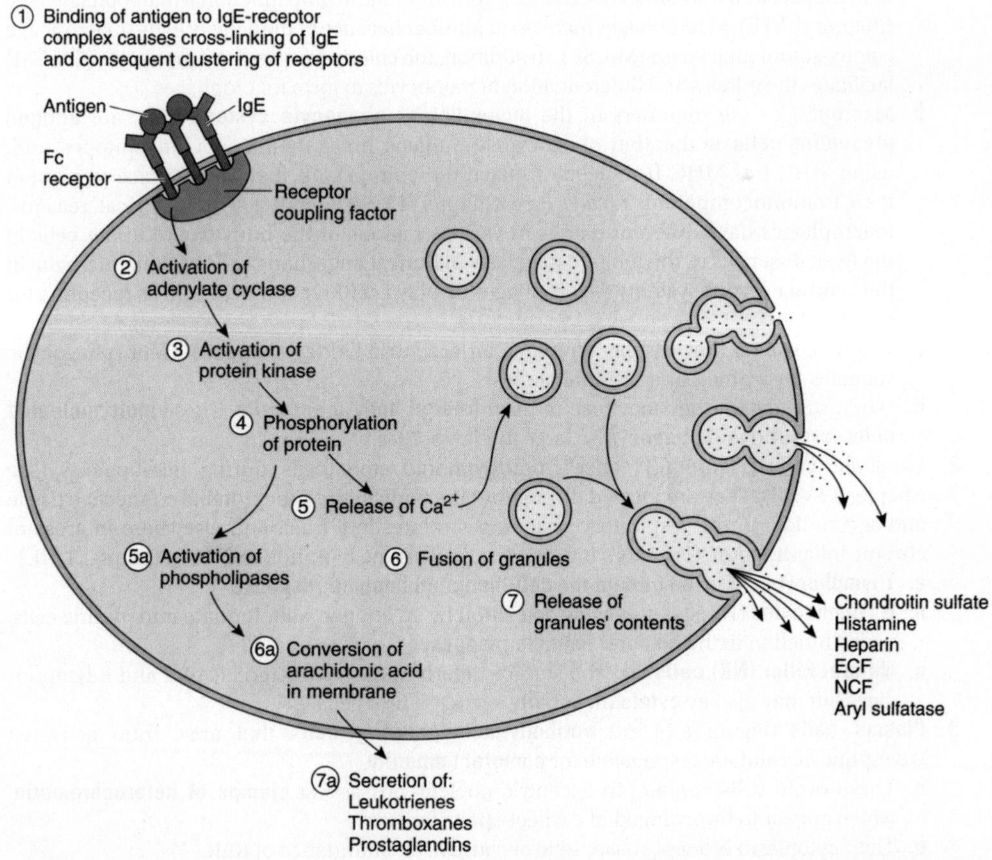

FIGURE 6.4. Activation and degranulation of the mast cell. ECF, eosinophil chemotactic factor; NCF, neutrophil chemotactic factor. (Adapted with permission from Gartner LP, Hiatt JL. *Color Textbook of Histology*. 3rd ed. Philadelphia, PA: Saunders; 1997:120.)

Hay fever and asthma

Hay fever is characterized by nasal congestion caused by localized edema in the nasal mucosa. This edema results from the increased permeability of small blood vessels because of excessive release of **histamine** from mast cells in the nasal mucosa.

People with **asthma** have difficulty breathing due to bronchospasms resulting from **leukotrienes** released in the lungs.

Anaphylactic shock results from the effects of powerful mediators released during an **immediate hypersensitivity reaction** following a second exposure to an allergen.

1. This reaction can occur within seconds or minutes after contact with an allergen.
2. Signs and symptoms include shortness of breath, decreasing blood pressure, and other signs and symptoms of shock.
3. Anaphylactic shock may be life-threatening if untreated.

B. **Transient cells of connective tissue**
   1. **Macrophages** (Figure 6.1) are the principal **phagocytosing cells** of connective tissue. They are responsible for removing large particulate matter and assisting in the **immune response**. They also secrete substances that function in wound healing.
      a. Macrophages originate in the bone marrow as **monocytes**, circulate in the bloodstream, and then migrate into the connective tissue, where they mature into functional macrophages (see Chapter 10 VI E). Macrophages increase in number because of the activity of the macrophage colony-stimulating factor (M-CSF). In addition, the colony-forming unit monocyte (CFU-M) facilitates the mitosis and differentiation of monocytes to form macrophages.
      b. Macrophages are members of the **mononuclear phagocyte system**. They are **antigen presenting cells**, in that they phagocytose antigens, break them down into epitopes, and, using MHC I or MHC II molecules, place the epitopes on their cell surface to present it to immunocompetent T cells (see Chapter 12 Section III). For historical reasons, macrophages have different names in various regions of the body (e.g., Kupffer cells in the liver, dust cells in the lungs, osteoclasts in bone, Langerhans cells in skin, microglia in the central nervous system). Macrophages display FcεRI receptors as well as receptors for complement.
      c. When activated, they display filopodia, an eccentric kidney-shaped nucleus, phagocytic vacuoles, lysosomes, and residual bodies.
      d. When stimulated, they may fuse to form **foreign body giant cells**. These **multinucleated cells** surround and phagocytose large foreign bodies.
   2. **Lymphoid cells** (Figure 6.1) arise from lymphoid stem cells during hemopoiesis (see Chapter 10 VI G). They are located throughout the body in the subepithelial connective tissue and accumulate in the respiratory system, gastrointestinal tract, and elsewhere in areas of chronic inflammation. (For more information concerning lymphoid cells, see Chapter 12 II.)
      a. **T lymphocytes** (T cells) initiate the **cell-mediated immune response**.
      b. **B lymphocytes** (B cells), following activation by an antigen, differentiate into plasma cells, which function in the **humoral immune response**.
      c. **Natural killer (NK) cells** lack the surface determinants characteristic of T and B lymphocytes but may display **cytotoxic activity** against tumor cells.
   3. **Plasma cells** (Figure 6.1) are **antibody-manufacturing cells** that arise from activated B lymphocytes and are responsible for **humoral immunity**.
      a. These ovoid cells contain an eccentric nucleus possessing **clumps of heterochromatin**, which appear to be arranged in a wheel-spoke fashion.
      b. Their cytoplasm is deeply basophilic because of an abundance of RER.
      c. A prominent area adjacent to the nucleus appears pale and contains the Golgi complex (negative Golgi image).
      d. They are most abundant at wound entry sites or in areas of chronic inflammation.
   4. **Granulocytes** (Figure 6.1) are white blood cells that possess cytoplasmic granules and arise from myeloid stem cells during hemopoiesis. At sites of inflammation, they leave the

bloodstream and enter the loose connective tissue, where they perform their specific functions (see Chapter 10 II B 2 a).

a. **Neutrophils phagocytose, kill, and digest bacteria** at sites of acute inflammation. **Pus** is an accumulation of dead neutrophils, bacteria, extracellular fluid, and additional debris at an inflammatory site.

b. **Eosinophils** bind to antigen–antibody complexes on the surface of parasites (e.g., helminthes) and then release cytotoxins that damage the parasites.

   (1) They are most prevalent at sites of chronic or allergic inflammation.

   (2) Eosinophils are attracted by eosinophil chemotactic factor (ECF), which is secreted by mast cells and basophils, to sites of allergic inflammation. There, eosinophils release enzymes that cleave histamine and leukotriene C, thus **moderating the allergic reaction**.

   (3) These cells also phagocytose antibody–antigen complexes.

c. **Basophils** are similar to mast cells in that they possess FcεRI receptors; their granules house the same primary mediators; and the same secondary mediators are manufactured de novo from the phospholipids of their plasmalemma. They differ, however, in that they circulate via the bloodstream, whereas mast cells do not.

IV. CLASSIFICATION OF CONNECTIVE TISSUE

Classification is based on the proportion of cells to fibers and on the arrangement and type of fibers (embryonic connective tissue, connective tissue proper, or specialized connective tissue).

A. **Embryonic connective tissue**

   1. **Mucous tissue (Wharton jelly)** is a loose connective tissue that is the main constituent of the umbilical cord. It consists of a jellylike matrix with some collagen fibers in which large stellate fibroblasts are embedded.

   2. **Mesenchymal tissue** is found only in **embryos**. It consists of a gel-like amorphous matrix containing only a few scattered reticular fibers, in which star-shaped, pale-staining mesenchymal cells are embedded. Mitotic figures are often observed in these pluripotential cells.

B. **Connective tissue proper**

   1. **Loose connective tissue (areolar tissue)** possesses fewer fibers but more cells than dense connective tissue.

   a. This tissue is **well vascularized**, **flexible**, and **not very resistant to stress**.

   b. It is **more abundant** than dense connective tissue and is the connective tissue that fills in the spaces just deep to the skin.

CLINICAL CONSIDERATIONS **Edema** is a pathologic process resulting in an **increased volume of tissue fluid**.

Edema may be caused by venous obstruction or decreased venous blood flow (as in congestive heart failure), increased capillary permeability (due to injury), starvation, excessive release of histamine, and obstruction of lymphatic vessels.

Edema that is responsive to localized pressure (i.e., depressions persist after release of pressure) is called **pitting edema**.

---

   2. **Dense connective tissue** contains more fibers but fewer cells than loose connective tissue. It is classified by the orientation of its fiber bundles into two types:

   a. **Dense, irregular connective tissue** (most common), which contains fiber bundles that have no definite orientation. This tissue is characteristic of the **dermis** and **capsules of many organs**.

   b. **Dense, regular connective tissue,** which contains fiber bundles and attenuated fibroblasts that are arranged in a uniform parallel fashion.

      (1) It is present only in **tendons** and **ligaments**.

      (2) This tissue may be collagenous or elastic.

3. Elastic tissue is composed of coarse, branching elastic fibers with a sparse network of collagen fibers and some fibroblasts filling the interstitial spaces. It is present in the dermis, lungs, elastic cartilage, and elastic ligaments and in large (conducting) blood vessels, where it forms fenestrated sheaths.

4. Reticular tissue consists mostly of a network of branched reticular fibers (**type III collagen**) (Figure 6.5).

    a. This tissue invests liver sinusoids, smooth muscle cells, and fat cells and forms the stroma of lymphatic organs, bone marrow, and endocrine glands.

    b. It also forms the reticular lamina of basement membranes.

5. Adipose tissue is the primary site for storage of energy (in the form of **triglycerides**) and has a rich neurovascular supply. It acts as an insulator, as a body cushion by filling in certain spaces, and as a shock absorber. Insulin and prostaglandins assist in the control of lipid storage in adipose tissue.

    a. White adipose tissue is composed of **unilocular** adipose cells.

        (1) This tissue constitutes nearly all of the adult adipose tissue throughout the body. White adipose tissue controls the body's fatty acid homeostasis by accumulating free fatty acids during an excess of caloric ingestion and releasing free fatty acids during a scarcity of caloric intake.

        (2) It **stores and releases lipids** as follows:

            (a) Adipose cells synthesize the enzyme **lipoprotein lipase**, which is transferred to the luminal aspect of the capillary endothelium.

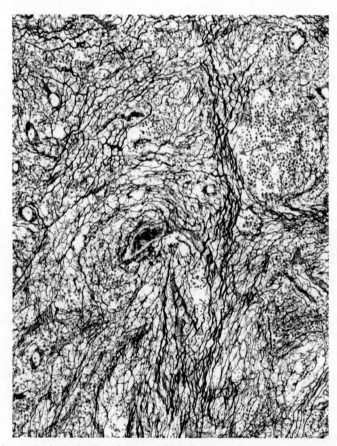

FIGURE 6.5. Light micrograph of reticular tissue (silver stain) (×132). Observe the reticular fibers at the tips of the *arrows*.

(b) Dietary fat is transported to adipose tissue as **very-low-density lipoproteins** and **chylomicrons**. Lipoprotein lipase then hydrolyzes these substances into fatty acids and glycerol.

(c) The free fatty acids enter the adipose cells, where they are re-esterified and stored as triglycerides (in fat droplets). Adipose cells also synthesize fatty acids from glucose.

(d) Lipid storage is stimulated by **insulin**, which increases the rate of synthesis of lipoprotein lipase and the uptake of glucose by adipose cells.

(e) Release of lipids is affected by neural impulses and/or adrenaline. Stored triglycerides are hydrolyzed by **hormone-sensitive lipase**, which is activated by cyclic adenosine monophosphate. The free fatty acids are released into the ECM and then enter the capillary lumen.

(3) **White adipose tissue** is also an **endocrine organ** that produces a number of hormones known as **adipokines**. Some of these hormones, **leptin, adiponectin, resistin**, and **retinol-binding protein-4**, are manufactured by adipocytes, whereas other hormones/factors, namely **tumor necrosis factor-α** and **interleukin-6**, are produced by the macrophages that reside in adipose tissue of obese individuals. It has been reported that obesity is always accompanied by **chronic inflammation**, and inflammatory agents released in response to inflammation-damaged tissue elicit a recruitment of macrophages into the connective tissue stroma among the enlarged adipocytes.

(a) **Leptin** is a protein hormone, produced primarily by adipocytes, which inhibits appetite for extended periods of time by binding to the appetite increasing neuropeptide Y, thus suppressing the area of the hypothalamus that control feeding, and induces the regions of the hypothalamus that controls the disbursement of energy. Additionally, leptin also induces the synthesis and release of the appetite-repressing neuropeptide α-melanocyte–stimulating hormone. Individuals who have mutations in the leptin gene or in the receptors for leptin exhibit uncontrollable hunger and become obese as a result. The volume of each adipocyte and the number of adipocytes are greater in obese than in thin individuals; therefore, the blood leptin levels of obese individuals may be as much as seven times greater than those of thin individuals.

(b) **Adiponectin** is also a protein hormone produced only by unilocular adipocytes. This hormone increases insulin sensitivity, therefore, facilitates the uptake of glucose and the oxidation of fatty acids in skeletal muscle cells, and decreases gluconeogenesis and glucose release by hepatocytes. Thus, adiponectin regulates the body's energy metabolism and facilitates weight loss. The blood levels of this hormone are greater in thin than in obese individuals.

(c) **Resistin** is a peptide hormone that is manufactured by adipocytes in rodents but by macrophages in humans. It is suggested that this hormone induces **insulin resistance**, resulting in hyperglycemia and type II diabetes mellitus in obese patients. Additionally, resistin contributes to the inflammatory response, a common finding in insulin resistance, obesity, and type II diabetes mellitus.

(d) **Retinol-binding protein-4** is also produced by unilocular adipocytes, and it has been demonstrated to elevate insulin resistance, inflammation, and fatty liver disease with a concomitant increase in glucose output by hepatocytes.

(e) **Tumor necrosis factor-α (TNF-α)** is manufactured by macrophages that reside in adipose tissues of obese individuals and is believed to be the principal cause of insulin resistance. Additionally, TNF-α also depresses liver cell's ability to oxidize fatty acids.

(f) **Interleukin-6 (IL-6)** is also manufactured and released by macrophages in the connective tissue interstices of unilocular adipose tissue of obese individuals. Similar to tumor necrosis factor-α interleukin-6 increases insulin resistance but also enhances skeletal muscle cells' ability to take up glucose and oxidize fatty acids.

OBESITY has been recently reclassified as a disease. Individuals are said to be obese if their adipose tissue buildup is great enough that their body mass index is greater than 30 kg/m^2 with a resultant decrease in life span and an increase in the possibility of acquiring a group of health problems referred to as **metabolic syndrome**. Insulin resistance, type II diabetes mellitus, fatty liver disease, and cardiovascular disease are commonly included under the rubric of metabolic syndrome.

Obesity occurs as either **hypertrophic obesity**, characterized by an increase in adipose cell **size** resulting from increased fat storage (**adult onset**), or **hypercellular (hyperplastic) obesity**, characterized by an increase in the **number** of adipose cells that begins in childhood and is usually lifelong.

A genetic basis for obesity is the result of mutations in the gene for the hormone leptin or in the genes for leptin receptors, thus preventing the production of leptin or producing an inactive form of the hormone or producing inactive leptin receptors. Since leptin functions in the regulation of appetite, persons affected by either of these two conditions possess an insatiable appetite, bringing about unrestrained weight gain. The volume of each adipocyte and the number of adipocytes are greater in obese than in thin individuals; therefore, the blood leptin levels of obese individuals may be as much as seven times greater than in thin individuals.

   b. **Brown adipose tissue** is composed of **multilocular** adipose cells, which contain many large mitochondria.
      (1) This tissue is capable of **generating heat** by **uncoupling oxidative phosphorylation**. **Thermogenin**, a transmembrane protein in mitochondria, causes the release of protons away from adenosine triphosphate synthesis, resulting in heat production.
      (2) This tissue is found in infants (also in hibernating animals) and is much reduced in adults.

1. **Adipose tumors** may be either benign or malignant. **Lipomas** are benign fatty tissue tumors usually found in subcutaneous connective tissues of the neck, back, and proximal regions of the limbs of middle-aged and elderly persons.
   2. **Liposarcomas** are the most common malignant adipose tumors. Although liposarcomas are most frequently located in the leg and/or the retroperitoneal tissues, they are not restricted to these sites. Liposarcomas are difficult to diagnose since they resemble lipomas. Adipocytes of the malignant tissue resemble either unilocular or multilocular adipocytes. Presently, chromosome markers are used to differentially diagnose liposarcomas.

Irisin. When an individual is doing physical exercises, his/her skeletal muscle cells release the hormone **irisin** that not only converts certain unilocular adipocytes into multilocular adipocytes but also enhances the maintenance of neuromuscular synapses.

C. **Specialized connective tissue**
   1. Cartilage and bone are discussed in Chapter 7.
   2. Blood is discussed in Chapter 10.

Review Test

Directions: Each of the numbered items or incomplete statements in this section is followed by answers or by completions of the statement. Select the ONE lettered answer or completion that is BEST in each case.

1. Which one of the following statements regarding collagen is true?

(A) It is composed of tropocollagen.
(B) Reticular fibers are composed of type II collagen.
(C) It is synthesized mostly by mast cells.
(D) Elastic fibers are composed of type IV collagen.
(E) Type II collagen is most common in connective tissue proper.

2. Dense regular connective tissue is present in

(A) capsules of organs.
(B) basement membrane.
(C) tendons.
(D) skin.
(E) dermis.

3. Of the following cell types found in connective tissue, which is most often present along capillaries and resembles fibroblasts?

(A) Plasma cell
(B) Lymphocyte
(C) Macrophage
(D) Mast cell
(E) Pericyte

4. Synovial fluids of normal joints are usually devoid of collagen. Patients with rheumatoid diseases have various types of collagen in their synovial fluid, depending on the tissue being damaged. If a patient has type II collagen in the synovial joint, which of the following tissues is being eroded?

(A) Vascular endothelium
(B) Compact bone
(C) Vascular smooth muscle
(D) Articular cartilage
(E) Synovial membrane

5. Which one of the following cell types arises from monocytes?

(A) Plasma cells
(B) Fibroblasts
(C) Lymphocytes
(D) Macrophages
(E) Mast cells

6. Foreign body giant cells are formed by the coalescence of

(A) macrophages.
(B) lymphocytes.
(C) fibroblasts.
(D) adipose cells.
(E) plasma cells.

7. Which one of the following cell types in the connective tissue arises from myeloid stem cells?

(A) Pericytes
(B) Eosinophils
(C) Fibroblasts
(D) Osteoblasts
(E) Adipocytes

8. Which of the following cell types is responsible for anaphylactic shock?

(A) Fibroblasts
(B) Eosinophils
(C) Pericytes
(D) Mast cells
(E) Macrophages

9. Which one of the following statements regarding proteoglycans is true?

(A) They consist of a core of fibrous protein covalently bound to glycoproteins.

(B) They are attached to ribonucleic acid.

(C) They are binding sites for deoxyribonucleic acid.

(D) They are composed of a protein core to which glycosaminoglycans are attached.

(E) They are the exclusive substance of the ECM along with collagen.

10. Which one of the following statements concerning loose connective tissue is true?

(A) It is less abundant than dense connective tissue.

(B) It has a lower proportion of cells to fibers than does dense connective tissue.

(C) It acts as a medium for exchange of nutrients and wastes between the blood and tissues.

(D) It provides structural support for organs.

(E) It consists of many fibers in which various types of cells are embedded.

Answers and Explanations

1. **A.** Collagen is composed of closely packed tropocollagen molecules. Reticular fibers are composed of type III collagen, whereas elastic fibers are composed of elastin microfibrils rather than collagen. Fibrocytes are inactive nonsecreting fibroblasts that synthesize the procollagen molecules (see Chapter 6 II B 1).

2. **C.** Tendons are composed of dense regular connective tissue containing collagen fibers arranged in a uniform parallel fashion (see Chapter 6 IV B 2).

3. **E.** Pericytes are pluripotential cells that resemble fibroblasts, although they are smaller, and are adjacent to capillaries (see Chapter 6 III B).

4. **D.** Type II collagen is present only in hyaline and elastic cartilages; therefore, finding type II collagen in the synovial fluid of a joint indicates erosion of the articular cartilage (see Chapter 6 II B 1).

5. **D.** Monocytes leave the bloodstream and migrate into the connective tissue, where they mature into functional macrophages (see Chapter 6 III E).

6. **A.** Foreign body giant cells result when macrophages coalesce (see Chapter 6 III E 3).

7. **B.** Eosinophils arise from myeloid stem cells during hemopoiesis and migrate to sites of inflammation within the connective tissue. Pericytes, fibroblasts, osteoblasts, and adipocytes arise from undifferentiated mesenchymal cells (see Chapter 6 III H 2).

8. **D.** After first exposure to an allergen, plasma cells make IgE antibodies that bind to FceRI receptors on mast cells (and basophils), sensitizing them. At the second exposure, the allergen binds to IgE, initiating degranulation of mast cells and releasing several mediators that give rise to type I hypersensitivity reaction (see Chapter 6 III D 4).

9. **D.** Proteoglycans consist of a protein core to which glycosaminoglycans are attached (see Chapter 6 II A).

10. **C.** Both loose and dense connective tissues are composed of three elements: an amorphous ground substance, fibers, and various types of cells. The amorphous ground substance of loose connective tissue is the medium of exchange between the connective tissue cells and the bloodstream (see Chapter 6 IV B 1).

chapter 7

Cartilage and Bone

I. OVERVIEW—CARTILAGE

Cartilage is an **avascular** specialized **fibrous connective tissue**. It has a **firm extracellular matrix** that is less pliable than that of connective tissue proper, and it contains **chondrocytes** embedded in matrix. Surrounding the cartilage is the **perichondrium** housing **chondroblasts** and **chondrogenic cells**. Cartilage **functions** primarily to support soft tissues and assists in the development and growth of long bones. The three types of cartilage—**hyaline cartilage, elastic cartilage**, and **fibrocartilage**—vary in certain matrix components (Table 7.1).

A. **Hyaline cartilage** (Figures 7.1 and 7.2; Table 7.1) is the most abundant cartilage in the body, and it also serves as a temporary skeleton in the fetus until it is replaced by bone.
   1. **Structure**
      a. **Matrix**
         (1) The matrix is composed of an amorphous ground substance containing **proteoglycan aggregates** and **chondronectin**, in which **type II collagen** is embedded (see Tables 4.2 and 7.1).

table **7.1** Cartilage Types, Characteristics, and Locations

Type of Cartilage	Identifying Characteristics	Perichondrium	Location
Hyaline	Type II collagen, basophilic matrix, chondrocytes usually arranged in groups (isogenous groups)	Perichondrium usually present except on articular surfaces	Articular ends of long bones, nose, larynx, trachea, bronchi, ventral ends of ribs, template for endochondral bone formation
Elastic	Type II collagen; elastic fibers	Perichondrium present	Pinna of ear, auditory canal and tube, epiglottis, some laryngeal cartilages
Fibrocartilage	Type I collagen, acidophilic matrix, chondrocytes arranged in parallel rows between bundles of collagen, always associated with dense collagenous connective tissue and/or hyaline cartilage	Perichondrium absent	Intervertebral discs, articular discs, pubic symphysis, insertion of tendons, meniscus of knee

Adapted with permission from Gartner LP, Hiatt JL. *Color Textbook of Histology*. Philadelphia, PA: Saunders; 1997;133.

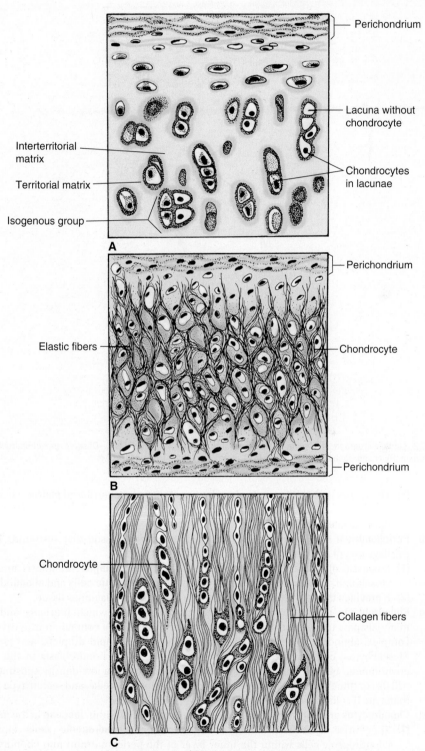

FIGURE 7.1. The three types of cartilage. **A.** Hyaline cartilage. **B.** Elastic cartilage. **C.** Fibrocartilage. (Reprinted with permission from Borysenko M, Berringer T. *Functional Histology*. 2nd ed. Little Brown and Co., Boston, 1984, p 102)

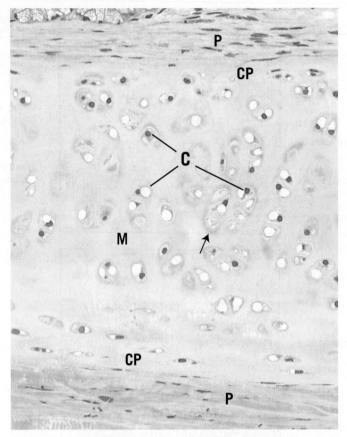

FIGURE 7.2. Light micrograph of hyaline cartilage of the monkey trachea (×270). Observe the chondrocytes (C), perichondrium (P), chondrogenic perichondrium (CP), matrix (M), and the lacuna (*arrow*).

      (2) The matrix that is adjacent to chondrocytes is called the **territorial matrix**. This part of the matrix is poor in collagen but rich in proteoglycans, and it stains more deeply than does the **interterritorial matrix**.

  b. Perichondrium is a layer of dense, irregular connective tissue that surrounds hyaline cartilage except at articular surfaces.

      (1) It consists of an **outer fibrous layer** containing **type I collagen**, fibroblasts, and blood vessels and an **inner cellular layer** containing **chondrogenic cells** and **chondroblasts**.

      (2) It **provides the nearest blood supply** to the avascular cartilaginous tissue.

  c. Chondroblasts manufacture the cartilage matrix through which nutrients and waste materials pass to and from the cells, respectively. These cells contain an extensive Golgi complex, abundant rough endoplasmic reticulum (RER), lipid droplets, and glycogen. Mesenchymal cells can be induced to become secreting chondroblasts in the proper environment, but if removed and grown as a monolayer in a low-density substrate, they will discontinue secreting cartilage matrix, become fibroblast-like, and secrete type I rather than type II collagen.

  d. Chondrocytes are mature cartilage cells that are embedded within **lacunae** in the matrix.

      (1) They arise by differentiation of mesenchymal **chondrogenic cells** and from chondrogenic cells within the inner layer of the perichondrium into chondroblasts, which are the earliest cells to produce cartilage matrix. Once these cells become totally enveloped by matrix, they are referred to as **chondrocytes** (see Figure 6.1).

      (2) Chondrocytes located **superficially** are ovoid and positioned with their longitudinal axis parallel to the cartilage surface. Those located **deeper** are more nearly spherical and may occur in groups of four to eight cells (**isogenous groups**).

table 7.2	Effects of Hormones and Vitamins on Hyaline Cartilage
Hormones	**Function**
Thyroxine, testosterone, somatotropin	Stimulate cartilage histogenesis
Cortisone, hydrocortisone, estradiol	Inhibit cartilage histogenesis
Vitamins	
Hypovitaminosis A	Diminishes thickness of epiphyseal plates
Hypervitaminosis A	Accelerates ossification of epiphyseal plates
Hypovitaminosis C	Stops matrix production, distorts cartilage columns in epiphyseal plates; scurvy develops
Hypovitaminosis D	Deficient absorption of calcium and phosphorus: epiphyseal cartilage cells proliferate, but matrix fails to calcify, and growing bones become deformed; rickets develops

2. **Histogenesis of hyaline cartilage** is similar to that of elastic cartilage and fibrocartilage and is affected by certain hormones and vitamins (Table 7.2). It occurs by the following two processes:
   a. **Interstitial growth** results from cell **division of preexisting chondrocytes**. This type of growth occurs only during the early stages of cartilage formation and in articular cartilage and the epiphyseal plates of long bones.
   b. **Appositional growth** results from differentiation of chondrogenic cells in the perichondrium. This type of growth results in the formation of chondroblasts and/or new chondrocytes, which elaborate a new layer of cartilage matrix at the periphery.
3. **Degeneration of hyaline cartilage** occurs when chondrocytes undergo hypertrophy and die and the matrix becomes calcified, a process that becomes more frequent with age. Degeneration of hyaline cartilage is a normal part of endochondral bone formation (discussed later).

CLINICAL CONSIDERATIONS

Arthritis, one of the processes of aging, is the degeneration of hyaline cartilage, especially as it covers the articulating surfaces of the members of bony joints. Over time, this causes joint pain, redness, swelling, stiffness, and restricts joint mobility.

Osteoarthritis is usually caused by wear and tear on the joint where the hyaline cartilage is worn away, resulting in bone grinding on bone. Other causes include joint injury or infection within the joint.

Rheumatoid arthritis is a very severe form of arthritis, where the immune system attacks the joint, including the cartilage, bone, and the synovial membrane. If left untreated, it may destroy the joint, including the cartilage and the bone.

B. **Elastic cartilage** (Figure 7.1; Table 7.1) possesses a perichondrium and is nearly identical to hyaline cartilage except for a network of elastic fibers, which impart **a yellowish** color. Although it contains type II collagen, it is less prone to degeneration than hyaline cartilage and does not calcify in aging. It is located in areas where **flexible support** is required. Elastic cartilage exists as in the cartilage of the auditory tube, external ear, and epiglottis.

C. **Fibrocartilage** (Figure 7.1; Table 7.1) **lacks** an identifiable perichondrium. It is characterized by alternating rows of fibroblast-derived chondrocytes surrounded by scant matrix and thick parallel bundles of **type I collagen** fibers. Fibrocartilage is located in areas where **support and tensile strength** are required and where tissues are exposed to compressive and shear forces. It is located in the intervertebral disks, menisci of the knees, sternoclavicular joints, and the pubic symphysis.

II. OVERVIEW—BONE

Bone is the primary constituent of the adult skeleton. It is a specialized type of connective tissue with a calcified extracellular matrix in which characteristic cells are embedded. Bone functions to support and protect vital organs, and fleshy structures, as a hemopoiesis organ, and provides a storage site for phosphate and calcium (bone contains about 99% of the body's calcium). Secondarily, it functions to regulate blood calcium levels via input from two separate nonbony tissues. Parathyroid hormone (PTH) from the parathyroid gland acts to increase calcium levels in the blood, whereas calcitonin secreted by the parafollicular cells (C cells) of the thyroid gland decreases calcium levels in the blood. Thus, the activities of these two substances on the calcium levels in bone are responsible for maintaining the proper blood calcium level. Bone is also a dynamic tissue that constantly undergoes changes in shape, such that applied pressure results in bone resorption, whereas applied tension results in bone formation.

A. **Structure**
  1. **Bone matrix**
     a. The **inorganic (calcified) portion of the bone matrix** (about 65% of the dry weight) is composed of calcium, phosphate, bicarbonate, citrate, magnesium, potassium, and sodium. It consists primarily of **hydroxyapatite crystals**, which have the composition $Ca_{10}(PO_4)_6(OH)_2$.
     b. The **organic portion of the bone matrix** (about 35% of the dry weight) consists primarily of **type I collagen** (95%) and a minor contribution of **type V collagen**. It has a ground substance that contains **chondroitin sulfate, keratan sulfate, and hyaluronic acid**.
        (1) Osteocalcin, stimulated by vitamin D, inhibits osteoblast function, and osteopontin, both glycoproteins, binds to hydroxyapatite and to integrins on osteoblasts and osteoclasts. Osteonectin, produced mostly by osteoblasts, is located in bone undergoing remodeling. Cytokines, growth hormones, and bone morphogenic proteins (BMPs), among others contribute to the bone matrix.
        (2) Bone sialoprotein is a matrix protein that also binds to integrins of the osteoblasts and osteocytes and is thus related to adherence of bone cells to bone matrix.
  2. The **periosteum** is a layer of **noncalcified** connective tissue covering bone on its **external** surfaces, except at synovial articulations and muscle attachments.
     a. It is composed of an outer dense **fibrous** collagenous layer and an inner cellular **osteoprogenitor (osteogenic)** layer.
     b. **Sharpey fibers** (type I collagen) attach the periosteum to the bone surface.
     c. The periosteum functions to distribute blood vessels to bone.
  3. The **endosteum** is a thin specialized connective tissue that lines the **marrow cavities** and supplies **osteoprogenitor cells** and **osteoblasts** for bone growth and repair.

B. **Bone cells**
  1. **Osteoprogenitor cells**
     a. These spindle-shaped cells are derived from embryonic mesenchyme and are **located in the periosteum and the endosteum, and persist throughout life as stem cells that line bone. They can be activated later for bone repair of fractures or other repair.**
     b. They are capable of differentiating into osteoblasts. However, at **low oxygen tensions, they may change into chondrogenic cells**.
  2. **Osteoblasts**
     a. Osteoblasts are derived from osteoprogenitor cells under the influence of members of the **BMP family** and also **transforming growth factor-β**. They possess receptors for PTH (see Chapter 13 V). Osteoblasts are responsible for the synthesis of organic protein components of bone matrix, including type I collagen, proteoglycans, and glycoproteins, which they secrete as **osteoid** (uncalcified bone matrix), which is mineralized under the influence and control by the osteoblasts. Additionally, they produce macrophage colony-stimulating factor **(M-CSF)**, a receptor for the activation of nuclear factor kappa B **(RANKL)**,

osteoprotegerin, osteocalcin (for bone mineralization), **osteopontin** (for formation of sealing zone between osteoclasts and the subosteoclastic compartment), **osteonectin** (related to bone mineralization), and **bone sialoprotein** (binding osteoblasts to extracellular matrix).

b. On bony surfaces, they resemble a layer of cuboidal, basophilic cells as they secrete organic matrix (see Figure 6.1).

c. They possess cytoplasmic processes with which they contact the processes of other osteoblasts and osteocytes and form **gap junctions**.

d. **When synthetically active**, they have a well-developed RER and Golgi complex.

e. These cells become entrapped in **lacunae**, but maintain contact with other cells via their cytoplasmic processes. Entrapped osteoblasts are known as osteocytes.

3. Osteocytes (Figure 7.3)

a. Osteocytes are **mature bone cells** housed in their own lacunae.

b. They have narrow cytoplasmic processes that extend through **canaliculi** in the calcified matrix (see Figures 6.1 and 7.3).

c. They maintain communication with each other via **gap junctions** between their processes.

d. They are nourished and maintained by nutrients, metabolites, and signal molecules carried by the extracellular fluid that flows through the lacunae and canaliculi. In addition, calcium released from bone enters the extracellular fluid located within these spaces.

e. They contain abundant heterochromatin, a paucity of RER, and a small Golgi complex.

4. Osteoclasts

a. Overview. Osteoclasts are large, motile, multinucleated cells (up to 50 nuclei) that resorb bone. They are derived from cells of the **mononuclear-phagocyte system**, comprising blood-borne **monocytes** that enter the connective tissue spaces where they differentiate into various types of macrophages and osteoclasts (see Section **(3)**).

(1) Osteoclasts possess cell surface receptors: colony-stimulating factor-1 receptor, calcitonin receptor, and RANK (nuclear factor kappa B).

(2) Osteoblasts that have been stimulated by PTH promote osteoclast formation, whereas osteoblasts that have been stimulated by calcitonin inhibit osteoclast formation by stimulating osteoid synthesis and calcium deposition.

(3) Via a series of three osteoblast signals, osteoclast precursors (macrophages) are stimulated by **M-CSF** to undergo mitosis. Another signaling molecule, **RANKL**, binds to the precursor, inducing it to differentiate into the multinucleated osteoclast, thus activating it to commence bone resorption. A third signal, **osteoprotegerin (OPG)**, a member of the **tumor necrosis factor receptor (TNFR)** family produced by osteoblasts and other cells, can prohibit RANKL from binding to the macrophage, thus prohibiting osteoclast formation.

b. Osteoclast cytoplasm is **acidophilic**. Osteoclasts function in the **resorption of bone** (osteolysis). They form and reside in depressions known as **Howship lacunae**, which represent areas of bone resorption.

c. Morphology. Osteoclasts activated by **osteoclast-stimulating factor** produced and released by osteoblasts display four regions in electron micrographs.

(1) Basal zone is that part of the osteoclast housing most of the organelles and is the farthest from the subosteoclastic compartment.

(2) The **ruffled border** is the site of active bone resorption. It is composed of irregular fingerlike cytoplasmic projections extending into the **subosteoclastic compartment**, a slight depression that deepens as the osteoclast resorbs bone and then that depression is referred to as **Howship lacuna**. The ruffled border of an inactive osteoclast is collapsed as the cell is in a resting stage.

(3) The **clear zone** surrounds the ruffled border. It contains actin filaments at the periphery that help osteoclasts maintain contact with the bony surface. This isolates and seals the region of osteolytic activity. Further, **osteopontin**, secreted by osteoblasts, is used to seal the zone between osteoclasts and the subosteoclastic compartment.

(4) The **vesicular zone** contains exocytotic vesicles that transfer lysosomal enzymes to Howship lacunae and endocytotic vesicles that transfer degraded bone products from Howship lacunae to the interior of the cell.

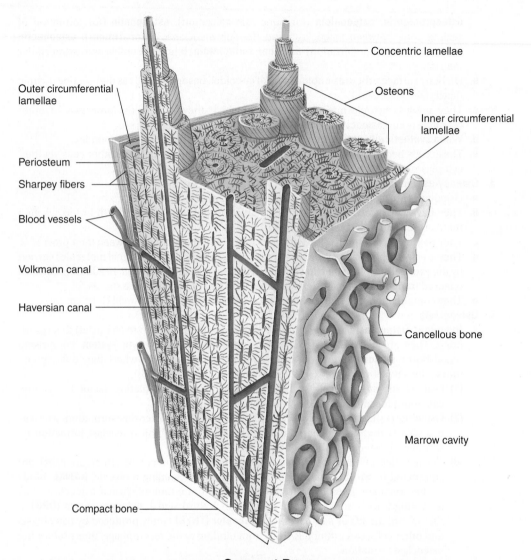

Outer circumferential lamellae

Periosteum

Sharpey fibers

Blood vessels

Volkmann canal

Haversian canal

Compact bone

Concentric lamellae

Osteons

Inner circumferential lamellae

Cancellous bone

Marrow cavity

Compact Bone

Compact bone is surrounded by dense irregular collagenous connective tissue, the **periosteum**, which is attached to the **outer circumferential lamellae** by **Sharpey fibers**. Blood vessels of the periosteum enter the bone via larger nutrient canals or small **Volkmann canals**, which not only convey blood vessels to the **Haversian canals** of **osteons** but also interconnect adjacent Haversian canals. Each osteon is composed of concentric lamellae of bone whose collagen fibers are arranged so that they are perpendicular to those of contiguous lamellae. The **inner circumferential lamellae** are lined by endosteal lined cancellous bone that protrudes into the marrow cavity.

FIGURE 7.3. Histological aspects of a long bone. Inset: cross section of an osteon. (Reprinted with permission from Gartner LP, Hiatt JL. *Color Atlas and Text of Histology.* 6th ed. Baltimore, MD: Wolters Kluwer Health/Lippincott, Williams & Wilkins; 2013:88.)

Osteopetrosis, unlike osteoporosis, is a genetic disorder affecting osteoclasts so that they do not possess ruffled borders; therefore, these osteoclasts cannot resorb bone, which creates an imbalance between bone formation and bone resorption. Thus, persons with osteopetrosis display increased bone density. This condition leads to anemia because of decreased marrow space, blindness, deafness, and damage to the cranial nerves as the foramina of the skull become narrow and impinge on the nerves.

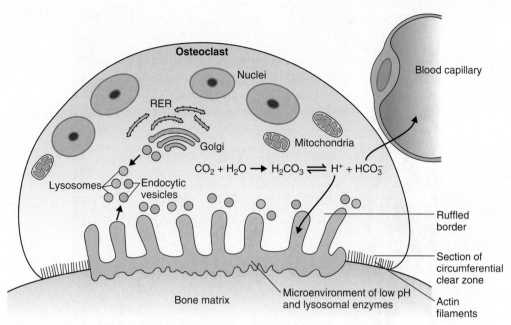

FIGURE 7.4. Osteoclastic function. RER, rough endoplasmic reticulum.

In the figure: Osteoclast; Nuclei; RER; Golgi; Mitochondria; Blood capillary; Lysosomes; Endocytic vesicles; $CO_2 + H_2O \rightarrow H_2CO_3 \rightleftharpoons H^+ + HCO_3^-$; Ruffled border; Section of circumferential clear zone; Bone matrix; Microenvironment of low pH and lysosomal enzymes; Actin filaments

    d. Bone resorption (Figure 7.4) involves the following events:

      (1) Osteoclasts secrete **acid**, which decalcifies the surface layer of bone.

      (2) Acid hydrolases, collagenases, and proteolytic enzymes, and the acid environment within Howship lacuna release the mineral content of bone. Cathepsin K secreted by the osteoclasts is released into Howship lacuna to **degrade the organic portion** of the bone.

      (3) Osteoclasts resorb the organic and inorganic residues of the bone matrix and release them into connective tissue capillaries.

      (4) At the conclusion of the bone resorption function, osteoclasts undergo apoptosis.

      (5) Increases in PTH stimulate osteoclastic activity, thereby promoting bone resorption, whereas calcitonin, secreted by C cells (parafollicular cells) in the thyroid gland, inhibits osteoclastic activity. However, evidence indicates that PTH, under certain conditions, may stimulate bone formation although the mechanism for this is not known.

C. Classification of bone is based on both gross and microscopic properties.

    1. Gross observation (Figure 7.3) of cross sections of bone reveals two types:

    a. Spongy (cancellous) bone, which is composed of interconnected trabeculae. Bony trabeculae surround cavities filled with bone marrow. The trabeculae contain osteocytes and are lined on both surfaces by a single layer of osteoblasts. Spongy bone is always surrounded by compact bone.

    b. Compact (dense) bone has no trabeculae or bone marrow cavities.

    2. Microscopic observation of bone reveals two types:

    a. Primary bone, also known as **immature** or **woven** bone

      (1) Primary bone contains many osteocytes and large, irregularly arranged type I collagen bundles.

      (2) It has a low mineral content.

      (3) It is the first compact bone produced during fetal development and bone repair.

      (4) It **is remodeled and replaced by secondary bone** except in a few places (e.g., tooth sockets, near suture lines in skull bones, and at insertion sites of tendons).

    b. Secondary bone, also known as **mature** or **lamellar** bone

      (1) Secondary bone is the compact bone of adults.

      (2) It has a **calcified matrix arranged in regular layers**, or **lamellae**. Each lamella is 3 to 7 μm thick.

      (3) It contains osteocytes in lacunae between, and occasionally within, lamellae.

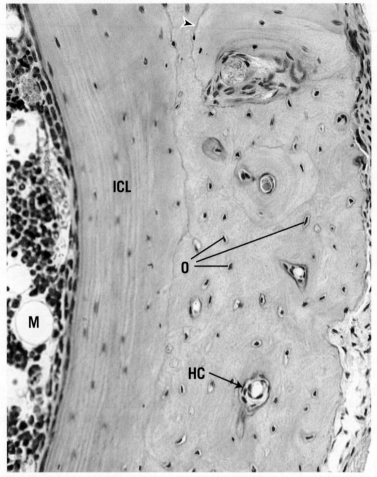

FIGURE 7.5. Light micrograph of bone and bone marrow from the rib (×270). M, bone marrow; ICL, inner circumferential lamellae; O, osteocytes; HC, haversian canal.

D. **Organization of lamellae** in compact bone (e.g., diaphysis of long bones) is characteristic and consists of the following elements (Figure 7.5):
  1. **Haversian systems (osteons)** are long cylindrical structures that run approximately parallel to the long axis of the diaphysis.
     a. Haversian systems are composed of 4 to 20 lamellae surrounding a central haversian canal, which contains blood vessels, nerves, and loose connective tissue. They are lined by osteoprogenitor cells and osteoblasts.
     b. They are often surrounded by an amorphous **cementing substance**.
     c. They are interconnected by **Volkmann canals**, which also connect to the periosteum and endosteum and **carry the neurovascular supply**.
  2. **Interstitial lamellae** are irregularly shaped lamellae between haversian systems. They are remnants of remodeled haversian systems.
  3. **Outer and inner circumferential lamellae** are located at the external and internal surfaces of the diaphysis, respectively (Figure 7.6).

E. **Histogenesis of bone** occurs by two processes, **intramembranous** and **endochondral bone formation**. Both processes produce bone that appears histologically identical. Bone histogenesis is accompanied by bone resorption. The combination of bone formation and resorption, termed **remodeling**, occurs throughout life, although it is slower in secondary than in primary bone.

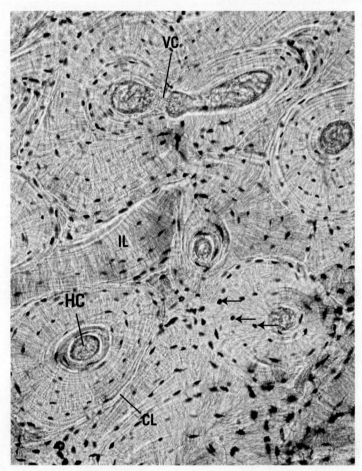

FIGURE 7.6. Light micrograph of ground bone (×132). Observe the haversian canal (HC), cementing line (CL), interstitial lamellae (IL), Volkmann canal (VC), and osteocytes within lamellae (*arrows*).

1. **Intramembranous bone formation** (Figure 7.7) is the process by which most of the **flat bones** (e.g., parietal bones of the skull) are formed. It involves the following events:
   a. Mesenchymal cells, in the presence of a vascular zone, condense into **primary ossification centers**, differentiate into osteoblasts, **and** begin secreting **osteoids** in a rather haphazard form, known as **woven bone**.
   b. As appositional bone growth continues and calcification occurs, osteoblasts become trapped in their own matrix and become osteocytes. These centers of developing bone are called **trabeculae** (fused spicules).
   c. Fusion of the bony trabeculae produces **spongy bone** as blood vessels invade the area and other undifferentiated mesenchymal cells become hematopoietic cells forming blood cells of the bone marrow.
   d. The periosteum and endosteum develop from portions of the mesenchymal layer that do not undergo ossification.
   e. Mitotic activity of the mesenchymal cells gives rise to osteoprogenitor cells, which undergo cell division and form more osteoprogenitor cells or differentiate into osteoblasts within the inner layer of the developing periosteum.
   f. Finally, intramembranous bone may then be converted to lamellar bone.
2. **Endochondral bone formation** (Figure 7.8) is the process by which **long bones** are formed. It begins in a segment of **hyaline cartilage** that serves as a small **model** for the bone. The two

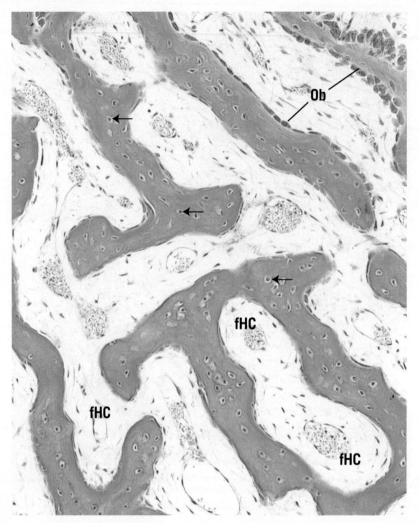

FIGURE 7.7. Light micrograph of membranous bone formation (×132). Observe the forming haversian canals (fHC), osteo-blasts (Ob), and osteocytes (*arrows*).

stages of endochondral bone formation involve the development of primary and secondary centers of ossification.

a. The **primary center of ossification** develops at the **midriff of the diaphysis** of the hyaline cartilage model, containing type II collagen, by the following sequence of events:

   (1) Vascularization of the perichondrium at this site causes the transformation of chondrogenic cells to osteoprogenitor cells, which differentiate into osteoblasts. This region of the perichondrium is now called the **periosteum**.

   (2) Osteoblasts elaborate matrix deep to the periosteum, and via **intramembranous bone formation**, form the **subperiosteal bone collar**.

   (3) Chondrocytes within the core of the cartilaginous model undergo **hypertrophy** and degenerate, and their lacunae become confluent, forming large cavities that eventually become marrow spaces.

   (4) Osteoclasts create perforations in the bone collar that permit the **periosteal bud** (blood vessels, osteoprogenitor cells, and mesenchymal cells) to enter the newly formed spaces in the cartilaginous model. The cartilage that constitutes the walls of these spaces then becomes calcified.

   (5) Newly developed osteoblasts elaborate bone matrix that becomes calcified on the surface of the calcified cartilage, forming a **calcified cartilage–calcified bone complex**.

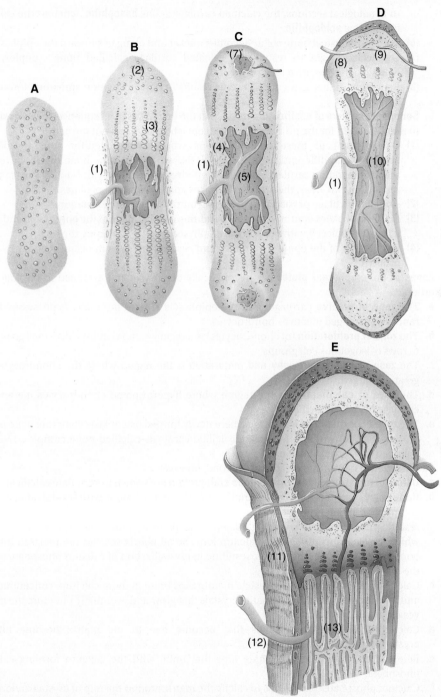

FIGURE 7.8. Endochondral bone formation. **A.** Endochondral bone formation requires the presence of a hyaline cartilage model. **B.** Vascularization of the diaphysis perichondrium (2) results in the transformation of chondrogenic cells to osteogenic cells, hence formation via intramembranous bone formation of a subperiosteal bone collar (1) that quickly becomes perforated by osteoclastic activity. Chondrocytes in the center of the cartilage hypertrophy (3) and their lacunae become confluent. **C.** The subperiosteal bone collar (1) increases in length and width. The confluent lacunae are invaded by the periosteal bud (4). Osteoclastic activity forms a primitive marrow cavity (5) whose walls are composed of calcified cartilage—calcified bone complex. The epiphyses display the beginning of secondary ossification centers (7). **D** and **E.** The subperiosteal bond collar (1) is now large enough to support the developing long bone, so that much of the cartilage has been resorbed except for the epiphyseal plate (8) and the covering of the epiphyses (9). Ossification in the epiphyses occurs from the center (10); thus, the vascular periosteum (11) does not cover the cartilaginous surface. Blood vessels (12) enter the epiphyses, without vascularizing the cartilage, to constitute the vascular network (13) around which spongy bone will form. (Reprinted with permission from Gartner LP, Hiatt JL. *Color Atlas of Histology.* 5th ed. Baltimore, MD: Lippincott Williams & Wilkins; 2009.)

In histological sections, the calcified cartilage stains **basophilic**, whereas the calcified bone stains **acidophilic**.

(6) The subperiosteal bone collar becomes thicker and elongates toward the epiphysis.

(7) Osteoclasts begin to resorb the calcified cartilage–calcified bone complex, thus enlarging the primitive marrow cavity.

(8) Repetition of this sequence of events results in bone formation spreading toward the **epiphyses**.

   b. Secondary centers of ossification develop at the **epiphyses** in a sequence of events similar to that described for the primary center, except a bone collar is not formed.

      (1) Development of these centers begins when osteoprogenitor cells invade the epiphysis and differentiate into osteoblasts, which elaborate bone matrix to replace the disintegrating cartilage. When the epiphyses are filled with bone tissue, cartilage remains in two areas, the articular surfaces and the epiphyseal plates.

      (2) Articular cartilage persists and does not contribute to bone formation.

      (3) Epiphyseal plates continue to grow by adding new cartilage at the epiphyseal end while it is being replaced with bone at the diaphyseal end (lengthening the bone).

      (4) Ossification of the epiphyseal plates and cessation of growth occur at about 20 years of age.

3. Zones of the epiphyseal plates are histologically distinctive and arranged in the following order:

   a. The **zone of reserve** cartilage is at the epiphyseal side of the plate. It possesses small, randomly arranged inactive chondrocytes.

   b. The **zone of proliferation** (of chondrocytes) is a region of rapid mitotic divisions giving rise to rows of isogenous cell groups.

   c. The **zone of cell hypertrophy and maturation** is the region where the chondrocytes are greatly enlarged.

   d. The **zone of calcification** is the region where hypertrophied chondrocytes die and the cartilage becomes calcified.

   e. The **zone of ossification** is the area where newly formed osteoblasts elaborate bone matrix on the calcified cartilage, forming a calcified cartilage–calcified bone complex, which is resorbed and replaced by bone.

4. Calcification of bone is not clearly understood, however.

   a. Osteonectin, proteoglycans, and **bone sialoprotein** are known to stimulate calcification.

   b. Bone matrix contains high concentrations of calcium Ca^{2+} along with several other organic compounds and enzymes. Osteocalcin and sialoproteins further concentrate the calcium, resulting in osteoblasts secreting alkaline phosphatase, thus concentrating PO_4^{3-} ions, which further concentrates the calcium ions. Small matrix vesicles are released into the bone matrix from the osteoblasts, resulting in crystallization of calcium phosphate within the matrix vesicles.

   c. Calcium pumps in the matrix vesicle membranes bring in more calcium, concentrating it and forming calcium hydroxyapatite crystals that grow and eventually puncture the matrix vesicle expelling its contents.

   d. Calcium hydroxyapatite crystals that become free in the matrix become **nidi of crystallization**.

   e. Released enzymes free phosphate ions that unite with the calcium forming calcium phosphate.

   f. Calcium phosphate then begins to calcify the matrix around the nidi of crystallization.

   g. Water is removed from the matrix, permitting hydroxyapatite crystals to be deposited into gaps within the collagen fibrils.

   h. Nidi of mineralization enlarge and fuse with neighboring nidi, eventually calcifying the entire matrix.

F. Bone remodeling. Bone is constantly being remodeled as necessary for growth and to alter its structural makeup to adapt to changing stresses in the environment throughout life.

   1. Early on, bone development outpaces bone resorption as new haversian systems are added and fewer are resorbed.

2. Later, when the epiphyseal plates are closed, ending bone growth, bone development and resorption are balanced.

Several factors, including **calcitonin** and PTH, are responsible for this phenomenon regarding compact bone (see Section II J). Remodeling of cancellous bone is under the control of many factors within the bone marrow.

G. **Repair of a bone fracture.** A bone fracture damages the matrix, bone cells, and blood vessels in the region and is accompanied by localized hemorrhaging and blood clot formation.

1. **Proliferation of osteoprogenitor cells** occurs in the periosteum and endosteum in the vicinity of the fracture. As a result of this proliferation, cellular tissue surrounds the fracture and penetrates between the ends of the damaged bone.

2. **Formation of a bony callus** occurs both internally and externally at a fracture site.
   a. Fibrous connective tissue and hyaline cartilage are formed in the fracture zone.
   b. Endochondral bone formation replaces the cartilage with primary bone.
   c. Intramembranous bone formation also produces primary bone in the area.
   d. The irregularly arranged trabeculae of primary bone join the ends of the fractured bone, forming a **bony callus**.
   e. The primary bone is resorbed and replaced with secondary bone as the fracture heals.

CLINICAL CONSIDERATIONS **Bone Repair.** After severe injury where segments of bone have been lost or must be removed, the remaining bone is prevented from forming a bony union followed by a bony callus that over time would result in completed bone repair. When the bony union is not possible, a bone graft is required. For this purpose, bone fragments that are stored frozen to maintain osteogenic potential may then may be utilized in bone grafts.

Autographs are most successful since the bone donor is the recipient.

Homographs are of bone donated from a different individual.

Heterographs are the least successful because the donor bone comes from another species. However, calf bone that has been frozen can serve as a viable bone graft when necessary.

H. **Role of vitamins in bone formation**

1. **Vitamin D** is necessary for **absorption of calcium** from the small intestine. Vitamin D deficiency results in poorly calcified (soft) bone, a condition known as **rickets** in children and **osteomalacia** in adults. Vitamin D is also necessary for **bone formation** (ossification), whereas an excess of vitamin D causes bone resorption.

2. **Vitamin A** deficiency inhibits proper bone formation and growth, whereas an excess accelerates ossification of the epiphyseal plates. Deficiency or excess of vitamin A results in small stature.

3. **Vitamin C** is necessary for **collagen formation**. Deficiency results in **scurvy**, characterized by poor bone growth and inadequate fracture repair.

CLINICAL CONSIDERATIONS **Rickets** occurs in children deficient in vitamin D, which results in calcium deficiency. It is characterized by deficient calcification in newly formed bone and is generally accompanied by deformation of the bone spicules in epiphyseal plates; as a result, bones grow more slowly than normal and are deformed by the stress of weight bearing. **Osteomalacia** (rickets of adults) results from calcium deficiency.

1. It is characterized by deficient calcification in newly formed bone and decalcification of already calcified bone.
2. This disease may be severe during pregnancy because the calcium requirements of the fetus may lead to calcium loss from the mother.

I. Role of hormones in bone formation
   1. **PTH** activates osteoblasts to secrete **osteoclast-stimulating factor**, which then activates osteoclasts to **resorb bone**, thus **elevating blood calcium levels**. Excess PTH (hyperparathyroidism) renders bone **more susceptible to fracture** and subsequent deposition of calcium in arterial walls and certain organs, such as the kidney.
   2. **Calcitonin** is produced by parafollicular cells (C cells) of the thyroid gland. It eliminates the ruffled border of osteoclasts and **inhibits bone matrix resorption**, preventing the release of calcium.
   3. **Pituitary growth hormone (somatotropin)** is produced in the pars distalis of the pituitary gland. It stimulates overall growth, especially that of epiphyseal plates, and influences bone development via insulin-like growth factors (somatomedins), especially stimulating growth of the epiphyseal plates. Children deficient in this hormone exhibit dwarfism, whereas adults with an excess of somatotropin in their growing years display **pituitary gigantism** and **acromegaly**.

CLINICAL CONSIDERATIONS

Osteoporosis is a disease characterized by **low bone mass (low bone mineral density)** and structural deterioration of bone tissue, making the bone fragile and susceptible to fracture. Osteoporosis is associated with an abnormal ratio of mineral to matrix.

   1. It results from increased bone resorption, decreased bone formation, or both.
   2. Estrogen activates bone formation by osteoblasts, and in its absence an imbalance causes osteoclastic activity to render bones fragile and susceptible to fracture.
      a. Osteoporosis is most common in postmenopausal women because of diminished estrogen secretion, and in immobile patients because of lack of physical stress on the bone.
      b. Estrogen therapy was employed for decades to minimize the onset of osteoporosis. Recently, it was determined that estrogen replacement therapy increases the risk of heart disease, stroke, breast cancer, and blood clots. Now, instead of estrogen, a recent new group of drugs, the bisphosphonates, has been developed that reduces the incidence of osteoporosis.
      c. Preventive measures include a balanced diet rich in calcium and vitamin D and weight-bearing exercise.

Acromegaly

Acromegaly results from an **excess of pituitary growth hormone** in adults. It is characterized by **very thick bones** in the extremities and in portions of the facial skeleton.

III. JOINTS

A. Synarthroses are immovable joints composed of connective tissue, cartilage, or bone. These joints unite the first rib to the sternum and connect the skull bones to each other.

B. Diarthroses (synovial joints) permit **maximum movement** and generally unite long bones. These joints are surrounded by a two-layered **capsule**, enclosing and sealing the articular cavity. The articular cavity contains **synovial fluid**, a colorless, viscous fluid that is rich in hyaluronic acid and proteins.
   1. The **external (fibrous) capsular layer** is a tough, fibrous layer of dense connective tissue.
   2. The **internal (synovial) capsular layer** is also called the **synovial membrane**. It is lined by a layer of squamous to cuboidal epithelial cells on its internal surface. Two cell types are displayed in electron micrographs of this epithelium.
      a. **Type A cells** are intensely phagocytic and have a well-developed Golgi complex, many lysosomes, and sparse RER.
      b. **Type B cells** resemble fibroblasts and have a well-developed RER; these cells probably secrete synovial fluid.

Review Test

Directions: Each of the numbered items or incomplete statements in this section is followed by answers or by completions of the statement. Select the ONE lettered answer or completion that is BEST in each case.

1. Which of the following statements characterizes osteoclasts?

(A) They are enucleated cells.
(B) They produce collagen.
(C) They secrete osteoid.
(D) They are derived from osteoprogenitor cells.
(E) They occupy Howship lacunae.

2. Which one of the following statements is correct concerning the periosteum?

(A) It is devoid of a blood supply.
(B) It produces osteoclasts.
(C) It is responsible for interstitial bone growth.
(D) Its inner layer contains osteoprogenitor cells.
(E) Its outer layer is devoid of fibers.

3. Which one of the following statements is characteristic of osteocytes?

(A) They communicate via gap junctions between their processes.
(B) They contain large amounts of RER.
(C) They are immature bone cells.
(D) They are housed as isogenous groups in lacunae.
(E) They give rise to osteoclasts.

4. Which one of the following statements concerning hyaline cartilage is correct?

(A) It is vascular.
(B) It contains type IV collagen.
(C) It undergoes appositional growth only.
(D) It is located at the articular ends of long bones.
(E) Its chondrocytes are aligned in rows.

5. A 7-year-old boy is seen by his pediatrician because the child broke his humerus as he tripped and fell while walking. The pediatrician asked about the child's diet and learned that he might have a dietary deficiency. Which of the following may be lacking in his diet?

(A) Potassium
(B) Calcium
(C) Iron
(D) Carbohydrates
(E) Protein

6. A 22-year-old woman is seen for the first time by her new physician, who notes that she has very thick bones in her extremities and face. The physician suspects acromegaly, caused by which of the following?

(A) Hypervitaminosis A
(B) Excess growth hormone
(C) Hypovitaminosis A
(D) Hypervitaminosis D
(E) Hypovitaminosis D

7. Which of the following statements is characteristic of bone?

(A) Bone matrix contains primarily type II collagen.
(B) About 65% of the dry weight of bone is organic.
(C) Haversian canals are interconnected via Volkmann canals.
(D) Bone growth occurs via interstitial growth only.
(E) Bone growth occurs via appositional growth only.

121

8. Which one of the following inhibits histogenesis of cartilage?

(A) Thyroxine
(B) Hypervitaminosis A
(C) Hypovitaminosis D
(D) Hydrocortisone
(E) Hypovitaminosis C

9. Which one of the following stimulates cartilage histogenesis?

(A) Thyroxine
(B) Hypervitaminosis A
(C) Hypovitaminosis D
(D) Hydrocortisone
(E) Hypovitaminosis C

10. Which one of the following accelerates epiphyseal ossification?

(A) Thyroxine
(B) Hypervitaminosis A
(C) Absence of vitamin D
(D) Hydrocortisone
(E) Hypovitaminosis C

11. Which one of the following makes epiphyseal cartilage matrix fail to calcify?

(A) Thyroxine
(B) Hypervitaminosis A
(C) Hypovitaminosis D
(D) Hydrocortisone
(E) Hypovitaminosis C

12. A 25-year-old patient, anemic for several years, complains of failing eyesight and hearing loss. During a physical examination, it is determined that the patient has lost function of some of the cranial nerves. The diagnosis could be which one of the following?

(A) Osteoporosis
(B) Osteomalacia
(C) Rickets
(D) Acromegaly
(E) Osteopetrosis

Answers and Explanations

1. **E.** Osteoclasts are multinucleated cells that produce proteolytic enzymes and occupy Howship lacunae. They are not derived from osteoprogenitor cells but from monocyte precursors (see Chapter 7 II C 4).

2. **D.** The inner layer of the periosteum possesses osteoprogenitor cells, whereas the outer layer of the periosteum is fibrous. The periosteum functions to distribute blood vessels to the bone; thus, appositional bone growth takes place here (see Chapter 7 II B 2).

3. **A.** Osteocytes communicate with each other via gap junctions on narrow cytoplasmic processes that extend through canaliculi. They are mature bone cells that occupy individual lacunae as mature resting bone cells (see Chapter 7 II C 3).

4. **D.** Hyaline cartilage is avascular, contains type II collagen, and grows both interstitially and appositionally. It is located at the articulating ends of long bones (see Chapter 7 I A).

5. **B.** Because calcium must be maintained at a constant level in the blood and the tissues, a diet deficient in calcium leads to calcium loss from the bones. As a result, the bones become fragile (see Chapter 7 II C 4 Clinical Considerations).

6. **B.** Excessive growth hormone causes acromegaly. Excessive vitamin D causes bone resorption. Both an excess and a deficiency of vitamin A result in short stature (see Chapter 7 II J Clinical Considerations).

7. **C.** Haversian canals run longitudinally, parallel to the long axis of bone. They are connected to one another by Volkmann canals that run perpendicular (or obliquely) to them (see Chapter 7 II E 1).

8. **D.** Hydrocortisone inhibits cartilage growth and matrix formation (see Chapter 7 I A 2).

9. **A.** Thyroxine, testosterone, and somatotropin stimulate cartilage growth and matrix formation (see Chapter 7 I A 2).

10. **B.** Hypervitaminosis A accelerates ossification of epiphyseal plates, whereas hypovitaminosis A reduces the width of the epiphyseal plates (see Chapter 7 II I).

11. **C.** In the absence of vitamin D, epiphyseal chondrocytes continue to proliferate, but their matrix does not calcify, which leads to rickets (see Chapter 7 II I Clinical Considerations).

12. **E.** Osteopetrosis is a genetic defect involving the osteoclasts. Persons with this defect possess osteoclasts without ruffled borders, which prohibit them from resorbing bone. Therefore, bone forms but is not resorbed. This leads to increased bone density, anemia, blindness, deafness, and cranial nerve involvement because the nerves are impinged upon as they exit the cranium via their foramina (see Chapter 7 II B Clinical Considerations).

8 Muscle

I. OVERVIEW—MUSCLE

A. Muscle is classified into two types: **striated** and **smooth**, and striated muscle has two subdivisions: **skeletal** and **cardiac muscles**.

B. Muscle cells possess **contractile filaments** whose major components are **actin** and **myosin**.

C. Contraction may be **voluntary** (skeletal muscles) or **involuntary** (cardiac and smooth muscles).

II. STRUCTURE OF SKELETAL MUSCLE

A. **Connective tissue investments** convey neural and vascular elements to muscle cells and provide a vehicle that harnesses the forces of muscle contraction.
  1. **Epimysium** surrounds an entire muscle and forms **aponeuroses**, which connect skeletal muscle to muscle, and **tendons**, which connect skeletal muscle to bone.
  2. **Perimysium** surrounds **fascicles** (small bundles) of muscle cells.
  3. **Endomysium** surrounds individual muscle cells and is composed of **reticular fibers** and an **external lamina**.

B. **Types of skeletal muscle cells**
  1. Types of skeletal muscle cells (also known as **muscle fibers**) include **red** (slow contraction but does not fatigue easily), **white** (fast contraction but fatigues easily), and **intermediate**. All three types may be present in a given muscle.
  2. These three types differ from each other in their content of **myoglobin** (a protein that is similar to hemoglobin in that it binds O_2), **number of mitochondria, concentration of various enzymes**, and **rate of contraction** (Table 8.1).
  3. A change in **innervation** can change a fiber's type. If a red fiber is denervated and its innervation replaced with that of a white fiber, the red fiber will change its characteristics and will become a white fiber.

C. **Skeletal muscle cells** (Figures 8.1 and 8.2) are long, cylindrical, **multinucleated** and are enveloped by an external lamina and reticular fibers. Their cytoplasm is called **sarcoplasm**, and their plasmalemma is called the **sarcolemma** and forms deep tubular invaginations, or **T (transverse)**

| table 8.1 | Characteristics of Red and White Muscle Fibers |

Type	Myoglobin Content	Number of Mitochondria	Enzyme Content	Contraction	Primary Method of ATP Generation
Red (slow; type I)	High	Many	High in oxidative enzymes; low in ATPase	Slow but repetitive; not easily fatigued	Slow oxidative phosphorylation
Intermediate (type IIa)	Intermediate	Intermediate	Intermediate in oxidative enzymes and ATPase	Fast but not easily fatigued	Oxidative phosphorylation and anaerobic glycolysis
White (fast; type IIb)	Low	Few	Low in oxidative enzymes; high in ATPase and phosphorylases	Fast and easily fatigued	Anaerobic glycolysis

ATP, adenosine triphosphate; ATPase, adenosine triphosphatase.

tubules, which extend into the cells. Skeletal muscle cells possess cylindrical collections of **myofibrils**, 1 to 2 μm in diameter, which extend the entire length of the cell.

1. **Myofibrils** are composed of longitudinally arranged, cylindrical bundles of **thick** and **thin myofilaments** observable by transmission electron microscopy (see Figure 8.1).

   a. Precise alignment of myofibrils results in a characteristic banding pattern visible by light microscopy as alternating dark **A bands** and light **I bands**; the latter are bisected by **Z disks** (see Figure 8.1).

   b. Myofibrils are held in alignment by the intermediate filament **desmin** (and during embryonic development also **vimentin**); desmin filaments, bound to each other by **plectin**, tether Z disks of adjacent myofibrils to one another.

   c. Desmin has also been shown to connect the cytoskeleton, nucleus, motor end plates, and mitochondria to the myofibrils, and in this fashion distribute the force of contraction throughout the entire cell, protecting the structural integrity of the muscle fiber.

CLINICAL CONSIDERATIONS **Desmin-related myopathy (DRM)** is a rare, inherited disease where a mutation is responsible for the formation of desmin molecules that form desmin aggregates rather than the normal desmin filaments. The absence of filamentous desmin results in disorganized myofilaments and skeletal muscle fibers. The symptoms of the disease begin as progressive weakness in the muscles of the legs, followed by weakness in the trunk and the rest of the body. Because DRM affects cardiac and smooth muscles also, respiratory insufficiency, heart failure, and gastrointestinal dysfunctions follow with possibly fatal consequences.

2. The **sarcomere** is the regular repeating region between successive Z disks and constitutes the **functional unit of contraction** in skeletal muscle.

3. The **sarcoplasmic reticulum (SR)** is a modified smooth endoplasmic reticulum (SER) that surrounds myofilaments and forms a meshwork around each myofibril.

   a. The SR forms a pair of dilated **terminal cisternae**, which encircle the myofibrils at the junction of each A and I band.

   b. It **regulates muscle contraction** by sequestering calcium ions (leading to relaxation) or releasing calcium ions (leading to contraction).

4. **Triads** are specialized complexes consisting of a narrow central T tubule flanked on each side by terminal cisternae of the SR. They are located at the A–I junction in mammalian skeletal muscle cells and **help provide uniform contraction** throughout the muscle cell.

5. **Myofilaments** include **thick** filaments (15 nm in diameter and 1.5 μm long) and **thin** filaments (7 nm in diameter and 1.0 μm long). They lie parallel to the long axis of the myofibril in a precise arrangement that is responsible for the sarcomere banding pattern.

D. **Satellite cells** (**myoblast-like cells, regenerative cells**) that are probably residual cells from embryonic development lie within the external lamina (basal lamina) of skeletal muscle cells and

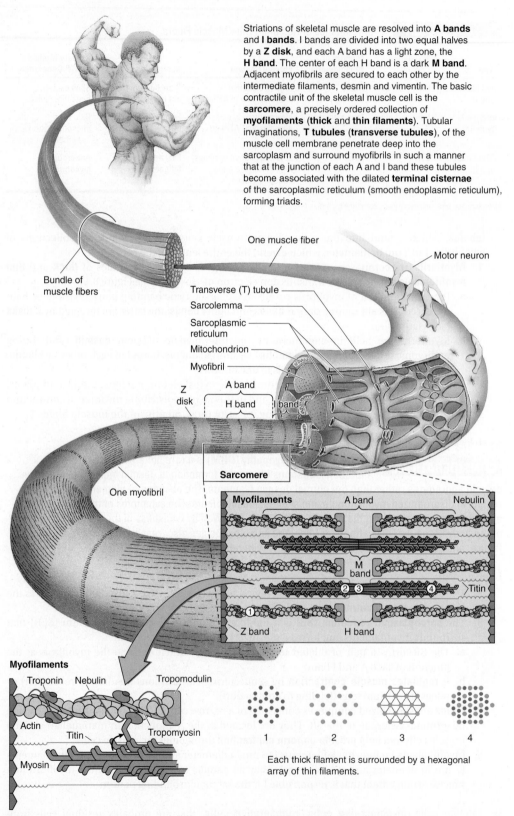

Striations of skeletal muscle are resolved into **A bands** and **I bands**. I bands are divided into two equal halves by a **Z disk**, and each A band has a light zone, the **H band**. The center of each H band is a dark **M band**. Adjacent myofibrils are secured to each other by the intermediate filaments, desmin and vimentin. The basic contractile unit of the skeletal muscle cell is the **sarcomere**, a precisely ordered collection of **myofilaments** (**thick and thin filaments**). Tubular invaginations, **T tubules** (**transverse tubules**), of the muscle cell membrane penetrate deep into the sarcoplasm and surround myofibrils in such a manner that at the junction of each A and I band these tubules become associated with the dilated **terminal cisternae** of the sarcoplasmic reticulum (smooth endoplasmic reticulum), forming triads.

One muscle fiber

Motor neuron

Bundle of muscle fibers

Transverse (T) tubule

Sarcolemma

Sarcoplasmic reticulum

Mitochondrion

Myofibril

Z disk

A band

H band

I band

One myofibril

Sarcomere

Myofilaments

A band

Nebulin

M band

Titin

Z band

H band

Myofilaments

Troponin　　Nebulin　　　　Tropomodulin

Actin

Titin　　　　　　　Tropomyosin

Myosin

Each thick filament is surrounded by a hexagonal array of thin filaments.

FIGURE 8.1. Diagram of skeletal muscle and its components as observed by light and electron microscopy. (Reprinted with permission from Gartner LP, Hiatt JL. *Color Atlas of Histology.* 5th ed. Baltimore, MD: Lippincott Williams & Wilkins; 2009:116.)

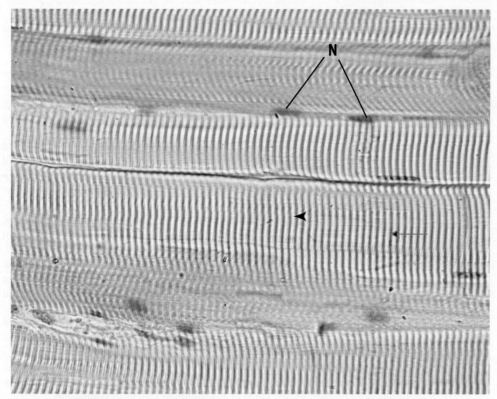

FIGURE 8.2. Light micrograph of a longitudinal section of monkey skeletal muscle fibers. N, nuclei of skeletal muscle cells; arrowhead, I band; red arrow, A band. Plastic section (×540).

adhere to these cells via M-cadherin molecules. In order to be able to form new skeletal muscle cells, satellite cells have to become activated, by damage to the muscle or possibly by mechanical stresses placed on the skeletal muscle. The activated satellite cells, under the influence of myogenic regulatory factors such as Myo-D become myoblasts that fuse with each other to form myotubes, and differentiate into mature skeletal muscle cells.

CLINICAL CONSIDERATIONS In order to ensure that muscle cells do not become overly long or broad, they manufacture and release a protein, **myostatin**, a member of the tumor growth factor β superfamily, which restricts the size of individual skeletal muscle cells.

Anabolic steroid use is prevalent among athletes and high school–aged male students. It is estimated that almost 10% of high school–aged male students use anabolic steroids (similar to testosterone) to increase their muscle mass. Approximately 65% of the abusers of anabolic steroids are football and baseball players, weight lifters, and wrestlers. Of the two forms, tablets and injected, the tablets are more insidious because they may cause jaundice and liver damage as well as aspermia, reduction in testis size, and breast induction in males. In females, anabolic steroid use may result in a decrease in breast size, irregular menstrual cycles, and male-pattern baldness. Additional side effects are increased libido, increased acne, and mood swings and aggressive behavior that may become violent. The presence of anabolic steroids is detectable in the body fluids for 6 months after the last dose was taken.

E. **Skeletal muscle cross-striations** (see Figure 8.1)
1. **A bands** are anisotropic with polarized light; they usually stain dark. They contain **both thin** and **thick filaments**, which overlap and interdigitate. Six thin filaments surround each thick filament (see Figures 8.1 and 8.2).
2. **I bands** are isotropic with polarized light and appear lightly stained in routine histologic preparations. They contain only **thin filaments**.

3. **H bands** are light regions transecting A bands; they consist of **thick filaments** only.
4. **M lines** are narrow, dark regions at the center of H bands formed by several cross-connections (**M-bridges**) at the centers of adjacent thick filaments.
5. **Z disks (lines)** are dense regions bisecting each I band.
   a. Z disks contain α-**actinin** and **Cap Z**, two proteins that bind to thin filaments and anchor them to Z disks with the assistance of **nebulin**.
   b. **Desmin**, aided by **plectin**, anchors Z disks to each other. Peripherally located Z disks are anchored to regions of the sarcolemma, known as **costameres**, **dystrophin-associated glycoprotein complexes**.
      (1) **Costameres** are specialized areas of the sarcolemma located at regions that correspond to the Z-lines of myofibrils that are situated just beneath the striated muscle cell membrane. Costameres are defined by the presence of peripheral and transmembrane protein complexes whose principal moieties are localized on the sarcoplasmic aspect of the striated muscle cell membrane.
      (2) **Dystrophin-associated glycoprotein complexes** are composed of several protein groups, including dystrophin, sarcoglycan complex, dystroglycan complex, syntrophins, and dystrobrevin.
         (a) **Dystrophin** is a pencil-shaped molecule that is the lynchpin between the extracellular matrix and the cytoskeleton attached to the peripheral-most myofibril of the striated muscle fiber. It is dystrophin that plays the greatest role in strengthening and maintaining the integrity of the sarcolemma during the process of contraction.
         (b) **Sarcoglycan complex** is composed of several transmembrane proteins localized at the costameres of the sarcolemma. They form attachments to and reinforce the dystroglycan complex.
         (c) **Dystroglycan complex** is a complex of two transmembrane proteins whose extracellular domains bind to **laminin** of the external lamina of the muscle cells. Intracellularly dystroglycan binds to dystrophin as well as to **syntrophins**.
         (d) **Syntrophins** are relatively small proteins, approximately 60 kDa, that form bonds not only with dystrophins but also with desmin and dystrobrevin.
         (e) The protein **dystrobrevin** has binding sites with syntrophins and desmin.
            Therefore, the dystrophin-associated glycoprotein complex forms a series of bonds centered around dystrophin. These function to affix the desmin intermediate filaments to laminin of the extracellular matrix, allowing them to maintain the precise orientation and arrangement of the Z-lines of adjacent myofibrils throughout the entire skeletal muscle cell. These attachments to the glycoprotein laminin of the extracellular matrix occur in the costamere regions of the sarcolemma.

CLINICAL CONSIDERATIONS **Duchenne muscular dystrophy (DMD)** is caused by a **sex-linked**, recessive genetic defect that results in the inability to synthesize **dystrophin**, an actin-binding protein normally present in small amounts in the sarcoplasm. Dystrophin also stabilizes the sarcolemma and acts as a link between the cytoskeleton and the extracellular matrix.

1. This common, serious degenerative disorder occurs in young men and results in death usually before 20 years of age.
2. DMD is characterized by the replacement of degenerating skeletal muscle cells by fatty and fibrous connective tissue, but it may also affect cardiac muscle.

Facioscapulohumeral muscular dystrophy (FSHMD or Landouzy–Dejerine syndrome) is not sex-linked, but is an **autosomal dominant** genetic defect that results in "wasting" of the skeletal muscles of the face, those around the scapula, and those of the upper arm, initially, but as the disease progresses it affects skeletal muscles of other areas of the body. It is one of the most common forms of muscular dystrophy and manifests itself in the late teens and early twenties.

1. Many affected patients suffer hearing loss, abnormal heart rhythm, and dilations of the blood vessels in the retina of the eye (retinal telangiectasia).
2. The disease does not impinge on life expectancy, and 85% of affected individuals do not become wheelchair bound.

F. **Molecular organization of myofilaments**
   1. **Thin filaments** are composed of F-actin, tropomyosin, troponin, and associated proteins.
      a. **F-actin** (see Figure 8.1) is a polymer of G-actin monomers arranged in a double helix.
         (1) Each monomer possesses an **active site** that can interact with myosin.
         (2) F-actin is present as filaments (with a diameter of 5–7 nm) that exhibit **polarity**, having a plus (+) and a minus (−) end, where the plus end is tethered to **Cap Z** of the Z disk and the minus end, capped by **tropomodulin**, is located at the H band and is the growing end of the F-actin.
         (3) **F-actin** loses and gains back G-actin molecules at both its plus and minus ends, but this turnover rate is very slow, occurring over a period of several days, whereas in other cells this turnover occurs every few minutes.
      b. **Tropomyosin** molecules are about 40 nm in length. They bind head to tail, forming filaments that are located in the grooves of the F-actin helix.
      c. **Troponin** is associated with each tropomyosin molecule and is composed of the following:
         (1) **Troponin T (TnT)**, which forms the tail of the molecule and functions in binding the troponin complex to tropomyosin.
         (2) **Troponin C (TnC)**, which possesses four binding sites for calcium. It may be related to calmodulin.
         (3) **Troponin I (TnI)**, which binds to actin, inhibiting interaction of myosin and actin.
      d. **Nebulin** is a long, inelastic protein. Two nebulin molecules wrap around each thin filament and assist in anchoring it to the Z disk (see Figure 8.1).
         (1) Each nebulin molecule is embedded in the Z disk by its carboxy terminal but does not span the entire Z disk.
         (2) The amino terminal of each nebulin molecule ends in the A band, at or near the free end of its thin filament.
         (3) Nebulin in skeletal muscle is thought to determine the length of its associated thin filament, although in cardiac muscle it extends only one-quarter of the length of the thin filament.
      e. **Tropomodulin** caps the minus end of each thin filament and prevents the addition of more G-actin molecules to the growing end; thus, it limits the length of the F-actin filament.
   2. Each **thick filament** contains approximately 250 **myosin II** molecules arranged in an anti-parallel fashion and associated proteins—myomesin, titin, and C protein and the enzyme creatine kinase.
      a. **Myosin II** (see Figure 8.1) is composed of two identical heavy chains and two pairs of light chains. There are at least 18 different subtypes of myosin, and the one present in skeletal muscle is myosin II. This particular type of myosin molecule resembles a double-headed golf club, and from this point on it will be referred to as "myosin" without its numerical appellation in this textbook.
         (1) Myosin **heavy chains** consist of a long rod-like "tail" and a globular "head." The tails of the heavy chains wind around each other in an α-helical configuration.
            (a) Tails function in the self-assembly of myosin molecules into bipolar thick filaments.
            (b) Actin-binding sites of the heads function in contraction.
         (2) Myosin **light chains** are of two types; one molecule of each type is associated with the globular head of each heavy chain.
         (3) **Digestion of myosin**
            (a) The enzyme **trypsin** cleaves myosin into **light meromyosin** (part of the tail portion) and **heavy meromyosin** (the two heads and the remainder of the tail) (see Figure 8.1).
            (b) The enzyme **papain** cleaves the heavy meromyosin, releasing the short tail (**S2 fragment**) and the two globular heads (**S1 fragments**). These S1 fragments have adenosine triphosphatase (ATPase) activity but require interaction with actin to release the noncovalently bound adenosine diphosphate (ADP) and P_i.
      b. **Myomesin** and **creatine kinase** are located at the M line. The former is a protein that cross-links adjacent thick filaments to one another to maintain their spatial relations, whereas the latter is an enzyme that is responsible for removing a phosphate group from creatine phosphate and phosphorylating ADP converting it to the energy-rich compound adenosine triphosphate (ATP).

   c. **C protein** binds to thick filaments in the vicinity of M lines along much of their lengths (between the M line and the end of the thin filament in the vicinity of the A–I junction). This region of the A band is referred to as the **C zone**.

   d. **Titin** is a large linear protein that displays axial periodicity. It forms an elastic lattice that parallels the thick and thin filaments, and two titin filaments anchor each thick filament to the Z disk, thus maintaining their architectural relationships to each other (see Figure 8.1).

     (1) The amino terminal of the titin molecule spans the entire thickness of the Z disk and binds to α-actinin and Z proteins.

     (2) Within the Z disk, titin overlaps with other titin molecules from the neighboring sarcomere and probably forms bonds with them or with unidentified linker proteins.

     (3) The carboxyl terminal of the titin molecule spans the entire M line and overlaps with titin molecules from the other half of the same sarcomere, and binds to the protein **myomesin**.

     (4) Within the I band, in the vicinity of the Z disk, titin interacts with thin filaments.

     (5) Within the A band, titin interacts with **C protein**.

III. CONTRACTION OF SKELETAL MUSCLE

The contraction cycle (Figure 8.3) involves the binding, hydrolysis, and release of ATP.

A. Huxley sliding-filament model (Table 8.2)
1. During contraction, thick and thin filaments do not shorten but increase their overlap.
2. Thin filaments slide past thick filaments and penetrate more deeply into the A band, which remains constant in length.
3. I bands and H bands shorten as Z disks are drawn closer together.

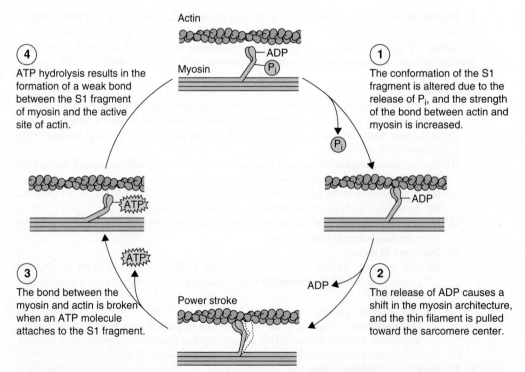

FIGURE 8.3. Contraction cycle in skeletal muscle cells. This sequence of steps is repeated many times, leading to extensive overlay of thick and thin filaments, which shortens the sarcomere and consequently the entire skeletal muscle fiber. ADP, adenosine diphosphate; ATP, adenosine triphosphate. (Copyright 1994 from *Molecular Biology of the Cell*, 3rd ed., by Alberts et al. Adapted with permission from Garland Science/Taylor & Francis LLC.)

table	**8.2**	Effects of Contraction on Skeletal Muscle Cross-Bands	
Bands	**Myofilament Component**		**Change in Bands During Contraction**
I	Thin only		Shorten
H	Thick only		Shorten
A	Thick and thin		N change in length
Z disks	Thin only (attached by α-actinin)		Move closer together

B. Initiation and regulation of contraction

   1. Depolarization, accompanied by the release of Ca^{2+}, triggers the binding of actin and myosin, leading to muscle contraction.

      a. The **sarcolemma** is depolarized at the myoneural junction.

      b. **T tubules** convey the wave of depolarization to the myofibrils. **Voltage-sensitive dihydropyridine (DHP) receptors** alter their conformation as a function of membrane depolarization.

      c. **Ca^{2+}** is released into the cytosol at the A–I junctions via **Ca^{2+}-release channels (junctional feet, ryanodine receptors)** of the SR terminal cisternae that are opened by activated DHP receptors. As long as the Ca^{2+} level is sufficiently high, the contraction cycle will continue.

   2. **Activation of actin by Ca^{2+}**

      a. In the **resting state**, the myosin-binding sites on thin (actin) filaments are partially covered by tropomyosin. Also, TnI is bound to actin and hinders myosin–actin interaction.

      b. Ca^{2+} binding by TnC results in a **conformational change** that breaks the TnI-actin bond; tropomyosin shifts its position slightly and uncovers the myosin-binding sites (**active state**).

   3. **Contraction cycle (Figure 8.3)**

      a. The **S1 fragment of myosin II** releases a phosphate group (P_i), but the ADP remains attached to the S1 fragment; the release of the P_i causes a conformational change leading to a strong bond between the actin filament and the S1 fragment.

      b. The ADP molecule is released from the S1 fragment of myosin II, which results in an alteration of the myosin II molecule and the thin filament is pulled toward the middle of the sarcomere for a distance of 5 nm; this is known as the **power stroke**.

      c. An ATP molecule becomes attached to the S1 fragment, resulting in the release of the S1 fragment from the thin filament.

      d. The ATP is hydrolyzed and a weak bond is formed between the actin filament and the S1 fragment of myosin II. If the contraction continues, then the cycle continues as the S1 fragment of myosin II releases a phosphate group (P_i) but the ADP remains attached to the S1 fragment; the release of the P_i causes a conformational change leading to a strong bond between the actin filament and the S1 fragment.

      e. For a complete contraction where a sarcomere is shortened by approximately 1 μm, the cycle just described for a single myosin II molecule must be repeated approximately 200 times.

C. Relaxation occurs when Ca^{2+} concentration in the cytosol is reduced enough that TnC loses its bound Ca^{2+}.

   1. As a result, tropomyosin returns to its resting position, covering actin's binding sites and restoring the resting state.

   2. Relaxation depends on a **Ca^{2+} pump** in the SR, which pumps Ca^{2+} from the cytosol to the inner surface of the SR membrane to be bound by **calsequestrin**.

CLINICAL CONSIDERATIONS   **Rigor mortis** is a temporary postmortem rigidity appearing as hardening of skeletal muscles caused by the inability of muscle cells to synthesize ATP. As a result, myosin remains bound to actin, and the muscles remain contracted because ADP remains attached to the S1 fragment; the release of the P_i causes a conformational change leading to a strong bond between the actin filament and the S1 fragment.

D. A **motor unit** consists of a neuron and every muscle cell it innervates. A **muscle** may contract with varying degrees of strength because only some of the muscle cells contract, but an individual muscle cell obeys the "**all or none law**" (i.e., it either contracts or does not contract). All muscle cells of a single motor unit contract in unison, and a large muscle such as the trapezius may have thousands of muscle cells in a motor unit, whereas a muscle such as the superior oblique muscle of the eye may have as few as 10 to 15 muscle cells in a motor unit.

CLINICAL CONSIDERATIONS Normally, as a muscle contracts the sarcomeres shorten and, consequently, the entire muscle becomes shorter. This type of contraction is referred to as **concentric contraction**, as in picking up a dumbbell and doing curls. Another type of contraction is **isometric contraction**, where the sarcomeres do not shorten; thus, the entire muscle remains the same length, as in squeezing a hard object such as a solid metal ball.

IV. INNERVATION OF SKELETAL MUSCLE

Innervation consists of **motor** nerve endings (myoneural junctions) and two types of **sensory** nerve endings (muscle spindles and Golgi tendon organs). Both types of sensory nerve endings function in **proprioception**.

A. The **myoneural junction** (neuromuscular junction) is a **synapse** between a branch of a motor nerve axon and a skeletal muscle cell.
  1. **Structural components**
     a. The **axon terminal** lacks myelin but has a **Schwann cell** on its nonsynaptic surface.
        (1) The membrane on the synaptic surface of the axon terminal is called the **presynaptic membrane**.
        (2) The axon terminal contains mitochondria, **synaptic vesicles** (containing the neurotransmitter **acetylcholine**), and SER elements.
     b. The **synaptic cleft** is a narrow space between the presynaptic membrane of the axon terminal and the **postsynaptic membrane** (also known as the **motor end plate**) of the muscle cell. The synaptic cleft contains an amorphous **external lamina**, a basal lamina-like material, derived from the muscle cell.
     c. **Muscle cell near the myoneural junction**
        (1) Sarcolemmal invaginations (of the postsynaptic membrane), called **junctional folds**, are lined by an external lamina and extend inward from the synaptic cleft.
        (2) **Acetylcholine receptors** are located in the postsynaptic membrane at the peaks of the junctional folds.
        (3) The sarcoplasm is rich in mitochondria, ribosomes, and rough endoplasmic reticulum (RER).
  2. **Conduction of a nerve impulse across a myoneural junction**
     a. The presynaptic membrane (i.e., the axon's end foot membrane) is depolarized and **voltage-gated Ca^{2+} channels** open, permitting the entry of extracellular Ca^{2+} into the axon terminal.
     b. The rise in cytosolic Ca^{2+} triggers the synaptic vesicles to release acetylcholine in multimolecular quantities (**quanta**) into the synaptic cleft. A quantum is approximately equivalent to 20,000 acetylcholine molecules.
     c. The released acetylcholine binds to acetylcholine receptors located on the peaks of the postsynaptic membrane.
     d. These acetylcholine receptors are **transmitter-gated Na^+ ion channels**, and the binding of acetylcholine results in a conformational change of the gate, permitting the influx of Na^+ ions, resulting in **depolarization** of the sarcolemma and generation of an **action potential**.
     e. The enzyme **acetylcholinesterase**, located in the external lamina lining the junctional folds of the motor end plate, degrades acetylcholine, thus ending the depolarizing signal to the muscle cell.

    f. Acetylcholine is recycled as **choline** and is returned to the axon terminal to be recombined with acetyl coenzyme A (CoA) (from mitochondria) under the influence of the enzyme **choline acetyl transferase** to form acetylcholine, which is then stored in synaptic vesicles.

    g. Membranes of the emptied synaptic vesicles are recycled via **clathrin-coated endocytic vesicles** (see Figure 3.5 in Chapter 3, Cytoplasm and Organelles).

CLINICAL CONSIDERATIONS   **Amyotrophic lateral sclerosis (or Lou Gehrig disease)** is marked by degeneration of motor neurons of the spinal cord, resulting in muscle atrophy. Death is usually due to respiratory muscle failure.

    Myasthenia gravis is an **autoimmune disease** in which **antibodies block acetylcholine receptors** of myoneural junctions, reducing the number of sites available for initiation of sarcolemma depolarization.

    1. Myasthenia gravis is characterized by gradual weakening of skeletal muscles, especially the most active ones (e.g., muscles of the eyes, tongue, face, and extremities). Death may result from respiratory compromise and pulmonary infections.

    2. Clinical signs include thymic hyperplasia (thymoma) and the presence of circulating antibodies to acetylcholine receptors.

    Botulism is a form of **food poisoning** caused by ingestion of *Clostridium botulinum* toxin, which inhibits acetylcholine release at myoneural junctions. Botulism is marked by muscle paralysis, vomiting, nausea, and visual disorders and is fatal if untreated.

B. The **muscle spindle (neuromuscular spindle)** is an elongated, fusiform sensory organ within skeletal muscle that functions primarily as a **stretch receptor**.

    1. Structure

        a. It is bounded by a connective tissue capsule enclosing the fluid-filled **periaxial space** and 8 to 10 modified skeletal muscle fibers (**intrafusal fibers**).

        b. Normal skeletal muscle fibers (**extrafusal fibers**) surround it.

        c. It is anchored via the capsule to the perimysium and endomysium of the extrafusal fibers.

    2. Function

        a. Stretching of a muscle also stretches the muscle spindle and thus stimulates the afferent nerve endings to send impulses to the central nervous system. The response is to both the **rate (phasic response)** and the **duration (tonic response)** of stretching.

        b. Depolarization of γ-efferent neurons also stimulates the intrafusal nerve endings; the rate and duration of the stimulation are monitored in the same way as stretching.

        c. Muscle overstimulation results from stretching at too great a frequency or for too long a time. Overstimulation causes stimulation of α-**efferent neurons** to the muscle, initiating contraction and thus counteracting the stretching.

C. The **Golgi tendon organ**, located in tendons, counteracts the effects of muscle spindles.

    1. Structure. It is composed of encapsulated **collagen fibers** that are surrounded by terminal branches of **type Ib sensory nerves**.

    2. It is stimulated when the muscle contracts too strenuously, increasing tension on the tendon. Impulses from type Ib neurons **inhibit** α-efferent (motor) neurons to the muscle, preventing further contraction.

V. CARDIAC MUSCLE

A. General features—cardiac muscle cells (Table 8.3). Cardiac muscle cells have the following features:

    1. Contract spontaneously and display a rhythmic beat, which is modified by hormonal and neural (sympathetic and parasympathetic) stimuli.

    2. May branch at their ends to form connections with adjacent cells.

table 8.3	Comparison of Skeletal, Cardiac, and Smooth Muscle		
Property	Skeletal Muscle	Cardiac Muscle	Smooth Muscle
Shape and size of cells	Long, cylindrical	Blunt-ended, branched	Short, spindle shaped
Number and location of nucleus	Many, peripheral	One or two, central	One, central
Striations	Yes	Yes	No
T tubules and SR	Has triads at A–I junctions	Has dyads at Z disks	Has caveolae (but no T tubules) and some SER
Gap junctions	No	Yes (in intercalated disks)	Yes (in sarcolemma); known as the nexus
Sarcomere	Yes	Yes	No
Regeneration	Restricted	None	Extensive
Voluntary contraction	Yes	No	No
Distinctive characteristics	Peripheral nuclei	Intercalated disks	Lack of striations

SR, sarcoplasmic reticulum; SER, smooth endoplasmic reticulum.

3. Contain one centrally located nucleus, or occasionally two nuclei.
4. Contain **glycogen granules**, especially at either pole of the nucleus, and the sarcoplasm is rich in **myoglobin**.
5. Possess thick and thin filaments arranged in **poorly defined myofibrils**.
6. Exhibit a cross-banding pattern identical to that in skeletal muscle.
7. **Do not regenerate**; injuries to cardiac muscle are repaired by the formation of fibrous connective (scar) tissue by fibroblasts (but note Clinical Considerations, below).

B. **Structural components of cardiac muscle cells** differ from those of skeletal muscle as follows:
1. **T tubules** are larger than those in skeletal muscle and are lined by external lamina. They invaginate from the sarcolemma at Z disks, not at A–I junctions as in skeletal muscle.
2. **SR** is poorly defined and contributes to the formation of **dyads**, each of which consists of one T tubule and one profile of SR. SR is also present in the vicinity of Z disks as small, basketlike saccules known as **corbular SR**, a region rich in **Ca^{2+}-release channels (junctional feet)** and, therefore, analogous to the SR terminal cisternae of skeletal muscles.
3. **Calcium ions**
   a. During relaxation, **Ca^{2+} leaks** into the sarcoplasm at a slow rate, resulting in automatic rhythm. Ca^{2+} also enters cardiac muscle cells from the extracellular environment via voltage-gated Ca^{2+} channels of T tubules and sarcolemma.
   b. In response to calcium entering through the voltage-gated Ca^{2+} channels, Ca^{2+} is released from the SR and corbular SR (both via **ryanodine receptors**) to cause contraction of cardiac muscle.
   c. The force of cardiac muscle contraction is directly dependent on the availability of Ca^{2+} in the sarcoplasm. During basal cardiac contraction, only 50% of the available calcium-binding sites of TnC are occupied.
   d. Subsequent to contraction, Ca^{2+} ions are returned into the SR by the activity of an integral sarcoplasmic membrane protein, known as **phospholamban**, which is the primary regulator of the sarcoplasmic Ca^{2+} pump and, thereby, of diastole (relaxation) of the ventricles and atria of the heart.
      (1) In the dephosphorylated state, phospholamban inhibits the sarcoplasmic Ca^{2+} pump, but when phosphorylated by the action of **cAMP-dependent protein kinase**, phospholamban becomes active and the sarcoplasmic Ca^{2+} pumps open.
4. **Mitochondria** are more abundant than in skeletal muscle; they lie parallel to the I bands and often are adjacent to lipids.
5. **Atrial granules** are present in the atrial cardiac muscle cells and contain the precursors of **atrial natriuretic peptide (ANP)** and **B-type natriuretic peptide (BNP)**, both of which act to *decrease* resorption of sodium and water in the kidneys, thus decreasing blood volume and,

thereby, reducing blood pressure. ANP and BNP act by inhibiting the release of renin from the juxtaglomerular cells of the kidney and aldosterone from the suprarenal cortex. Additionally, both ANP and BNP hinder vascular smooth muscle contraction, further reducing blood pressure. Ventricular cardiac muscle cells, if stretched much greater than under normal conditions, release both peptides.

6. **Intercalated disks** (Figures 8.4a, 8.4b, and 8.5) are complex step-like junctions forming end-to-end attachments between adjacent cardiac muscle cells.
   a. The **transverse portion of intercalated disks** runs across muscle fibers at right angles and possesses three specializations: **fasciae adherentes** (analogous to zonula adherentes) to which actin filaments attach, **desmosomes** (macula adherentes), and **gap junctions** (see Chapter 5 II).
   b. The **lateral portion of intercalated disks** has desmosomes and numerous large gap junctions, which facilitate **ionic coupling** between cells and aid in coordinating contraction; thus, cardiac muscle behaves as a **functional syncytium**.
7. Their thin filaments are secured to the Z disk by α-actinin as well as by **nebulette**, a nebulin-like molecule that, unlike nebulin in skeletal muscle, extends only as far as the proximal 25% of the length of the thin filament.
8. **Connective tissue elements** support a rich capillary bed that supplies sufficient nutrients and oxygen to maintain the high metabolic rate of cardiac muscle. At least 90% of the energy production of cardiac muscle cells is generated by aerobic respiration.
9. **Purkinje fibers** are **modified** cardiac muscle cells located in the **bundle of His**. They are specialized for **conduction** and contain a few peripheral myofibrils.
   a. These large, pale cells are rich in glycogen and mitochondria.
   b. They form gap junctions, fasciae adherentes, and desmosomes with cardiac muscle cells (but not through typical intercalated disks).

CLINICAL CONSIDERATIONS　Although it was mentioned earlier that no new cardiac muscle cells can be generated in the adult human, recent studies performed on tissue sources procured from the Karolinska Institute in Sweden and from the UK Human Tissue Bank in Great Britain, based on the ^{14}C levels in the DNA of heart muscles of individuals who were born before the nuclear bomb testing began, showed otherwise. It appears that approximately 1% of the heart muscle fibers of 20-year-old individuals and almost 50% of the cardiac muscle cells of 50-year-old individuals were formed after these individuals were born.

Myocardial infarct is an irreversible necrosis of cardiac muscle cells due to prolonged ischemia (ischemia lasting for more than approximately 20 minutes). Dying and dead cardiac muscle cells release creatine phosphokinase, creatine phosphokinase MB isoenzyme, and cardiocyte specific troponin I, and these three substances—especially the last—are indicative of a myocardial infarct, a condition that may result in death if the cardiac muscle damage is extensive.

VI. SMOOTH MUSCLE

A. **Structure—smooth muscle cells** (see Table 8.3; Figures 8.6 and 8.7). Smooth muscle cells are **nonstriated, fusiform** cells that range in length from 20 μm in small blood vessels to 500 μm in the uterus of pregnant women. They contain a single nucleus and actively divide and **regenerate**. They are surrounded by an external lamina and a reticular fiber network and may be arranged in layers, small bundles, or helices (in arteries).
1. **Nucleus**
   a. The centrally located nucleus may not be visible in each cell in cross sections of smooth muscle because some nuclei lie outside the plane of section.
   b. The nucleus in longitudinal sections of contracted smooth muscle has a **corkscrew shape** and is **deeply indented**.

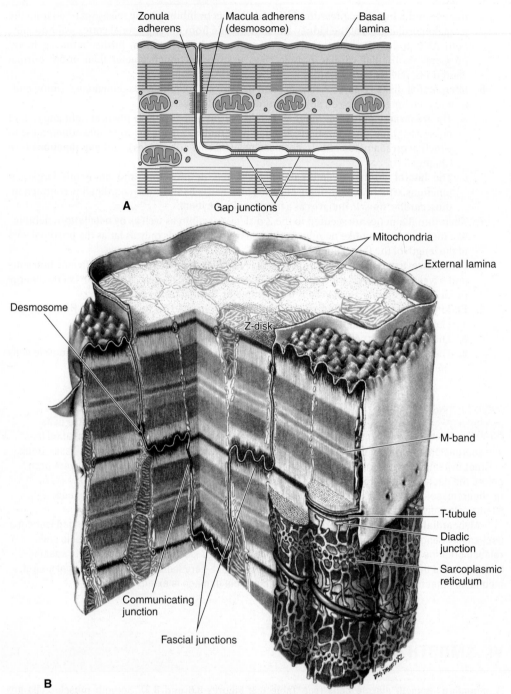

FIGURE 8.4. A. An intercalated disk's two regions, the transverse and lateral portions. (Adapted with permission from Junqueira LC, Carneiro J, Kelley RO. *Basic Histology*. 8th ed. Norwalk, CT: Appleton & Lange; 1995:197.) **B.** The principal characteristics of intercalated disks are illustrated in this diagram of cardiac muscle cells. The three types of junctions, gap junctions, fascia adherents, and desmosomes, are clearly delineated. Moreover, the relationships between the sarcoplasmic reticulum, T tubule, and the Z-lines of the sarcomeres are also emphasized. (Reprinted with permission from Kelly DE, Wood RL, Enders AC. *Bailey's Textbook of Microscopic Anatomy*. 18th ed. Baltimore, MD: Williams & Wilkins; 1984:292.)

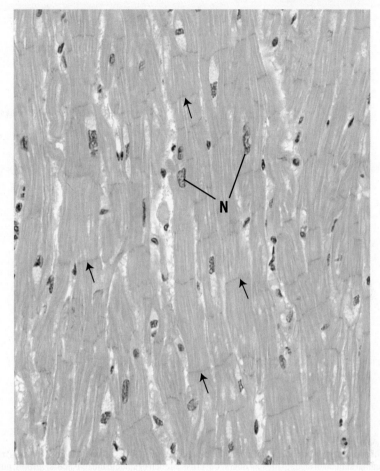

FIGURE 8.5. Light micrograph of a longitudinal section of monkey cardiac muscle fibers. N, nuclei of cardiac muscle cells; *arrows*, intercalated disks. Plastic section (×270).

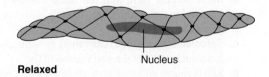

Nucleus

Relaxed

FIGURE 8.6. Relaxed and contracted smooth muscle cells: cytoplasmic and peripheral densities. The nucleus of the smooth muscle cell assumes a corkscrew shape. (Adapted with permission from Gartner LP, Hiatt JL. *Color Textbook of Histology.* Philadelphia, PA: Saunders; 1997:151.)

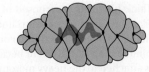

Contracted

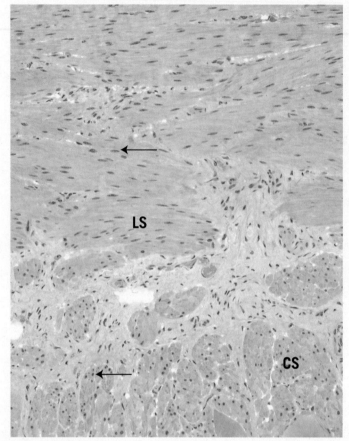

FIGURE 8.7. Light micrograph of a longitudinal section and cross sections of smooth muscle cells from the monkey duodenum. LS, longitudinal section of smooth muscle fibers; CS, cross section of smooth muscle fibers; *arrows*, nuclei of smooth muscle cells. Plastic section (×270).

2. **Cytoplasmic organelles**
   a. **Mitochondria, RER, and the Golgi complex** are concentrated near the nucleus and are involved in synthesis of type III collagen, elastin, glycosaminoglycans, external lamina, and growth factors.
   b. **Sarcolemmal vesicles (caveolae),** present along the periphery of smooth muscle cells, may function in the uptake and release of Ca^{2+}.
   c. **SER** is sparse and may be associated with caveolae.
3. **Filaments in smooth muscle**
   a. **Contractile filaments (actin and myosin)** are **not** organized into myofibrils. They are attached to peripheral and cytoplasmic densities and aligned obliquely to the longitudinal axis of smooth muscle cells.
      (1) **Thick filaments** (composed of **myosin II**) are each surrounded by as many as 15 thin filaments. In contrast to striated muscle, the heads of the myosin molecules all point in the same direction. Prior to contraction, the myosin II molecule is **inactive** and cannot bind to the actin filament because the tail of the myosin molecule (light meromyosin) is attached to the heavy meromyosin, so that the molecule resembles a golf club whose handle is folded to contact its head.
      (2) **Thin filaments** are composed of **actin, caldesmon, tropomyosin,** and **calponin.** Caldesmon functions similarly to TnT and TnI in that it masks the sites where myosin binds to effect muscle contraction.
   b. Intermediate filaments are attached to cytoplasmic densities and include **vimentin** and **desmin** in **vascular** smooth muscle cells and **desmin** only in **nonvascular** smooth muscle cells.

4. **Cytoplasmic densities**, believed to be **analogous to Z disks**, contain α-actinin, and function as **filament attachment sites**.

5. **Gap junctions** between smooth muscle cells facilitate the spread of excitation. These gap junctions are collectively called the **nexus**.

B. **Contraction of smooth muscle occurs more slowly and lasts longer** than contraction of skeletal muscle because the rate of ATP hydrolysis is slower. Contraction of smooth muscle is regulated by a mechanism different from that of skeletal muscle contraction.

1. The **contraction cycle** is stimulated by a transient increase in cytosolic Ca^{2+}.

   a. Ca^{2+} binds to **calmodulin**, altering its conformation.

   b. The Ca^{2+}–calmodulin complex activates the enzyme **myosin light-chain kinase**, which catalyzes phosphorylation of one of the light chains, the **regulatory light chain**, of myosin.

   c. Phosphorylated regulatory light chain of myosin permits the myosin molecule to unfold so that it can interact with other myosin II molecules to form a thick filament.

   d. In the presence of Ca^{2+}, the inhibitory effect of the caldesmon–tropomyosin complex on the actin–myosin interaction is eliminated (caldesmon masks the active site of G-actin). Another inhibitor of contraction is **calponin**, which, when phosphorylated, loses its inhibitory capability.

   e. The globular head of phosphorylated myosin interacts with actin and stimulates myosin ATPase, resulting in **contraction**. As long as myosin is in its phosphorylated form, the contraction cycle continues.

   f. **Dephosphorylation** of myosin disturbs the myosin–actin interaction and leads to relaxation.

2. **Initiation of contraction**

   a. In **vascular smooth muscle**, contraction is usually triggered by a **nerve impulse**, with little spread of the impulse from cell to cell.

   b. In **visceral smooth muscle**, it is triggered by stretching of the muscle itself **(myogenic)**; the signal spreads from cell to cell.

   c. In the **uterus** during labor, it is triggered by **oxytocin**.

   d. In smooth muscle elsewhere in the body, it is triggered by **epinephrine**.

C. **Innervation of smooth muscle** is by **sympathetic** (noradrenergic) nerves and **parasympathetic** (cholinergic) nerves of the autonomic nervous system, which act in an antagonistic fashion to stimulate or depress activity of the muscle.

VII. CONTRACTILE NONMUSCLE CELLS

A. **Myoepithelial cells**

1. In certain glands, these cells share basal laminae of secretory and duct cells.

2. They arise from **ectoderm** and can **contract** to express secretory material from glandular epithelium into the ducts and out of the gland.

3. Although generally similar in morphology to smooth muscle cells, they have a **basketlike shape** and several radiating **processes**.

4. They are attached to the underlying basal lamina via hemidesmosomes.

5. They contain **actin**, **myosin**, and intermediate filaments, as well as cytoplasmic and peripheral densities to which these filaments attach.

6. Contraction is similar to that of smooth muscle and occurs via a **calmodulin-mediated process**. In lactating **mammary glands**, they contract in response to **oxytocin**. In **lacrimal glands**, they contract in response to **acetylcholine**.

B. **Myofibroblasts**

1. Unlike myoepithelial cells, **myofibroblasts** arise from mesenchymal cells and possess vimentin as their characteristic intermediate filaments as well as caldesmon and cytokeratins.

2. Although they resemble fibroblasts, they possess higher amounts of **actin** and **myosin** and are capable of **contraction**.

3. They may contract during wound healing to decrease the size of the defect (**wound contraction**).

Review Test

Directions: Each of the numbered items or incomplete statements in this section is followed by answers or by completions of the statement. Select the ONE lettered answer or completion that is BEST in each case.

1. Which of the following is true for mammalian skeletal muscle?

(A) T tubules are located at the Z disk.
(B) T tubules are absent.
(C) Troponin is absent.
(D) It possesses triads.
(E) It possesses caveolae.

2. Which of the following is true for cardiac muscle?

(A) T tubules are located at the Z disk.
(B) T tubules have a smaller diameter than those of skeletal muscle.
(C) Troponin is absent.
(D) It possesses triads.
(E) Oxytocin triggers contraction.

3. Which of the following is true for smooth muscle?

(A) T tubules are located at the Z disk.
(B) It possesses dyads.
(C) Caveolae store and release calcium ions.
(D) It possesses triads.
(E) T tubules are located at the A–I interface.

4. Contraction in all types of muscle requires calcium ions. Which of the following muscle components can bind or sequester calcium ions?

(A) Rough endoplasmic reticulum
(B) Tropomyosin
(C) Troponin
(D) Active sites on actin
(E) Titin

5. Each smooth muscle cell

(A) has triads associated with its contraction.
(B) has dyads associated with its contraction.
(C) possesses a single central nucleus.
(D) is characterized by the absence of sarcolemmal vesicles.
(E) contains troponin.

6. Thick filaments are anchored to Z disks by

(A) C protein.
(B) nebulin.
(C) titin.
(D) myomesin.
(E) α-actinin.

7. The endomysium is a connective tissue investment that surrounds

(A) individual muscle fibers.
(B) muscle fascicles.
(C) individual myofibrils.
(D) an entire muscle.
(E) small bundles of muscle cells.

8. Which of the following statements concerning triads in mammalian skeletal muscle is true?

(A) They are located in the Z disk.
(B) They consist of two terminal cisternae of the SR separated by a T tubule.
(C) They can be observed with the light microscope.
(D) They are characterized by a T tubule that sequesters calcium ions.
(E) They consist of two T tubules separated by a central terminal cisterna.

9. Which one of the following statements concerning cardiac muscle cells is true?

(A) They are spindle shaped.

(B) They require an external stimulus to undergo contraction.

(C) They are multinuclear cells.

(D) They are joined together end to end by intercalated disks.

(E) They possess numerous caveolae.

10. A 19-year-old male patient and his mother arrive in the emergency department, both with nausea, vomiting, and visual disorders. The physician taking their history notes that they both had canned green beans that tasted funny. Which of the following possibilities should the physician consider?

(A) Duchenne muscular dystrophy

(B) Amyotrophic lateral sclerosis

(C) Botulism

(D) Myasthenia gravis

(E) Myocardial infarct

Answers and Explanations

1. **D.** The T tubules of skeletal muscle cells are positioned so that they form triads with the terminal cisternae of the SR at the interface of the A and I bands (see Chapter 8 II C).

2. **A.** The T tubules of cardiac muscle cells are wider than those of skeletal muscle cells and are lined by external lamina (a basal lamina–like material). In contrast to skeletal muscle, the T tubules are located at the Z disk, where they often form dyads, not triads (see Chapter 8 V B 6).

3. **C.** Smooth muscle cells do not have T tubules. Contraction may be initiated by stretching, neural impulses, the intercellular passage of small molecules via gap junctions, or the action of hormones such as oxytocin. Contraction is not dependent on troponin, which is absent from the thin filament of smooth muscle. Instead, Ca^{2+} controlled by sarcolemmal vesicles known as caveolae is released into the cytosol, where it binds with calmodulin. The calcium–calmodulin complex activates myosin light-chain kinase, which participates in the contraction process (see Chapter 8 VI A 2).

4. **C.** Binding of Ca^{2+} to the TnC subunit of troponin leads to the uncovering of myosin-binding sites on actin (thin filaments) (see Chapter 8 II F 1 c).

5. **C.** Smooth muscle cells contain one centrally located nucleus (see Chapter 8 VI A 1).

6. **C.** Titin forms an elastic lattice that anchors thick filaments to Z disks (see Chapter 8 II F 2 c).

7. **A.** The endomysium is a thin connective tissue layer composed of reticular fibers and an external lamina that invests individual muscle fibers (cells). The epimysium surrounds the entire muscle, and the perimysium surrounds bundles (fascicles) of muscle fibers (see Chapter 8 II A 3).

8. **B.** A triad in skeletal muscle is composed of three components: a T tubule and two terminal cisternae of the SR that flank it. The SR, not the T tubules, sequesters Ca^{2+} (see Chapter 8 II C 4).

9. **D.** Cardiac muscle cells are joined together end to end by a unique junctional specialization called the intercalated disk (see Chapter 8 V B 6).

10. **C.** Botulism is the only possible consideration, especially since they both had canned food. Duchenne muscular dystrophy is most common in young men but very rare in older women. It would be highly unlikely that both mother and son would show symptoms of amyotrophic lateral sclerosis or myasthenia gravis or have myocardial infarct at the same time (see Chapter 8 II E Clinical Considerations).

chapter **9** Nervous System

I. OVERVIEW—NERVOUS SYSTEM

The nervous system can be organized by anatomical or functional divisions.

A. Nervous system is divided **anatomically** into the **central nervous system** (CNS), which includes the brain and spinal cord encased in the skull and vertebral column, and the **peripheral nervous system** (PNS), which includes the nerves outside the CNS and their associated ganglia as well as connections to the CNS, including the receptors and motor components of the peripheral nerves of the body.

B. Nervous system is divided **functionally** into a **sensory** component, which transmits electrical impulses (signals) to the CNS, and a **motor** component, which transmits impulses from the CNS to various structures of the body. The motor component is further divided into the **somatic** and **autonomic** systems. The somatic nervous system (SNS), located within both the CNS and PNS, controls sensory and motor functions of all conscious voluntary actions. However, it does not control functions related to smooth or cardiac muscles, reflex arcs, or glands.

The autonomic nervous system (ANS) functions to regulate the internal organs. It is further subdivided into the **sympathetic, parasympathetic**, and **enteric systems**. The sympathetic nervous system readies the body for action against hostile situations, resulting in "flight or fight or freeze," whereas the parasympathetic nervous system is "calming" and supplies secretomotor innervation to most exocrine glands. The enteric nervous system, a very large component of the autonomic system, serves the digestive system. Although it operates independently, both the sympathetic and the parasympathetic components are utilized in modulating the functions of the enteric system.

C. Nervous tissue contains two types of cells: **nerve cells (neurons)**, which conduct electrical impulses, and supporting cells, which support, nurture, and protect the neurons within the CNS **(glial [neuroglial] cells)**, as well as cells located in the PNS **(satellite cells, capsule cells**, and **Schwann cells)**.

II. HISTOGENESIS OF THE NERVOUS SYSTEM (Figure 9.1)

A. **The neuroepithelium** thickens and differentiates to form the neural plate.

B. **The neural plate** invaginates and thickens to form the **neural groove**.

C. **The neural tube**, a cylindrical structure that results from fusion of the edges of the neural groove, enlarges at its cranial end to form the **brain**. The remaining portion gives rise to the **spinal cord**.

143

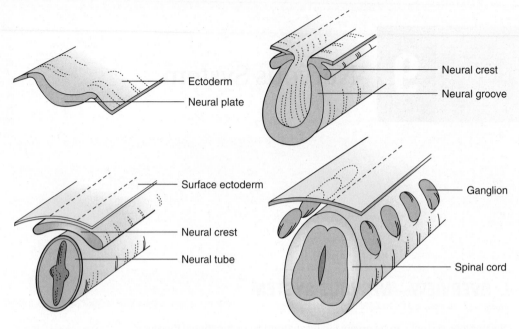

FIGURE 9.1. Early histogenesis of the nervous system. Notice how the neural crest forms and then fragments to migrate to its destinations.

D. **Neural crest cells** stream off the edges of the neural groove before formation of the neural tube. These cells migrate throughout the body and give rise to the following structures:
   1. Sensory neurons of cranial and spinal sensory ganglia
   2. Most sensory neurons and Schwann cells of the PNS
   3. Enteric and autonomic ganglia and their postganglionic neurons and associated glia
   4. Most of the mesenchymal (ectomesenchymal) cells of the head and anterior portion of the neck
   5. Melanocytes of the skin and oral mucosa
   6. Odontoblasts (cells responsible for the production of dentin)
   7. Cells of the arachnoid and pia mater (rostral to the mesencephalon)
   8. Chromaffin cells of the adrenal medulla

CLINICAL CONSIDERATIONS

1. Abnormal histogenesis of the CNS results in congenital malformations.
2. Congenital malformations
   a. **Spina bifida** is a defective closure of the spinal column. In severe cases, the spinal cord and meninges may protrude through the unfused areas. Very severe cases may be associated with defective development of the viscera of the thorax and abdomen.
   b. **Anencephaly** is failure of the developmental anterior neuropore to close. This produces a poorly formed brain without a cranial vault. It is usually not compatible with life.
   c. **Hirschsprung disease (congenital megacolon)** is the result of abnormal organogenesis in which neural crest cells fail to migrate into the wall of the gut. The disease is characterized by the absence of Auerbach plexus, a part of the parasympathetic system innervating the distal segment of the colon. This loss of motor function leads to dilation of the colon.
   d. **Neuroglial tumors** constitute 50% of intracranial tumors. CNS tumors are rarely associated with neurons; they are mostly derived from neuroglial cells (e.g., astrocytes, oligodendrocytes, and ependymocytes). These tumors range in severity from slowly growing **benign oligodendrogliomas** to rapidly growing fatal **malignant astrocytomas**.
   e. Brains of patients with AIDS and HIV-1 possess large populations of **microglial cells**. Although these microglia do not attack neurons, they produce cytokines that are toxic to neurons.

III. CELLS OF NERVOUS SYSTEM

A. **Neurons** consist of a **cell body (soma, perikaryon)**, and its processes, which usually include multiple **dendrites** and a single **axon**. Neurons comprise the smallest and largest cells of the body, ranging from 5 to 150 μm in diameter.

   1. **Morphologic classification of neurons** (Figure 9.2)

      a. Unipolar neurons possess a single process but are rare in vertebrates (see Section III A 1 d).

      b. Bipolar neurons possess a single axon and a single dendrite. These neurons are present in some sense organs (e.g., the vestibular–cochlear mechanism).

      c. Multipolar neurons possess a single axon and more than one dendrite. These neurons are the **most common type** of neuron in vertebrates.

      d. Pseudounipolar neurons possess a single process that extends from the cell body and subsequently branches into an axon and dendrite. They are present in spinal and cranial ganglia.

         (1) These neurons originate embryologically as bipolar cells whose axon and dendrite later fuse into a single process functionally categorized as an axon.

         (2) They are frequently referred to as unipolar neurons.

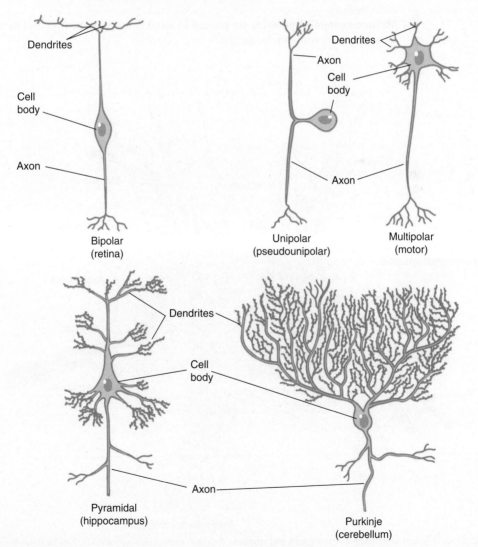

FIGURE 9.2. Various types of neurons. (Reprinted with permission from Gartner LP, Hiatt JL. *Color Textbook of Histology.* 2nd ed. Philadelphia, PA: Saunders; 2001:187.)

2. **Functional classification of neurons**
   a. **Sensory neurons** receive stimuli from the internal and external environments and conduct impulses **to the CNS** for processing and analysis.
   b. **Interneurons** (**intercalated neurons**) connect other neurons in a chain or sequence. They commonly connect sensory and motor neurons; they also regulate signals transmitted to neurons.
   c. **Motor neurons** conduct impulses **from the CNS** to other neurons, muscles, and glands.
3. **Neuron structure** (Figure 9.3)
   a. **Neuronal cell body (soma, perikaryon)** is the region of a neuron containing the nucleus, various cytoplasmic organelles and inclusions, and cytoskeletal elements.
      (1) The **nucleus** is large, spherical, and pale staining and is **centrally located** in the soma of most neurons. It contains abundant euchromatin and a large nucleolus (owl-eye nucleus).
      (2) Cytoplasmic organelles and inclusions
         (a) **Nissl bodies** are composed of polysomes and rough endoplasmic reticulum (RER). They appear as clumps under light microscopy and are most abundant in large motor neurons.
         (b) The **Golgi complex** is near the nucleus, and **mitochondria** are scattered throughout the cytoplasm.
         (c) **Melanin-containing granules** are present in some neurons in the CNS and in the dorsal root and sympathetic ganglia.

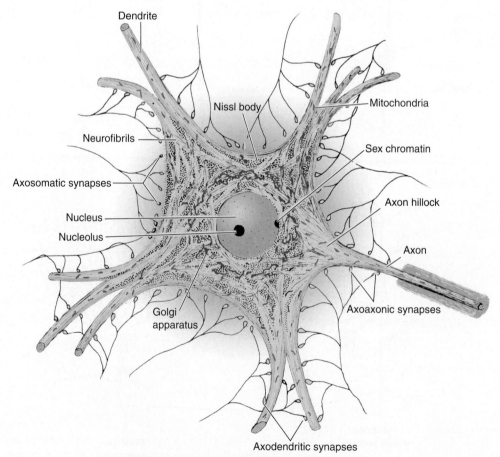

FIGURE 9.3. A typical neuron with its constituents and synapses. (Reprinted with permission from Kiernan JA. *Barr's The Human Nervous System: An Anatomical Viewpoint.* 8th ed. Baltimore, MD: Lippincott Williams & Wilkins; 2005:19.)

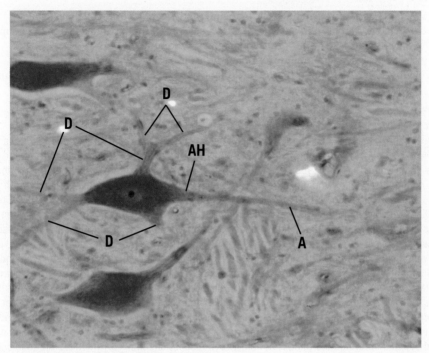

FIGURE 9.4. Light micrograph of the spinal cord in cross section (×540). Observe the multipolar neurons in the ventral horn of the spinal cord. D, dendrites; AH, axon hillock; A, axon.

      (d) Lipofuscin-containing granules are present in some neurons and increase in number with age.

      (e) Lipid droplets are occasionally present.

  (3) Cytoskeletal components (Figures 9.3 and 9.4)

      (a) Neurofilaments (10 nm in diameter) are abundant and run throughout the soma cytoplasm. They are intermediate filaments composed of three intertwining polypeptide chains.

      (b) Microtubules (24 nm in diameter) are also present in the soma cytoplasm.

      (c) Microfilaments (**actin filaments** 6 nm in diameter) are associated with the plasma membrane.

b. Dendrites receive stimuli (signals) from sensory cells, axons, or other neurons and convert these signals into small electrical impulses (action potentials) that are **transmitted toward** the soma.

  (1) Dendrites possess **arborized terminals** (except in bipolar neurons), which permit a neuron to receive stimuli simultaneously from many other neurons.

  (2) The dendrite cytoplasm is similar to that of the soma except that it lacks a Golgi complex.

  (3) Organelles are reduced in number or absent near the terminals except for mitochondria, which are abundant.

  (4) Spines on the surface of dendrites increase the area available for synapse formation with other neurons. These diminish with age and poor nutrition and exhibit altered configurations in individuals with trisomy 21 or trisomy 13.

c. Axons conduct impulses away from the soma to the axon terminals without any diminution in their strength.

  (1) The diameter and length of axons in different types of neurons vary. Some axons are as long as 100 cm.

  (2) Axons originate from the **axon hillock**, a specialized region of the soma that lacks RER, ribosomes, Golgi cisternae, and Nissl bodies but contains many microtubules and neurofilaments; abundance of the latter may regulate neuron diameter. Further, it permits passage of mitochondria and vesicles into the axon.

(3) Axons may have **collaterals**, branching at right angles from the main trunk.

(4) Axon cytoplasm (**axoplasm**) lacks a Golgi complex but contains smooth endoplasmic reticulum (SER), RER, and elongated mitochondria.

(5) A plasma membrane surrounding the axon is called the **axolemma**.

(6) Axons terminate in many small branches (**axon terminals**) from which impulses are passed to another neuron or other types of cells.

CLINICAL CONSIDERATIONS   **Alzheimer disease** is the most common cause of dementia. It is the sixth leading cause of death in the United States and is considered to be a disease of the aged. Currently, about 5.2 million persons in the United States have been diagnosed with Alzheimer disease, of whom five million are aged 65 and older and 200,000 are younger than 65 years of age. It is estimated that in 2013 Alzheimer disease is expected to cost the United States $203 billion, which is expected to rise to $1.2 trillion by 2050. Alzheimer disease starts with memory loss and confusion, loss of finding words, loss of abstract thinking, disorientation, and depression, followed by irritability and mood swings with aggression. Finally, there is withdrawal and decline of senses and the loss of bodily functions. It appears that a combination of genetics, lifestyle, and the environment plays a role in triggering the onset. The disease is characterized by the loss of neurons and synapses mainly within the cerebral cortex followed by atrophy of the individual cerebral lobes. Patients with Alzheimer disease develop β-amyloid plaques and neurofibrillary tangles that render the neurons nonfunctional. Recent studies have shown that β-amyloid protein can act as a prion and be transferred from infected neurons to noninfected neurons by traveling down the axon of the infected cell and entering the uninfected cell via synapses. Still other current investigations suggest that Alzheimer disease is a neuroendocrine disorder, specifically **type III diabetes mellitus**, resulting from specific deficiencies in insulin, insulin-like growth factor-1, and insulin-like growth factor-2 production, as well as in the scarcity of receptors for these three molecules confined to certain regions of the brain.

B. **The neuroglial cells,** astrocytes and oligodendroglia (as well as microglia and ependymal cells) are located only in the CNS. Schwann cells and capsule cells are their PNS equivalent cells.

  1. **General characteristics.** Neuroglial cells comprise several cell types and outnumber neurons by approximately a factor of 10. These cells are embedded in a web of tissue composed of modified ectodermal elements; the entire supporting structure is termed the **neuroglia**. They function to **support and protect neurons**, but they do not conduct impulses or form synapses with other cells; however, they do appear to provide some regulation of neurons in the process of neural transmissions. Neuroglia do that by actively monitoring synapses, removing neurotransmitter molecules from synapses, and delivering molecules known as **gliotransmitter substances**, such as glutamate and ATP into the synaptic vicinity. These gliotransmitters appear to suppress synaptic transmission in cultured hippocampal neurons. Additionally, neuroglial cells possess the capacity to undergo cell division. Neuroglia are revealed in histologic sections of the CNS only with special gold and silver stains.

  2. **Types of neuroglial cells** (Figure 9.5). Note that Schwann cells are also discussed in this section, but they are present only in the PNS.

  a. **Astrocytes**

    (1) Astrocytes are the largest of the neuroglial cells that reside in the CNS. They have many processes, some of which possess expanded pedicles (**vascular feet**) that surround blood vessels, whereas others exhibit processes that contact the pia mater.

    (2) Function

      (a) Astrocytes scavenge ions and debris from neuron metabolism and supply energy for metabolism.

      (b) Along with other components of the neuroglia, astroglia form a protective **sealed barrier** between the pia mater and the nervous tissue of the brain and the spinal cord.

      (c) They provide **structural support** for nervous tissue.

      (d) They proliferate to form **scar tissue** (**glial scar**) after injury to the CNS.

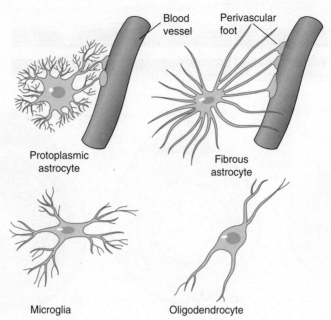

FIGURE 9.5. Various types of neuroglial cells. (Adapted with permission from Gartner LP, Hiatt JL. *Color Textbook of Histology.* 2nd ed. Philadelphia, PA: Saunders; 2001:192.)

(3) Types of astrocytes

(a) Protoplasmic astrocytes reside mostly in gray matter and have branched processes that envelop blood vessels, neurons, and synaptic areas. They contain some intermediate filaments composed of **glial fibrillar acidic protein** (GFAP). These astrocytes help establish the **blood–brain barrier** and may contribute to its maintenance.

(b) Fibrous astrocytes reside mostly in **white matter** and have long, slender processes with few branches. They contain many intermediate filaments composed of **GFAP**.

b. Oligodendrocytes

(1) Oligodendrocytes are neuroglial cells that live **symbiotically** with neurons (i.e., each cell type is affected by the metabolic activities of the other). These cells are necessary for the survival of neurons in the CNS.

(2) They are located in both **gray matter** and **white matter**.

(3) They possess a small, round, condensed nucleus and only a few short processes.

(4) Their electron-dense cytoplasm contains ribosomes, numerous microtubules, many mitochondria, RER, and a large Golgi complex.

(5) Oligodendrocytes produce **myelin**, a lipoprotein material organized into a sheath that insulates and protects axons in the CNS. Each oligodendrocyte forms several processes, and each process produces myelin for a single internode for a single axon. In this fashion, an oligodendroglion can myelinate an internode for several axons.

c. Schwann cells

(1) Schwann cells, located in the PNS, are flat cells with only a few mitochondria and a small Golgi region.

(2) Although Schwann cells are derived from neural crest cells, they are still considered neuroglial cells.

(3) These cells perform the same function in the PNS as oligodendrocytes in the CNS: they protect and insulate neurons. Schwann cells form either unmyelinated or myelinated coverings over neurons. However, a single Schwann cell can only insulate a single axon, whereas a single oligodendrocyte may insulate several axons. A myelin sheath consists of plasmalemmae of copious numbers of Schwann cells wrapped around a single axon (see Section V).

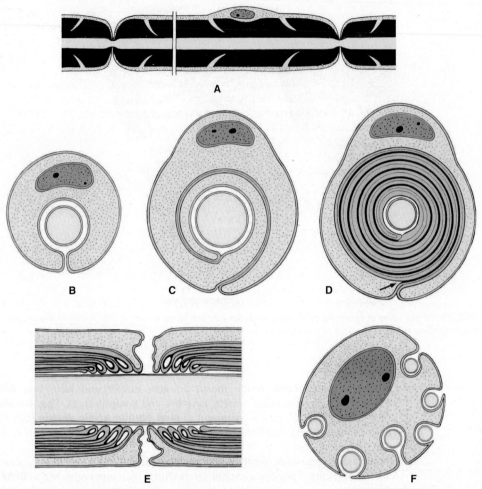

FIGURE 9.6. Myelin sheath formation. **A.** Myelin sheath and the Schwann cell as they are seen (ideally) by light microscopy. **B–D.** Successive stages in the development of the myelin sheath from plasma membrane of the Schwann cell. **E.** Ultrastructure of a node of Ranvier, sectioned longitudinally. **F.** Relation of the Schwann cell to several unmyelinated axons. (Reprinted with permission from Kiernan JA. *Barr's The Human Nervous System: An Anatomical Viewpoint.* 8th ed. Baltimore, MD: Lippincott Williams & Wilkins; 2005:22.)

    (4) Unmyelinated peripheral nerve fibers are surrounded by a large number of Schwann cells where each segment of the axon is enveloped by a single Schwann cell. Several axon segments may be embedded in each Schwann cell (see Figure 9.6F). Since impulses in myelinated axons jump from one node of Ranvier to another and in unmyelinated axons they move sequentially from ion channel to ion channel, propagation of the impulse is much faster in myelinated axons. It is interesting to note that, frequently, in the CNS unmyelinated axons, unlike in the PNS, are not enveloped by neuroglial cells.

  d. Microglia are small, **phagocytic** neuroglial cells that are derived from the mononuclear phagocytic cell population in the bone marrow. They have a condensed, elongated nucleus and many short, branching processes. Normally they are inactive but during injury or pathogen invasion they release interferon-γ which activates neighboring microglia. Activated microglial cells remove residues of cellular injury and secrete cytokines that attract T cells to the site of injury. Microglia also possess the ability to become antigen-presenting cells and present the antigens to the newly arrived T cells.

  e. Ependymal cells, derived from the neuroepithelium, are the **epithelial cells** that line the neural tube and ventricles of the brain. In certain regions of the brain, they possess **cilia**, which aid in moving the cerebrospinal fluid (CSF). Modified ependymal cells contribute to the formation of the **choroids plexus**.

IV. SYNAPSES

Synapses are sites of **functional apposition** where signals are transmitted from one neuron to another or from a neuron to another type of cell (e.g., muscle cell).

A. **Classification.** Synapses are classified according to the site of synaptic contact and the method of signal transmission (Figure 9.3).
   1. **Site of synaptic contact**
      a. **Axodendritic synapses** are located between an axon and a dendrite.
      b. **Axosomatic synapses** are located between an axon and a soma. The CNS primarily contains axodendritic and axosomatic synapses.
      c. **Axoaxonic synapses** are located between axons.
      d. **Dendrodendritic synapses** are located between dendrites.
   2. **Method of signal transmission**
      a. **Chemical synapses**
         (1) These synapses involve the release of a chemical substance (**neurotransmitter** or **neuromodulator**) by the presynaptic cell, which acts on the postsynaptic cell to generate an action potential.
         (2) Chemical synapses are the most common neuron–neuron synapse and the only neuron–muscle synapse.
         (3) Signal transmission across these synapses is **delayed** by about 0.5 ms, the time required for secretion and diffusion of neurotransmitter from the presynaptic membrane of the first cell into the synaptic cleft and then to the postsynaptic membrane of the receiving cell.
         (4) Neurotransmitters do not effect the change; they only activate a response in the receiving cell.

CLINICAL CONSIDERATIONS **Parkinson Disease**

Parkinson disease is a progressive degenerative disease characterized by tremors, muscular rigidity, difficulty in initiating movements, slow voluntary shuffling movement, and masklike facial expression. The cause is the loss of dopaminergic neurons from the substantia nigra of the brain. Although the cause of the loss of these cells is unclear, it is known that certain industrial toxins, such as those to which manganese miners are exposed, and the poisonous methyl-phenyl-tetrahydropyridine, a substance present in illegally manufactured heroin, cause Parkinson disease. Treatment modalities include administering levodopa, which gives some relief, although the cells continue to die. Transplanting fetal adrenal gland tissue has provided only transient relief. Advances in stem cell research may be applied some day to curing this deadly disease.

Deep brain stimulation is a technique that does not cure Parkinson disease, but can ease the symptoms and improve the patient's quality of life. Presently, it is used when routine medications either fail or produce severe side effects.

Huntington Chorea

Huntington chorea is a fatal hereditary disease that becomes evident during the third and fourth decades of life, first presenting as painful joints and progressing to uncontrolled flicking of joints, motor dysfunction, dementia, and death. The cause is thought to be the loss of neurons that produce the neurotransmitter γ-aminobutyric acid (GABA). The symptoms of dementia are thought to be related to the loss of the cells secreting acetylcholine.

      b. **Electrical synapses**
         (1) These synapses involve movement of ions from one neuron to another via **gap junctions**, which transmit the action potential of the presynaptic cell directly to the postsynaptic cell.

(2) Electrical synapses are much less numerous than chemical synapses.

(3) Signal transmission across these synapses is **nearly instantaneous**.

B. Synaptic morphology
1. **Axon terminals** may vary morphologically, depending on the site of synaptic contact.
   a. **Boutons terminaux** are bulbous expansions that occur singly at the end of axon terminals.
   b. **Boutons en passage** are swellings along the axon terminal; synapses may occur at each swelling.
2. The **presynaptic membrane** is the thickened axolemma of the neuron that is transmitting the impulse. It contains **voltage-gated Ca^{2+}** channels, which regulate the entry of calcium ions into the axon terminal. Synaptic vesicles fuse with and become incorporated into the presynaptic membrane before releasing their neurotransmitter substances.
3. The **postsynaptic membrane** is the thickened plasma membrane of the neuron or other target cell that is receiving the impulse.
4. The **synaptic cleft** is the narrow space (20–30 nm wide) between the presynaptic and postsynaptic membranes. Neurotransmitters diffuse across the synaptic cleft.
5. **Synaptic vesicles** are small, membrane-bound structures (40–60 nm in diameter) in the axoplasm of the transmitting neuron. They **discharge neurotransmitters** into the synaptic cleft by exocytosis.

C. Neurotransmitters (Table 9.1) are produced, stored, and released by presynaptic neurons. They diffuse across the synaptic cleft and bind to receptors in the postsynaptic membrane, leading to generation of an action potential.

V. NERVE FIBERS

Nerve fibers are individual axons enveloped by a myelin sheath, Schwann cells in the PNS, or oligodendrocytes in the CNS.

A. Myelin sheath (Figure 9.6)
1. The myelin sheath is produced by **oligodendrocytes** in the CNS and by **Schwann cells** in the PNS.

table 9.1	Common Neurotransmitters	
Neurotransmitter	Location	Function
Acetylcholine	Myoneural junctions; all parasympathetic synapses; preganglionic sympathetic synapses	Activates skeletal muscle, autonomic nerves, brain functions
Norepinephrine	Postganglionic sympathetic synapses	Increases cardiac output
Glutamate	CNS; presynaptic sensory and cortex	Most common excitatory neurotransmitter of CNS
GABA	CNS	Most common inhibitory neurotransmitter of CNS
Dopamine	CNS	Inhibitory and excitatory, depending on receptor
Glycine	Brainstem and spinal cord	Inhibitory
Serotonin	CNS	Pain inhibitor; mood control; sleep
Aspartate	CNS	Excitatory
Enkephalins	CNS	Analgesic; pain suppression
Endorphins	CNS	Analgesic; pain suppression

CNS, central nervous system; GABA, γ-aminobutyric acid.

2. It consists of several spiral layers of the plasma membrane of an oligodendrocyte or Schwann cell wrapping around the axon.
3. It is not continuous along the length of the axon but is interrupted by gaps called **nodes of Ranvier**.
4. Its thickness is constant along the length of an axon; however, thickness usually increases as the axonal diameter increases.
5. The myelin sheath can be extracted by standard histological techniques. Methods using **osmium tetroxide** preserve the myelin sheath and stain it black.
6. Under electron microscopy, the myelin sheath displays the following features:
   a. **Major dense lines** represent **fusions** between the cytoplasmic surfaces of the plasma membranes of Schwann cells (or oligodendrocytes).
   b. **Intraperiod lines** represent **close contact**, but not fusion, of the extracellular surfaces of adjacent Schwann cell (or oligodendrocyte) plasma membranes.
   c. **Clefts (incisures) of Schmidt–Lanterman** (observed in both electron and light microscopy) are cone-shaped oblique **discontinuities** of the myelin sheath due to the presence of Schwann cell (or oligodendrocyte) cytoplasm within the myelin.

B. **Nodes of Ranvier** are regions along the axon that **lack myelin** and represent discontinuities between adjacent Schwann cells or adjacent oligodendrocytes.
   1. In the PNS, the axon at the nodes of Ranvier is covered by interdigitated cytoplasmic processes of adjacent Schwann cells that protect the myelin-free surface of the axon. In the CNS, however, the axon is not covered by cytoplasmic processes of oligodendrocytes. Instead, the myelin-free surface of the axon at the node of Ranvier is covered by a foot plate of an astrocyte.
   2. The axolemma at the nodes contains **many Na$^+$** pumps, and in electron micrographs, it displays a characteristic electron density.

C. **Internodes** are the segments of a nerve fiber **between adjacent nodes of Ranvier**. They vary in length from 0.08 to 1 mm, depending on the size of the Schwann cells or oligodendrocytes associated with the fiber.

CLINICAL CONSIDERATIONS **Multiple Sclerosis**

Multiple sclerosis (MS) is an immune-mediated disease characterized by chronic and progressive dysfunction of the nervous system due to demyelination of the CNS, especially in the brain, spinal cord, and optic nerves. MS afflicts about 1 in 700 in this country, most commonly in the 20- to 40-year age group, affecting 2 females to 1 male. There are random episodes of inflammation, edema, and demyelination of axons followed by periods of remission that may last for months to years. Each episode may reduce the vitality of the patient and be sufficient to cause death within months. It is believed that, in the CNS, T lymphocytes mount an attack on myelin sheaths, demyelinate axons, and interfere with normal propagation of action potentials. However, recent studies have suggested that the true causative factor of MS is oligodendrogliopathy and the T-cell response is merely a secondary reaction. Present treatments include immunosuppression with corticosteroids.

VI. NERVES

Nerves are cordlike bundles of nerve fibers surrounded by connective tissue sheaths (Figure 9.7). They are **visible to the unaided eye** and usually appear **whitish** because of the presence of myelin.

A. **Connective tissue investments**
   1. **Epineurium** is the layer of dense fibrous connective tissue (**fascia**) that forms the external coat of nerve bundles and is often embedded in adipose tissue.

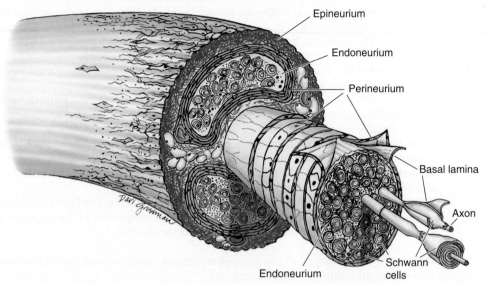

FIGURE 9.7. A peripheral nerve in cross section showing the various connective tissue sheaths. Each bundle of nerve fibers, or fascicle (one is extended in drawing), is covered by perineurium. (Reprinted with permission from Kelly DE, Wood RL, Enders AC. *Bailey's Textbook of Microscopic Anatomy.* 18th ed. Baltimore, MD: Williams & Wilkins; 1984:353.)

2. **Perineurium** surrounds each bundle of nerve fibers (**fascicle**). Its inner surface consists of layers of flattened cells joined by **tight junctions** (zonulae occludentes) that prohibit passage of most macromolecules, thus assisting in the formation of the blood–nerve barrier (Figure 9.8).
3. **Endoneurium** is a thin layer of reticular fibers, produced mainly by Schwann cells, that surrounds individual nerve fibers. This layer, difficult to observe without specialized stains, contains occasional mast cells and macrophages.

CLINICAL CONSIDERATIONS   **Meningitis**

Meningitis results from an inflammation of the meninges caused by viral or bacterial infection of the CSF. Viral meningitis is not severe, but bacterial meningitis is contagious and dangerous, leading to hearing loss, learning disability, brain damage, and death, sometimes within 24 hours if untreated. In the United States, children 4 years of age or younger have been vaccinated for the most prevalent form of the bacterium. Recently, because of so many outbreaks of meningitis on college campuses, several schools have chosen to vaccinate all students and those in close contact with them. Major symptoms include fever, headache, stiff neck, and alteration of consciousness with rapid onset and progression. Spinal tap and culture of CSF to determine the bacterial species is the only diagnosis. This is followed by treatment with a specific antibiotic. Bacterial meningitis can be spread by respiratory and throat secretions (i.e., coughing, sneezing, kissing).

B. **Functional classification of nerves**
1. **Sensory nerves** contain **afferent** fibers and carry sensory signals only from the internal and external environments to the CNS.
2. **Motor nerves** contain **efferent** fibers and carry signals only from the CNS to effector organs.
3. **Mixed nerves** are the most common type of nerve, containing both afferent and efferent fibers and thus carry both sensory and motor signals.

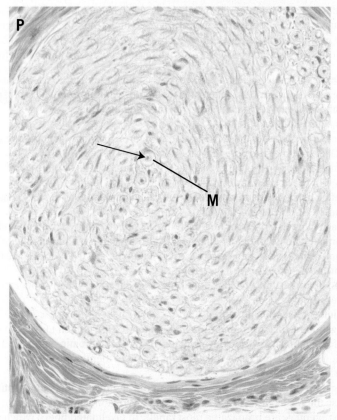

FIGURE 9.8. Light micrograph of peripheral nerve in cross section (×132). Note that an axon (*tip of arrow*) is located in the center of the myelin sheath (M). P, perineurium.

VII. GANGLIA

Ganglia are encapsulated aggregations of **neuronal cell bodies (soma)** outside the CNS.

A. **Autonomic ganglia** are **motor** ganglia in which axons of preganglionic neurons synapse on postganglionic neurons (**see Section IX B 1**).

B. **Craniospinal ganglia** are **sensory** ganglia associated with most cranial nerves and the dorsal roots of spinal nerves (**dorsal root ganglia**). Unlike autonomic ganglia, craniospinal ganglia **do not possess synapses**. These ganglia contain the cell bodies of sensory neurons, which are **pseudounipolar (unipolar)** and transmit sensory signals from receptors to the CNS.

VIII. HISTOPHYSIOLOGY OF NERVOUS SYSTEM

A. **Resting membrane potential**
   1. The resting membrane potential exists across the plasma membrane of all cells. The resting potential of most neuron plasmalemmae is negative –70 mV inside the cell compared to outside the cell.

2. It is established and maintained mostly by **K^+ leak channels** and to a lesser extent by the **$Na^+–K^+$ pump**, which actively transports three Na^+ ions out of the cell in exchange for two K^+ ions. The resting potential exists when there is no net movement of K^+ (i.e., when outward diffusion of K^+ is just balanced by the external positive charge acting against further diffusion).

B. **An action potential** is the electrical activity that occurs in a neuron as an impulse is propagated along the axon and is observed as a **movement of negative charges along the outside of an axon**. It is an **all-or-nothing event with a constant amplitude and duration**.

    1. **Generation of the action potential**

        a. An excitatory stimulus on a postsynaptic neuron partially **depolarizes** a portion of the plasma membrane (the potential difference is **less negative**).

        b. Once the membrane potential reaches a critical **threshold, voltage-gated Na^+ channels** in the membrane open, permitting Na^+ to enter the cell (Figure 9.9).

        c. The influx of Na^+ leads to **reversal of the resting potential** in the immediate area (i.e., the external side becomes negative).

        d. The Na^+ channels close spontaneously and are inactivated for 1 to 2 ms (**refractory period**).

        e. Opening of **voltage-gated K^+ channels** is also triggered by depolarization. Because these channels remain open longer than the Na^+ channels, exit of K^+ during the refractory period **repolarizes** the membrane to its resting potential.

        f. The ion channels then return to their normal states. The cell is now ready to respond to another stimulus.

    2. **Propagation of the action potential**

        a. Propagation results from longitudinal diffusion of Na^+ (which enters the cell at the initial site of excitation) toward the axon terminals (**orthodromic spread**). The longitudinal diffusion of Na^+ depolarizes the adjacent region of membrane, giving rise to a new action potential at this site.

        b. Propagation does **not** result from diffusion of Na^+ toward the soma (**antidromic spread**), because the Na^+ channels are inactivated in this region.

        c. Action potentials are propagated most rapidly in myelinated fibers, which exhibit **saltatory conduction**. In this type of conduction, the action potential jumps from one node of Ranvier to the next.

C. **Axonal transport** of proteins, organelles, and vesicles occurs at high, intermediate, and low velocities, depending on the nature of the transported materials.

    1. **Anterograde transport** carries material away from the soma.

    2. **Retrograde transport** carries material toward the soma for reuse, recycling, or degradation. However, some viruses (e.g., herpes simplex and rabies) spread in this fashion. Also, some toxins (e.g., tetanus) move from the periphery to the CNS in this manner.

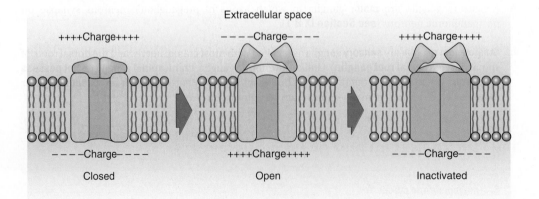

FIGURE 9.9. Model of the voltage-gated Na^+ channel showing the transition between its closed, open, and inactivated states. In the resting state, the channel-blocking segment and gating keep the channel closed to entry of extracellular Na^+. Depolarization of the membrane causes a conformational change that opens the channel to influx of Na^+. The channel closes spontaneously and becomes inactive within a millisecond after opening.

D. **Trophic function of nervous tissue**
  1. **Denervation** of a muscle or gland leads to its atrophy.
  2. **Reinnervation** of a muscle or gland restores its structure and function.

IX. SOMATIC NERVOUS SYSTEM AND AUTONOMIC NERVOUS SYSTEM

Somatic and autonomic are functional concepts relating to all the neural elements involved in the transmission of impulses from the CNS to the somatic and visceral components of the body, respectively. Neural crest cells give rise to neurons of both the parasympathetic and sympathetic divisions of the ANS whose **preganglionic cell bodies** are located in the CNS and **postganglionic cell bodies** are located in **autonomic ganglia** located outside the CNS.

A. **The somatic nervous system (SNS)** contains sensory fibers that bring information to the CNS and the motor fibers that originate in the CNS that innervate voluntary **skeletal muscles**.

B. **The autonomic nervous system (ANS)** is generally considered to be purely motor in function as it contains motor fibers that control and regulate **smooth muscle, cardiac muscle**, and some **glands**. It establishes and maintains **homeostasis** of the body's visceral functions. Anatomically and functionally, the ANS is divided into three parts: the **sympathetic, parasympathetic**, and **enteric nervous systems**. The sympathetic and parasympathetic nervous systems generally **function antagonistically** in a given organ (i.e., when the sympathetic system stimulates an organ, the parasympathetic inhibits it, and vice versa). The enteric nervous system is confined to the digestive system, where it controls digestive processes; however, it is modulated by the sympathetic and parasympathetic nervous systems.
  1. **Autonomic nerve chains**
    a. Cell bodies of **preganglionic neurons** are located in the CNS and extend their **preganglionic fibers** (axons) to an **autonomic ganglion** located outside of the CNS.
    b. In the ganglion, the preganglionic fibers synapse with postganglionic neurons, which typically are multipolar and are surrounded by satellite cells.
    c. **Postganglionic fibers** leave the ganglion and terminate in the **effector organ** (smooth muscle, cardiac muscle, and glands).
  2. **Sympathetic system (thoracolumbar outflow)**
    a. Preganglionic cell bodies of the sympathetic nervous system are located in the thoracic and the first two lumbar segments of the spinal cord.
    b. **Function**. The sympathetic system effects **vasoconstriction**. In general, it functions to prepare the body for flight-or-fight-or-freeze responses by increasing heart rate, respiration, blood pressure, and blood flow to skeletal muscles; dilating pupils; and decreasing visceral function.
  3. **Parasympathetic system (craniosacral outflow)**
    a. Preganglionic cell bodies of the parasympathetic nervous system are located in certain cranial nerve nuclei within the brain and in some sacral segments of the spinal cord.
    b. **Function**. The parasympathetic system stimulates secretion (**secretomotor** function). In general, it functions to prepare the body for rest-or-digest functions by decreasing heart rate, respiration, and blood pressure; constricting pupils; and increasing visceral function.
  4. **Enteric nervous system**
    a. **Enteric nervous system** consists of two divisions of neurons located in the wall of the digestive tract: the **myenteric plexus of Auerbach** and the **submucosal plexus of Meissner**.
    b. **Function**. The enteric nervous system is a stand-alone system that is generally responsible for the proper course of digestion, including the control of digestive secretions and blood flow to and from the gut. Although the enteric system is considered to be an independent system, its functions are modulated by the sympathetic and parasympathetic components of the ANS.

X. CENTRAL NERVOUS SYSTEM

The **CNS** consists of the brain, located in the skull, and the spinal cord housed in the bony vertebral column.

A. **White matter and gray matter** are both present in the CNS.
   1. **White matter** contains mostly myelinated nerve fibers but also some unmyelinated fibers and neuroglial cells.
   2. **Gray matter** contains neuronal cell bodies, many unmyelinated fibers, some myelinated fibers, and neuroglial cells.
   3. **Spinal cord gray matter** appears in the shape of an H in cross sections of the spinal cord (Figure 9.10).
      a. A small **central canal**, lined by ependymal cells, is at the center of the crossbar in the H. This canal is a remnant of the embryonic neural tube.
      b. The dorsal vertical bars of the H (**dorsal horns**) consist of **sensory** fibers extending from the dorsal root ganglia and cell bodies of interneurons.
      c. The ventral vertical bars of the H (**ventral horns**) consist of cell bodies and fibers of large multipolar motor neurons.
   4. **Brain gray matter** is located at the periphery (cortex) of the cerebrum and cerebellum. White matter lies beneath the gray matter in these structures.
      a. The **Purkinje cell layer** (cerebellar cortex only) consists of flask-shaped Purkinje cells. These cells have a central nucleus, highly branched (arborized) dendrites, and a single myelinated axon. These cells may receive several hundred thousand excitatory and inhibitory impulses to sort and integrate (Figure 9.11).
      b. Brain gray matter also forms the **basal nucleus** (previously called **basal ganglia**) which are deep within the cerebrum and are surrounded by white matter.

B. **Meninges** are **membranous coverings of the brain and spinal cord**. They are formed from connective tissue. There are three layers of meninges: the outermost **dura mater**, lining the bony skull and spinal cord; the intermediate **arachnoid mater**, abutting the dura; and the innermost, highly vascular **pia mater** lying directly on the surface of the brain and spinal cord.

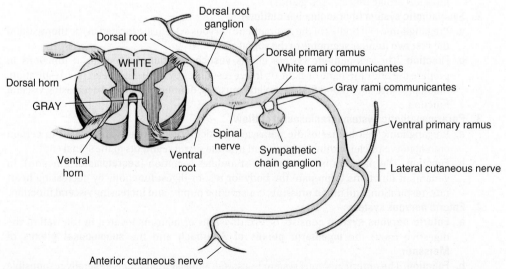

FIGURE 9.10. Typical thoracic spinal cord segment with spinal nerve. (Reprinted with permission from Hiatt JL, Gartner LP. *Textbook of Head and Neck Anatomy.* 4th ed. Baltimore, MD: Lippincott Williams & Wilkins; 2010:25.)

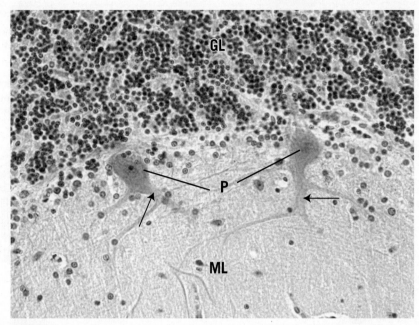

FIGURE 9.11. Light micrograph of the cerebellum (×132). Observe the Purkinje cells (P) with their dendritic trees (*arrows*) protruding into the molecular layer (ML). The heavily populated and deeply stained region is the granular layer (GL) of the cerebellum.

C. **Cerebrospinal fluid**
1. CSF is a clear fluid produced primarily by cells of the **choroid plexus** in the ventricles of the brain. The choroid plexus is composed of folds of pia mater and capillaries that are surrounded by cuboidal ependymal cells.
2. CSF circulates through the ventricles, subarachnoid space, and central canal, bathing and nourishing the brain and spinal cord; it also acts as a shock-absorbing cushion to protect these structures.
3. CSF is about 90% water and ions; it contains little protein, occasional white blood cells, and infrequent desquamated cells.
4. CSF is continuously produced and is reabsorbed by **arachnoid granulations** that transport it into the superior sagittal sinus. If reabsorption is blocked, **hydrocephalus** may occur.

CLINICAL CONSIDERATIONS   **Lumbar puncture**: A small amount of CSF can be extracted from the spinal cord for analysis via a needle inserted into the vertebral canal between the third and fourth lumbar vertebrae.

---

5. **Blood–brain barrier** functions to isolate the nervous tissue of the CNS from products carried by the blood vascular system. Tight junctions formed by adjacent endothelial cells lining the continuous capillaries supplying the neural tissues perform this function. Although this barrier permits the passage of certain molecules (i.e., O_2, H_2O, CO_2, lipids, and drugs), other substances such as vitamins, some drugs, and glucose are afforded access only via diffusion or receptor-mediated transport. Additionally, certain ions can also pass through the blood–brain barrier by the use of active transport. Protoplasmic astrocytes assist in the maintenance of the blood–brain barrier.

XI. DEGENERATION AND REGENERATION OF NERVE TISSUE

A. **Death of neurons** occurs as the result of injury to or disease affecting the somata.

   1. Neuronal death has been described until recently as resulting in degeneration and permanent loss of nerve tissue because it was believed that neurons of areas of the CNS could not divide.

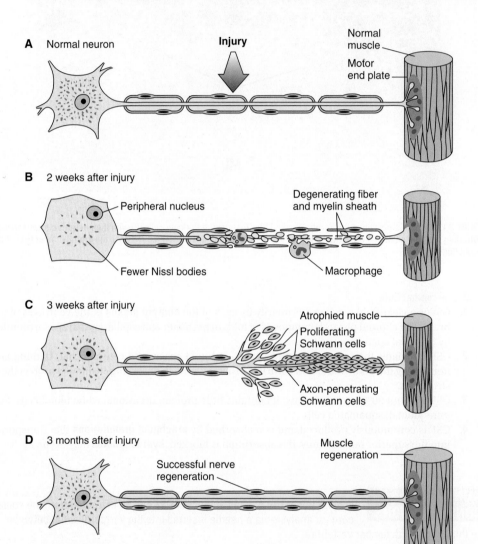

Unsuccessful nerve regeneration

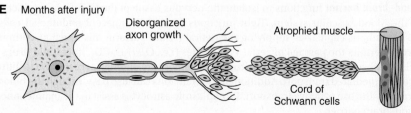

FIGURE 9.12. Peripheral nerve regeneration. (Adapted with permission from Gartner LP, Hiatt JL. *Color Textbook of Histology.* Philadelphia, PA: Saunders; 1997:185.)

However, there is now evidence that neuronal stem cells within certain regions of the brain exhibit multipotential capability and can be stimulated to differentiate into glial cells and neurons, replacing those that were lost or injured in the damaged tissue.

2. In the CNS, neuronal death may be followed by proliferation of the neuroglia, which fills in areas left by dead neurons.

B. Transection of peripheral axons induces changes in the soma, including **chromatolysis** (disruption of Nissl bodies with a concomitant loss of cytoplasmic basophilia), increase in soma volume, and movement of the nucleus to a peripheral position.

1. **Degeneration of distal axonal segment** (anterograde changes)

   a. The axon and its myelin sheath, which are separated from the soma, degenerate completely (**Wallerian degeneration**), and the remnants are removed by macrophages.

   b. Schwann cells proliferate, forming a **solid cellular column** that is distal to the injury and that remains attached to the effector cell.

2. **Regeneration of proximal axonal segment** (retrograde changes) (Figure 9.12)

   a. The distal end, closest to the wound, initially degenerates, and the remnants are removed by macrophages.

   b. Growth at the distal end then begins (0.5–3 mm/day) and progresses toward the columns of Schwann cells.

   c. Regeneration is successful if the sprouting axon penetrates a Schwann cell column and reestablishes contact with the effector cell.

Review Test

Directions: Each of the numbered items or incomplete statements in this section is followed by answers or by completions of the statement. Select the ONE lettered answer or completion that is BEST in each case.

1. Neural crest cells give rise to which of the following?

(A) Dorsal horns of the spinal cord
(B) Adrenal cortex
(C) Sympathetic ganglia
(D) Preganglionic autonomic nerves
(E) Somatic motor neurons

2. Which one of the following neurotransmitters functions to increase cardiac output?

(A) Dopamine
(B) Serotonin
(C) Norepinephrine
(D) Glutamate
(E) GABA

3. Which of the following statements regarding nerve cell membrane potentials is true?

(A) Membrane potentials are maintained at rest by Na^+ entering the cell.
(B) Entrance of K^+ causes the membrane to return to its resting potential.
(C) Depolarization triggers the opening of voltage-gated K^+ channels.
(D) Voltage-gated Na^+ channels become activated during the refractory period.
(E) The influx of K^+ reverses the resting potential.

4. Which of the following statements is characteristic of the perineurium?

(A) It is a fascia surrounding many bundles of nerve fibers.
(B) It is the fascia surrounding a single nerve fiber.
(C) It is a thin layer of reticular fibers covering individual nerve fibers.
(D) It is a fascia that excludes macromolecules and forms the external coat of nerves.
(E) It consists in part of epithelioid cells that surround a bundle (fascicle) of nerve fibers.

5. Acetylcholine is the only neurotransmitter in which of the following regions of the nervous system?

(A) Central nervous system
(B) Presynaptic sensory cortex
(C) Myoneural junctions
(D) Postganglionic sympathetic synapses
(E) Motor cortex

6. Nissl bodies are composed of

(A) synaptic vesicles and acetylcholine.
(B) polyribosomes and rough endoplasmic reticulum.
(C) lipoprotein and melanin.
(D) neurofilaments and microtubules.
(E) SER and mitochondria.

7. The axon hillock contains

(A) rough endoplasmic reticulum.
(B) ribosomes.
(C) microtubules.
(D) Golgi complex.
(E) synaptic vesicles.

8. Synaptic vesicles possess which of the following characteristics?

(A) Manufacture neurotransmitter
(B) Enter the synaptic cleft
(C) Become incorporated into the presynaptic membrane
(D) Become incorporated into the postsynaptic membrane
(E) Release neurotransmitter via endocytosis

9. A patient with Hirschsprung presents with which of the following symptoms?

(A) Absent cranial vault
(B) Exposed spinal cord
(C) Headache
(D) Large, dilated colon
(E) Absent small intestine

10. Myelination of peripheral nerves is accomplished by

(A) astrocytes.
(B) oligodendrocytes.
(C) Schwann cells.
(D) neural crest cells.
(E) basket cells.

11. Episodes of demyelination are associated with

(A) meningitis.
(B) Huntington chorea.
(C) spina bifida.
(D) Parkinson disease.
(E) multiple sclerosis.

12. Tremors, shuffling gate, and masklike facial expressions are associated with

(A) meningitis.
(B) Huntington chorea.
(C) spina bifida.
(D) Parkinson disease.
(E) multiple sclerosis.

13. Loss of neurotransmitter GABA is associated with

(A) meningitis.
(B) Huntington chorea.

(C) spina bifida.
(D) Parkinson disease.
(E) multiple sclerosis.

14. Rapid onset of fever, stiff neck, headache, and an altered state of consciousness are associated with

(A) meningitis.
(B) Huntington chorea.
(C) spina bifida.
(D) Parkinson disease.
(E) multiple sclerosis.

15. Deterioration and death of the dopaminergic neurons within the substantia nigra of the brain are associated with

(A) meningitis.
(B) Huntington chorea.
(C) spina bifida.
(D) Parkinson disease.
(E) multiple sclerosis.

Answers and Explanations

1. **C.** Neural crest cells migrate throughout the body and give rise to ganglia and other structures, including portions of the adrenal medulla, but they do not contribute to the development of preganglionic autonomic nerves, adrenal cortex, or the dorsal horns of the spinal cord (see Chapter 9 II D).

2. **C.** Norepinephrine increases cardiac output, whereas dopamine and GABA are CNS inhibitors. Glutamate is the most common excitatory neurotransmitter of the CNS. Serotonin functions as a pain inhibitor in mood control and in sleep (see Chapter 9 IV C).

3. **C.** Once the critical threshold is reached, voltage-gated Na^+ channels open and Na^+ enters the cell, which depolarizes the cell. Depolarization triggers the opening of voltage-gated K^+ channels, and K^+ then exits the cell (see Chapter 9 VIII A).

4. **E.** Each bundle of nerve fibers is surrounded by the perineurium, which consists primarily of several layers of epithelioid cells. Tight junctions between these cells exclude most macromolecules. The external coat of nerves, the epineurium, surrounds many fascicles but does not exclude macromolecules. The layer of reticular fibers that covers individual nerve fibers is the endoneurium; it also does not exclude macromolecules (see Chapter 9 VI A).

5. **C.** Acetylcholine is the neurotransmitter for myoneural junctions as well as for preganglionic sympathetic and preganglionic and postganglionic parasympathetic synapses (Table 9.1).

6. **B.** Nissl bodies are large, granular basophilic bodies composed of polysomes and RER. They are found only in neurons (in the soma cytoplasm) (see Chapter 9 III A 3).

7. **C.** The axon hillock is devoid of large organelles, such as Nissl bodies and Golgi cisternae, but it does contain microtubules arranged in bundles and permits passage of neurofilaments, mitochondria, and vesicles into the axon (see Chapter 9 III A 3 c).

8. **C.** Synaptic vesicles release neurotransmitter into the synaptic cleft by exocytosis. In this process, the vesicle membrane is incorporated into the presynaptic membrane. Although these vesicles contain neurotransmitter, they do not manufacture it (see Chapter 9 IV B 2).

9. **D.** Hirschsprung disease is characterized by a dilated colon caused by the absence of the parasympathetic myenteric ganglia known as Auerbach plexus (see Chapter 9 II D Clinical Considerations).

10. **C.** Schwann cells produce myelin in the PNS, whereas oligodendrocytes produce myelin in the CNS. Astrocytes, neural crest cells, and basket cells do not produce myelin (see Chapter 9 V A B).

11. **E. Multiple sclerosis** is an immune-mediated disease exhibiting chronic and progressive dysfunction of the nervous system due to demyelination of the CNS and optic nerves, striking the 20- to 40-year age group affecting 1.5 times more women than men. There are random episodes of inflammation, edema, and demyelination of axons followed by periods of remission. Each episode may reduce the vitality of the patient and be sufficient to cause death within months (see Chapter 9 V B Clinical Considerations).

12. **D. Parkinson disease** is a progressive degenerative disease characterized by tremors, muscular rigidity, difficulty in initiating movements, slow voluntary shuffling movement, and masklike face. The cause is the loss of dopaminergic neurons from the substantia nigra of the brain. Although the cause of the loss of these cells is unclear, it is known that certain poisons and environmental factors cause Parkinson disease (see Chapter 9 IV A Clinical Considerations).

13. **B. Huntington chorea is** a fatal heredity disease that becomes evident during the third and fourth decades of life. It progresses to uncontrolled flicking of joints, motor dysfunction,

dementia, and death. The cause is apparently the loss of neurons that produce the neurotransmitter GABA. Dementia symptoms are thought to be related to the loss of cells secreting acetylcholine (see Chapter 9 IV A Clinical Considerations).

14. **A. Meningitis** results from an inflammation of the meninges caused by viral or bacterial infection in the CSF. Although viral meningitis is not severe, bacterial meningitis is contagious and dangerous, leading to hearing loss, learning disability, brain damage, and death if untreated, sometimes within 24 hours. Major symptoms include fever, headache, stiff neck, and alteration of consciousness with rapid onset and progression. Spinal tap and culture of CFS to determine the bacterial species is the only diagnosis. Treatment is by species-specific antibiotic. Bacterial meningitis can be spread by respiratory and throat secretions (i.e., coughing, sneezing, kissing) (see Chapter 9 VI A Clinical Considerations).

15. **D. Parkinson disease** is a progressive degenerative disease characterized by tremors, muscular rigidity, difficulty in initiating movements, slow voluntary shuffling movement, and masklike face. It is caused by the loss of dopaminergic neurons from the substantia nigra of the brain (see Chapter 9 IV A Clinical Considerations).

I. OVERVIEW—BLOOD

A. Blood is a specialized connective tissue that consists of formed elements (**erythrocytes, leukocytes, and platelets**) and a fluid component called **plasma**.

B. The volume of blood in an average human adult is approximately **5 L**.

C. Blood circulates in a closed system of vessels and **transports** nutrients, waste products, hormones, proteins, ions, oxygen (O_2), carbon dioxide (CO_2), and formed elements.

D. It also **regulates body temperature** and assists in regulation of **osmotic** and **acid–base balance**.

E. Blood cells have short life spans and are continuously replaced by a process called **hemopoiesis**.

II. BLOOD CONSTITUENTS

A. **Plasma** consists of 90% **water;** 9% **organic compounds** (such as proteins, amino acids, and hormones); and 1% **inorganic salts**, dissolved **gases**, and **nutrients**.
   1. **Main plasma proteins**
      a. **Albumin**, a small protein (60,000 molecular weight), preserves the colloid osmotic pressure in the vascular system and helps transport some metabolites. Colloid osmotic pressure assists in maintaining proper blood volume by resisting the exit of plasma from the bloodstream. Recall that **plasma** that leaves blood vessels to enter the connective tissue spaces is known as **extracellular fluid (tissue fluid)**.
      b. **γ-Globulins** are **antibodies (immunoglobulins) (see Chapter 12)**.
      c. **α-Globulins** and **β-globulins** transport metal ions (e.g., iron and copper) and lipids (in the form of lipoproteins).
      d. Clotting proteins, including **fibrinogen**, a soluble protein that is converted into fibrin during blood clotting.
      e. **Complement proteins** (C1–C9) are part of the innate immune system, and they function in nonspecific host defense and initiate the inflammatory process.
   2. **Serum** is the **yellowish fluid** that remains after blood has clotted. It is similar to plasma but lacks fibrinogen and clotting factors.

table 10.1	Size and Number of Formed Elements in Human Blood			
	Diameter (μm)			
Cell Type	Smear	Section	Cells/mm³ of Blood	Leukocytes (%)
Erythrocyte	7–8	6–7	5×10^6 (men)	–
			4.5×10^6 (women)	
Agranulocytes				
Lymphocyte	8–10	7–8	1,500–2,500	20–25
Monocyte	12–15	10–12	200–800	3–8
Granulocytes				
Neutrophil	9–12	8–9	3,500–7,000	60–70
Eosinophil	10–14	9–11	150–400	2–4
Basophil	8–10	7–8	50–100	0.5–1
Platelet	2–4	1–3	250,000–400,000	–

Reprinted from Gartner LP, Hiatt JL. *Color Atlas of Histology.* 2nd ed. Baltimore, MD: Williams & Wilkins; 1994:84.

B. Formed elements of blood (Table 10.1 and Figure 10.1)

  1. Erythrocytes (red blood cells)

    a. General features

      (1) Red blood cells (RBCs) are round, **anucleate**, biconcave cells that **stain light salmon pink** with either Wright or Giemsa stains (Figure 10.1).

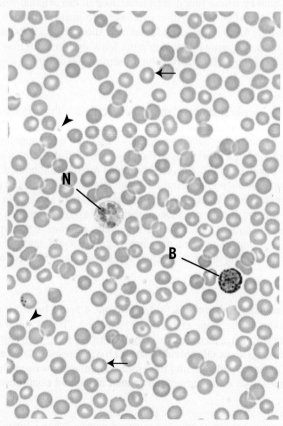

FIGURE 10.1. Light micrograph of a human blood smear. N, neutrophil; B, basophil; *arrows*, erythrocytes; *arrowheads*, platelets. Wright stain (×540).

(2) The average life span of an RBC is 120 days. Aged RBCs are fragile and express membrane surface oligosaccharides that are recognized by splenic, hepatic, and bone marrow macrophages, which destroy those erythrocytes.

(3) Carbohydrate determinants for the **A, B**, and **O blood groups** are located on the external surface of the erythrocyte's plasmalemma. A, B, and O antigens are short sequences of carbohydrate molecules that are almost identical to each other. All three are attached to the extracellular moiety of transmembrane proteins (**glycophorins**), and the only difference is that in types A and B there is an additional terminal sugar molecule attached to the carbohydrate chain of type O antigens. The addition of the terminal carbohydrate molecule requires enzymes whose presence is genetically determined.

　(a) In type A, the enzyme N-acetylgalactosamine transferase adds a terminal **N-acetylgalactosamine** to the type O antigen.

　(b) In type B, the enzyme **galactose transferase** adds a terminal **galactose** to the type O antigen.

　(c) In type AB, both enzymes are present; therefore, RBCs possess both A and B antigens on their cell membranes.

　(d) In type O, neither enzyme is present; therefore, only type O antigens are located on the RBC cell membrane.

　　Blood type AB is the **universal acceptor**, that is, an individual with AB blood type can receive a transfusion from individuals whose blood type is A or B or AB or O.

　　Blood type O is the **universal donor**, so that an individual with blood type O can give blood to individuals whose blood type is A or B or AB or O.

(4) Although there are more than 45 **Rh blood type antigens**, the most important one is the **D antigen** because it is prone to result in the greatest immunogenic response and is the one which is responsible for **erythroblastosis fetalis** in the newborn ("Rh" is for **Rhesus monkey** whose blood cells were used in the original work on this antigen). A particular individual's RBC either expresses (Rh positive, **Rh$^+$**) or does not express (Rh negative, **Rh$^-$**) the D antigen (**Rh factor**). If a mother who is Rh negative carries an Rh-positive fetus, it is quite possible that the fetus' erythrocytes may come in contact with the mother's blood either during the third trimester or during the birth process.

CLINICAL CONSIDERATIONS　**Erythroblastosis fetalis**, as described in the text, may occur in pregnancies where the mother's blood supply is exposed to D antigen (the **Rh factor**). If the mother is Rh negative, her immune system will produce IgM antibodies against D antigen, but these antibodies are too large to go through the placental barrier. During a subsequent pregnancy with another Rh-positive fetus, the mother will again produce antibodies, but this time IgG antibodies and these are small enough to penetrate the placental barrier and mount an immune response against the fetus. This condition is known as erythroblastosis fetalis and may be lethal to the fetus. In order to protect future fetuses, the Rh-negative mother who has an Rh-positive child is given anti-D globulin (**RhoGAM**) after the baby is born. The anti-D globulin attaches to the antigenic sites of the D antigen so that the mother's immune system does not recognize it and does not produce antibodies against the D antigens, protecting future Rh-positive fetuses from the mother's immune system.

---

(5) Several **cytoskeletal proteins** (ankyrin, band 4.1 and band 3 proteins, spectrin, and actin) maintain the shape of RBCs (see Chapter 1, Plasma Membrane, Section V A).

(6) Mature erythrocytes possess no organelles but are filled with **hemoglobin (Hb)**.

(7) Erythrocytes also contain **soluble enzymes** that are responsible for glycolysis, the hexose monophosphate pathway, and the production of adenosine triphosphate (ATP).

b. The **hematocrit** is an estimation of the **volume of packed erythrocytes per unit volume of blood**.

(1) The hematocrit is expressed as a percentage.

(2) Normal values are 40% to 50% in adult men, 35% to 45% in adult women, 35% in children up to 10 years of age, and 45% to 60% in newborns.

c. Hb is a protein composed of four polypeptide chains, each covalently linked to a heme group. The four chains that normally occur in humans are α, β, γ, and δ. Each chain differs in its amino acid sequence.

(1) Hb occurs in several normal forms that differ in their **chain composition**.

(a) The predominant form of adult Hb is **HbA$_1$** ($\alpha_2\beta_2$).

(b) A minor form is **HbA$_2$** ($\alpha_2\delta_2$).

(c) Fetal Hb is designated **HbF** ($\alpha_2\gamma_2$).

d. Transport of CO_2 and O_2 to and from the tissues of the body is carried out by erythrocytes and plasma.

(1) Every minute approximately 200 mL of CO_2 is formed by cells of the body. Since the partial pressure of CO_2 is higher in the tissue than in the capillaries, the CO_2 enters the capillaries via simple diffusion.

(a) Twenty milliliters of the CO_2 is transported in the plasma, 40 mL binds to the globin moiety of Hb (forming **carbaminohemoglobin**), and 140 mL enters the RBC cytosol.

(b) Within the cytosol, the enzyme **carbonic anhydrase** forms H_2CO_3 by combining CO_2 with H_2O. H_2CO_3 dissociates and the HCO_3^- leaves the RBC to enter the plasma, and Cl^- from the plasma enters the erythrocyte cytosol to maintain electrical equilibrium. This exchange of ions between the RBC cytosol and the plasma is referred to as the **chloride shift**.

(c) Meanwhile, since the partial pressure of O_2 is greater in the RBC than in the tissue, the O_2 is released from the Hb, forming **deoxyhemoglobin**, and the place of O_2 is taken up by the binding of **2,3-diphosphoglycerate**.

(2) The partial pressure of O_2 is greater in the alveolar airspace than in the alveoli of the lung than in the capillaries; therefore, O_2 enters the capillaries via simple diffusion.

(a) O_2 enters the erythrocyte cytosol and binds to the heme moiety of the Hb molecule to form **oxyhemoglobin**.

(b) Bicarbonate ions of the plasma reenter the RBC cytosol, and in exchange Cl^- ions leave the RBC to enter the plasma (a reversal of the chloride shift). The bicarbonate ion is combined with H^+ ions to form H_2CO_3, which is cleaved by carbonic anhydrase to form CO_2 and H_2O. The CO_2 enters the plasma, and from there the alveolar airspace via simple diffusion to be exhaled.

(3) Because carbon monoxide binds avidly to Hb, it can block binding of O_2 and cause **carbon monoxide asphyxiation** if it is inhaled in sufficient amounts.

(4) Nitric oxide is a neurotransmitter substance that binds to Hb; in areas that are poor in O_2, it facilitates dilation of blood vessels and a more efficacious exchange of O_2 for CO_2.

CLINICAL CONSIDERATIONS

1. **Sickle cell anemia** is caused by a point mutation in the deoxyribonucleic acid (DNA) encoding the Hb molecule, leading to the production of an **abnormal Hb** (HbS). In the β-chain of HbS, the amino acid **valine** is substituted for **glutamate**.

a. Although this disease occurs almost exclusively among people of African descent (1 in 500 is affected in the United States), among the US Hispanic population, 1 in 1,000 to 1,400 people is affected with sickle cell anemia.

b. Crystallization of Hb under low O_2 tension gives RBCs the characteristic sickle shape. **Sickle RBCs** are fragile and have a **higher rate of destruction** than normal cells.

c. Signs include hypoxia, increased bilirubin levels, low RBC count, and capillary stasis.

2. **Pernicious anemia** is caused by a severe **deficiency of vitamin B$_{12}$**, resulting from impaired production of **gastric intrinsic factor** by the parietal cells of the stomach. This factor is required for the proper absorption of vitamin B$_{12}$.

3. Newborns are frequently deficient in **vitamin K,** an essential cofactor for the clotting process, and if they do not receive exogenous administration of this vitamin, they may die of hemorrhagic disease of the newborn. Adults who are unable to absorb lipids may also suffer from excessive bleeding, but the supplemental injection of vitamin K improves this condition.

table 10.2	Selected Characteristics of Granulocytes		
Characteristic	Neutrophils	Eosinophils	Basophils
Nuclear shape	Lobulated (3 or 4 lobes)	Bilobed	S-shaped
Number of azurophilic granules	Many	Few	Few
Specific granules			
Size	Small	Large	Large
Color*	Light pink	Dark pink	Dark blue to black
Contents			
	Alkaline phosphatase Collagenase	Acid phosphatase Arylsulfatase	Eosinophil chemotactic factor
	Lactoferrin	β-Glucuronidase	Heparin
	Lysozyme	Cathepsin	Histamine
	Phagocytin	Major basic protein	Peroxidase
		Peroxidase	
		Phospholipase	
		Ribonuclease	
Life span	1 week	Few hours in blood, 2 weeks in connective tissue	Very long (1–2 years in mice)
Main functions	Phagocytose, kill, and digest bacteria	Moderate inflammatory reactions by inactivating histamine and leukotriene C	Mediate inflammatory responses in a manner similar to mast cells
Special properties	Form H_2O_2 during phagocytosis	Are decreased in number by corticosteroids	Have receptors for immunoglobulin E on their plasma membrane

*Cells stained with Giemsa or Wright stain.

2. **Leukocytes, or white blood cells (WBCs)** (Table 10.1 and Figure 10.1) possess varying numbers of **azurophilic granules.** These are lysosomes containing various hydrolytic enzymes. There are two main categories of leukocytes, **granulocytes** and **agranulocytes**, depending on the presence (in granulocytes) or absence (in agranulocytes) of **specific granules** in their cytoplasm. (**Azurophilic granules** are present in both categories of WBCs and are, in fact, **lysosomes.**)
   a. **Granulocytes** (Table 10.2) include **neutrophils, eosinophils**, and **basophils** (Figure 10.1).
      (1) Granulocytes possess **specific granules** with type-specific contents.
      (2) These cells generate ATP via the glycolytic pathway, Krebs cycle (eosinophils and basophils), and anaerobic pathways (neutrophils).
      (3) Destruction of phagocytosed microorganisms by neutrophils occurs in two ways.
         (a) Azurophilic granules release **hydrolytic enzymes** into phagosomes to destroy microorganisms.
         (b) Reactive O_2 compounds **superoxide (O_2^-)**, hydrogen peroxide (H_2O_2), and hypochlorous acid (HOCl) formed within phagosomes (catalyzed by **myeloperoxidase**) destroy microorganisms.
   b. **Agranulocytes** (Table 10.3) lack specific granules.
      (1) They include **lymphocytes and monocytes**.
      (2) There are three categories of lymphocytes: B lymphocytes, T lymphocytes, and null cells. (See Chapter 12, Lymphoid Tissue Section II Cells of the Immune System for a more complete discussion of lymphocytes and monocytes.) B lymphocytes are responsible for the humoral immune response, and T lymphocytes are responsible for the cellular immune response. Null cells constitute approximately 5% of the circulating lymphocytes and are of two types, pluripotential hemopoietic stem cells (PHSCs) and natural

table **10.3** Selected Characteristics of Agranulocytes

Characteristic	Monocytes	T Lymphocytes	B Lymphocytes
Plasma membrane	Form filopodia and pinocytic vesicles	Have T-cell receptors	Have Fc receptors and antibodies
Number of azurophilic granules	Many	Few	Few
Life span	Less than 3 days in blood	Several years	Few months
Main functions	Become macrophages in connective tissue	Generate cell-mediated immune response, secrete numerous growth factors	Generate humoral immune response

CLINICAL CONSIDERATIONS

1. **Infectious mononucleosis** is caused by the **Epstein–Barr virus (EBV)**, which is related to the herpes virus.
   a. This disease mostly affects young individuals of high school and college age.
   b. Signs and symptoms include fatigue, swollen and tender lymph nodes, fever, sore throat, and an increase in circulating lymphocytes.
   c. EBV may be transmitted by saliva (as in kissing).
   d. Infectious mononucleosis may be life-threatening in immunosuppressed or immunodeficient individuals, whose B cells can undergo intense proliferation leading to death.
2. **Burkitt lymphoma** is also caused by EBV.
   a. In central Africa, it causes a type of non-Hodgkin lymphoma that originates from B lymphocytes and invades nonlymph node regions, such as the brain, cerebrospinal fluid, blood, and bone marrow.
   b. It is not understood why the EBV causes infectious mononucleosis in the United States and this very serious lymphoma in central Africa.
   c. Unlike mononucleosis, Burkitt lymphoma is not infectious; it does not spread from infected to uninfected individuals.
   d. It is fatal if untreated, but aggressive chemotherapy can offer a cure in 70% of cases if caught early, 50% of cases if it has not involved the bone marrow or the central nervous system, but only 20% of cases if the central nervous system and bone marrow are involved.
3. **Leukemias** are characterized by the replacement of normal hemopoietic cells of the bone marrow by neoplastic cells and are classified according to the **type** and **maturity** of the cells involved.
   a. **Acute leukemias** occur mostly in children.
      i. These leukemias involve **immature cells.**
      ii. **Rapid onset** of the following signs and symptoms occur: anemia; high WBC count and/or many circulating immature WBCs; low platelet count; tenderness in bones; enlarged lymph nodes, spleen, and liver; vomiting; and headache.
   b. **Chronic leukemias** occur mainly in adults.
      i. These leukemias initially involve relatively **mature cells.**
      ii. Early signs include **slow onset** of a mild leukocytosis and enlarged lymph nodes; later, signs and symptoms include anemia, weakness, enlarged spleen and liver, and reduced platelet count.

killer (NK) cells. Null cells resemble lymphocytes but lack their characteristic surface determinants.

3. **Platelets (thrombocytes)** (Tables 10.1 and 10.4; Figure 10.1) are anucleated disk-shaped cell fragments that arise from megakaryocytes in bone marrow.
   a. A clear peripheral region, the **hyalomere**, and a region containing purple granules, the **granulomere**, are visible in stained blood smears.

table 10.4	Platelet Components					
Hyalomere		Granulomere				
Structure	Function	Granules	Size (nm)	Contents		Function
Actin and myosin	Platelet contraction	α	300–500	Fibrinogen, platelet thromboplastin, factors V and VIII, platelet-derived growth factor		Repair of vessel, platelet aggregation, coagulation
Microtubule bundles	Maintains platelet shape	δ (dense bodies)	250–300	Pyrophosphate, ADP, adenosine triphosphate, histamine, serotonin, Ca^{2+}		Vasoconstriction, platelet aggregation and adhesion
Surface opening tubule system	Facilitates exocytosis and endocytosis in activated platelets	λ	200–250	Lysosomal enzymes		Clot removal
Dense tubular system	Prevents platelet stickiness by sequestering Ca^{2+}					

(1) The **hyalomere** is occupied by a small bundle of 10 to 12 circularly disposed **microtubules** that mirror and assist in sustaining the discoid shape. Additional components are other cytoskeletal elements, such as **actin, myosin,** and various proteins that bind the cytoskeletal components to each other and the plasmalemma. There are two systems of cytoplasmic channels: one that communicates with the extracellular space, the **open canalicular system,** and the **dense tubular system** that does not communicate with the extracellular space.

(2) The **granulomere** is occupied by three types of granules, alpha, delta, and gamma granules, where the last of the three are lysosomes. (Table 10.4 describes the contents and functions of these thromboplastic elements.)

b. Platelets are surrounded by a **glycocalyx,** which coats the plasmalemma and is composed of the extracellular components of integral proteins (**glycoprotein Ib [GPIb]**), glycosaminoglycans, glycoproteins, and various coagulation factors. **Calcium ions** and **adenosine diphosphate** (ADP) increase the stickiness of the glycocalyx and enhance platelet adherence.

c. Platelets function in **blood coagulation** by aggregating at lesions in vessel walls and producing various factors that aid in clot formation.

d. They are also responsible for **clot retraction** and contribute to **clot removal**.

III. BLOOD COAGULATION

A. Blood coagulation contributes to hemostasis (stoppage of bleeding) and is normally controlled very stringently so that it occurs **only in regions where the endothelium is damaged**.

B. The process of hemostasis is basically a twofold interconnected phenomenon that involves **platelets** as a common denominator. If damage to the endothelial lining of a blood vessel is great enough to expose the lamina densa and the collagen-rich subendothelial connective tissue of the denuded area, then the glycoproteins, **von Willebrand factor (vWF),** become exposed to the circulating blood.

C. Platelet plasmalemma integrin molecules, **glycoprotein Ib (GPIb),** contact and adhere to **vWF,** which in turn adhere to the **collagen molecules** of the subendothelial connective tissue. Although this adherence occurs in the presence of coagulation factors V (proaccelerin) and IX (plasma thromboplastin), it is the vWF bond to both collagen and the GPIb of the platelets that offers the greatest resistance to the sheer forces of the blood flow and allows the firm anchorage of the platelets to the denuded area. The contact between the GPIb and the vWF initiates the **platelet reaction**, and platelets that adhere to the vWF are said to be **activated**.

D. **Activated platelets** become flattened (to cover a greater surface area of the denuded region) and degranulate, releasing **ADP** and **calcium ions**, and in the platelet membrane the enzyme thromboxane-A synthase converts membrane arachidonic acid to synthesize **thromboxane A$_2$**, an avid vasoconstrictor and platelet activator. Moreover, regions of the platelet plasma membrane become modified to display **phospholipid complexes** that facilitate the progression of the **coagulation cascade**. ADP and thromboxane A$_2$ attract additional platelets to the injury site and cause the platelets to be present, resulting in the aggregation of the platelets. The platelets are held together by unmasking another set of their integrin molecules, **glycoprotein IIb/IIIa (GPIIb/IIIa)**, that bind to fibrinogen, which then binds platelets to each other. As the platelet numbers adhering to each other increase in number and size, they block the injury site by the formation of a **primary hemostatic plug**.

E. The primary hemostatic plug is not a very strong barrier and is reinforced by the process of platelet contraction, which is initiated by its contact with fibrinogen, a protein present in circulating blood, and the primary hemostatic plug becomes a very dense, firm, and well-anchored **secondary hemostatic plug**. Since this process of contraction is completed in about 15 to 20 minutes after its initiation, this time lag provides ample opportunity for the coagulation cascade to reinforce the clot and anchor it in place, preventing further blood loss.

F. Once the secondary hemostatic plug is large enough to stop blood loss, it must not increase in size. This is controlled by the release of **NO** and **prostacyclins** by the endothelial cells, two substances that inhibit platelet aggregation. Additionally, the **anticoagulant pathways** inhibit the coagulation cascade. One anticoagulant pathway involves **Protein C complex** (a combination of thrombomodulin and thrombin) and **Protein S**, which inhibit factors Va and VIIIa. Another pathway involves antithrombin III, which not only inactivates thrombin but also acts as an enzyme, degrading factors IXa, Xa, XIa, and XIIa. A third pathway, **tissue factor pathway inhibitor**, secreted mostly by endothelial cells, binds to factor Xa and to tissue factor-VIIa complex, inactivating them and thereby inhibiting the coagulation cascade.

G. **Phospholipid complexes of activated platelet membranes** and **Ca^{2+}** ions (also known as factor IV) are also required for blood coagulation.

H. Blood coagulation occurs via two interrelated pathways, the **extrinsic** and **intrinsic pathways**. The final steps in both pathways, referred to as the **common pathway**, involve the transformation of prothrombin to **thrombin**, an enzyme that catalyzes the conversion of fibrinogen (factor I) to **fibrin monomers**, which, under the influence of **Ca^{2+} ions** and **factor XIIIa**, coalesce to form a **reticulum of clot**.
   1. The **extrinsic pathway** occurs in response to damaged blood vessels where the insult involves not only the endothelium but also the wall of the vessel. It is initiated within seconds (**rapid onset**) after trauma that releases **tissue thromboplastin** (factor III).
   2. The **intrinsic pathway** is initiated within several minutes (**slow onset**) after trauma to the **endothelial cells**, per se, of the blood vessels or when platelets or factor XII are exposed to collagen in the vessel wall. This pathway depends on **von Willebrand factor** and **factor VIII**.
   3. The **common pathway** involves the conversion of prothrombin to thrombin and that of fibrinogen to fibrin and, finally, the cross-linking of **fibrin monomers** to form the **fibrin reticulum**, which is deposited within and around the contracted platelet plug.

I. Once the blood vessel is repaired, the clot is no longer necessary and has to be removed. This process is initiated by **tissue plasminogen activator (tPA)** and by **urokinase-type plasminogen activator (u-PA)**, enzymes localized on the luminal cell membranes of endothelial cells and in blood plasma. Both enzymes activate **plasminogen**, an enzyme precursor synthesized by liver cells and released into the bloodstream, by converting it to the active enzyme **plasmin**. It is plasmin that in concert with macrophages dissolves the secondary hemostatic plug.

CLINICAL CONSIDERATIONS	**Coagulation disorders** frequently result from inherited or acquired defects of coagulation factors.

1. **Factor VIII deficiency (hemophilia A)** is an X-linked disorder that affects mostly men.
   a. Severity varies with the extent of reduction in the level of factor VIII (produced by hepatocytes).
   b. Hemophilia A results in excessive bleeding (into joints, in severe cases).
   c. Affected individuals have a normal platelet count, normal bleeding time, and no petechiae, but thromboplastin time is increased.
2. **von Willebrand disease** is an autosomal dominant genetic defect, resulting in a **decrease in the amount of von Willebrand factor**, which is required in the intrinsic pathway of coagulation.
   a. Most cases are mild and do not involve bleeding into the joints.
   b. Severe cases are characterized by excessive and/or spontaneous bleeding from mucous membranes and wounds.
3. **Bernard–Soulier syndrome** is an uncommon, autosomal disease that is distinguished by very large platelets (as large as 7 μm in diameter) that do not possess enough GPIb integrin molecules in their plasma membrane. Because of this defect, the platelets cannot form bonds with von Willebrand factor and, therefore, cannot form a primary hemostatic plug, resulting in exceptionally severe bleeding.
4. **Glanzmann's thrombasthenia** is also an uncommon bleeding disorder, an autosomal recessive trait, where the platelets of affected individuals possess defective **glycoprotein IIb/IIIa (GpIIb/IIIa)**. Since this platelet plasmalemma integrin molecule is responsible for binding to fibrinogen and thereby ensuring that platelets of a primary hemostatic plug adhere to each other, a defect in the integrin molecule prevents the formation of a **primary hemostatic plug**. Since hemostasis is not controlled properly, severe bleeding may occur with consequent death of the affected individual.

IV. BONE MARROW

A. **Yellow marrow** is located in the long bones of adults and is highly infiltrated with fat. It is **not** hemopoietic, but it has the potential to become so if necessary.

B. In adults, **red marrow** is located in the epiphyses of long bones and in flat, irregular, and short bones (Figure 10.2). It is highly vascular and composed of a **stroma**, irregular **sinusoids**, and islands of **hemopoietic cells**. Red marrow is the site of blood cell **differentiation** and **maturation**. The largest cells of bone marrow are the **megakaryocytes** (Figure 10.2), precursors of platelets.
   1. **Sinusoids** are large venous vessels with highly attenuated (very thin) endothelia. They are associated on their extravascular surfaces with reticular fibers and **adventitial reticular cells**, which manufacture these fibers.
   2. **Stromal cells** include macrophages, adventitial reticular cells, fibroblasts, and endothelial cells. These cells produce and release various **hemopoietic growth factors** (see Table 10.7).
      a. **Macrophages** are located in extravascular areas near sinusoids and extend processes between endothelial cells into sinusoidal lumina. These cells phagocytose cast off cytoplasm and extruded nuclei and also transfer iron to differentiating cells of the red blood cell lineage.
      b. **Adventitial reticular cells** (Figure 10.2) are believed to subdivide the bone marrow cavity into smaller compartments, which are occupied by **islands of hemopoietic cells**. Adventitial reticular cells may accumulate fat (instead of fat cells), thus transforming red marrow into yellow marrow.

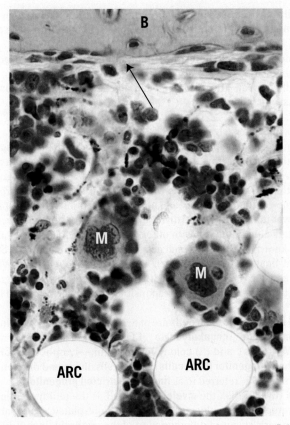

FIGURE 10.2. Light micrograph of a cross section of a human rib displaying its bone marrow. B, bone; M, megakaryocytes; ARC, adventitial reticular cells; *arrow*, endosteum (×540).

V. PRENATAL HEMOPOIESIS

This process occurs successively in the yolk sac, liver, spleen, and bone marrow.

A. The bone marrow first participates in hemopoiesis at about 6 months' gestation and assumes an increasingly large role thereafter.

B. The liver and spleen cease hemopoiesis at about the time of birth.

VI. POSTNATAL HEMOPOIESIS

This process involves three classes of cells: **stem, progenitor**, and **precursor cells**.

A. Comparison of stem, progenitor, and precursor cells
   1. **Stem cells** are capable of **self-renewal** and can undergo enormous proliferation.
      a. These cells can differentiate into **multiple** cell lineages.
      b. They are present in circulation (as null cells) and in bone marrow.

2. **Progenitor cells** have reduced potentiality and are committed to a single-cell lineage.
   a. They **proliferate** and **differentiate** into precursor cells in the presence of appropriate growth factors.
   b. They are morphologically indistinguishable from stem cells, and both appear similar to small lymphocytes.
3. **Precursor cells** are all the cells in each lineage that display **distinct morphological characteristics**.

B. Initial steps in blood formation (stem cells)
   1. **PHSCs** (also known as **hemopoietic stem cells [HSCs]**) give rise to **multipotential hemopoietic stem cells** in the bone marrow. Although PHSC cannot be recognized by their morphology, they *possess certain cell membrane markers* that assist in their recognition: **CD34** (permits adherence of this cell to other cells as well as to the extracellular matrix), **CD59** (inhibits the formation of the complement cascade known as membrane attack complex), **CD133** (whose function is as yet unknown), **Thy1** (thymocyte antigen 1, also known as **CD90**, is believed to function in interaction of the cell with other cells and with the extracellular matrix), and **C-kit receptor** (also known as **CD117**), which acts as a receptor molecule for **Stem Cell Factor** (also known as **C-kit ligand** and **steel factor**), and are *negative for other cell membrane markers* which further assist in their recognition: **lin** (lineage markers present on cells committed to a certain line of blood cells) and **CD38** (responsible for the mechanism of intracellular Ca^{2+} ion regulation).
   2. **Multipotential hemopoietic stem cells** are of two types: (1) **colony-forming unit—granulocyte, erythrocyte, monocyte, megakaryocyte (CFU-GEMM** also known as **common myeloid progenitor [GMP] cells)**, and (2) colony-forming unit—lymphocyte (**CFU-Ly**, also known as **common lymphoid progenitor [CLP] cells**). These cells divide and differentiate in bone marrow to form progenitor cells, referred to as **lineage-restricted progenitors**.
      a. **CFU-GEMM (GMP cells)**, the **myeloid stem cell**, is the multipotential stem cell that gives rise to erythrocytes, granulocytes, monocytes, and platelets. Probably, **Hox 2 genes** are active in the early stages of differentiation of the erythroid lines, and **Hox 1 genes** may be active in the early stages of differentiation of granulocytes, monocytes, and platelets.
      b. **CFU-Ly (CLP cells)**, the **lymphoid stem cell**, is the multipotential stem cell that gives rise to T and B lymphocytes and NK cells.

C. Erythrocyte formation (erythropoiesis) begins with the formation of two types of progenitor cells: **burst-forming unit—erythroid (BFU-E)**, derived from CFU-GEMM (GMP) under the influence of erythropoietin, IL-3 and IL-4, and **colony-forming unit—erythroid (CFU-E)**, which arises from BFU-E. Erythropoiesis yields about 1 trillion RBCs daily in a normal adult. **Erythropoietin receptors** on the surface of cells destined for the erythrocytic lineage bind erythropoietin activating a kinase, known as **Janus kinase 2 (JAK2)**, which is attached to the receptor's intracellular moiety. An intracellular protein, known as **signal transducer and activator of transcription 5 (STAT 5)**, binds to JAK2 and becomes phosphorylated. The process of phosphorylation activates the protein, and it becomes associated with another STAT 5, forming an activated dimer. The activated dimer is released from JAK2, enters the nucleus, and activates the genes that trigger erythropoiesis.
   1. **Erythroid progenitor cells**
      a. **BFU-E** has a high rate of mitotic activity and responds to high concentrations of **erythropoietin**.
      b. **CFU-E** responds to low concentrations of erythropoietin and gives rise to the first histologically recognizable erythrocyte precursor, the **proerythroblast**.
   2. **Erythrocyte precursor cells** include a series of cell types (the **erythroid series**) that differentiate sequentially to form mature erythrocytes (Table 10.5 and Figure 10.3).

D. Granulocyte formation begins with the production of three unipotential or bipotential cells, all of which are descendants of **CFU-GEMM (GMP)**. The process of forming CFU-GEMM from **PHSCs** requires high levels of **PU.1 transcription factor**, a protein that has an affinity for purine-rich segments of DNA present in the vicinity of promoter genes. By attaching to the purine-rich segment, the promoter gene is activated and PHSCs differentiate into GEMM cells. Other cytokines

table 10.5 Selected Characteristics of Erythrocyte Precursor Cells

Characteristic	Proerythroblast	Basophilic Erythroblast	Polychromatophilic Erythroblast (Normoblast)	Orthochromatophilic Erythroblast	Reticulocyte
Nucleus shape	Round	Round	Round and small	Round	None
Color*	Burgundy red	Burgundy red	Dense blue	Dark, may be extruding	None
Chromatin network	Very fine	Fine	Coarse	Pyknotic	None
Number of nucleoli	3–5 (very pale gray)	1–2	None	None	None
Mitosis	Yes	Yes	Yes	No	No
Cytoplasmic color*	Pale gray with blue clumps	Grayish pink with intensely blue clumps	Yellowish pink with bluish background	Pink with trace of blue	Pink†
Hemoglobin	None (ferritin is present)	Some	Abundant	Abundant	Abundant

*Cells stained with Giemsa or Wright stain.
†Cells stained supravitally with brilliant cresyl blue display a reticulum.

(see Table 10.7), such as **granulocyte–monocyte colony-stimulating factor** (**GM-CSF**), **granulocyte colony-stimulating factor** (**G-CSF**), and **interleukin 3** (**IL-3**), are responsible for the formation of granulocytes. The additional presence of **interleukin 5** (**IL-5**) directs the differentiation toward the

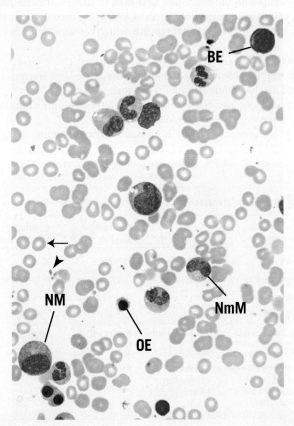

FIGURE 10.3. Light micrograph of a human bone marrow smear. BE, basophilic erythroblast; NM, neutrophilic myelocyte; NmM, neutrophilic metamyelocyte; OE, orthochromatophilic erythroblast; (*arrow*) erythrocyte; (*arrowhead*) platelet. Wright stain (×540).

eosinophil line, whereas if IL-5 is not present, the differentiation proceeds toward the formation of basophils. Granulocyte formation yields about 1 million granulocytes daily in a normal adult.

1. **Granulocyte progenitor** cells give rise to histologically identical **myeloblasts** and **promyelocytes** in all three cell lineages.
   a. **Colony-forming unit—eosinophil (CFU-Eo)** is the progenitor of the **eosinophil** lineage.
   b. **Colony-forming unit—basophil (CFU-Ba)** is the progenitor of the **basophil** lineage.
   c. **Colony-forming unit—granulocyte–monocyte (CFU-GM)**, the common progenitor of **neutrophils** and **monocytes**, gives rise to **CFU-G** (granulocyte, specifically neutrophil) and **CFU-M** (monocyte).
2. **Granulocyte precursor cells** are histologically similar in the early stages of all three lineages (myeloblasts and promyelocytes). They develop characteristic granules unique to each cell type during the myelocyte stage and a distinctive nuclear shape during the stab (band) stage (Table 10.6 and Figure 10.3).

E. **Monocyte formation (CFU-M)** begins with the common progenitor colony-forming unit–neutrophil–monocyte (CFU-NM) and involves only two precursor cells: **monoblasts** and **promonocytes**. Monocyte formation yields about 10 trillion monocytes daily in a normal adult.

1. **Promonocytes** are reported to be large cells (16–18 μm in diameter) and contain a kidney-shaped acentric nucleus, numerous azurophilic granules, an extensive rough endoplasmic reticulum (RER) and Golgi complex, and many mitochondria. They undergo cell division and subsequently develop into **monocytes**.
2. **Monocytes** leave the bone marrow to enter the circulation. From the bloodstream, they enter connective tissue, where they **differentiate into macrophages**.

F. **Platelet formation** begins with the progenitor **CFU-Meg** (also known as **megakaryocyte-committed progenitor [MKP] cells**), which arises from CFU-GEMM and involves a single precursor cell (the **megakaryoblast**), and the mature **megakaryocyte**, which remains in the bone marrow and sheds platelets.

1. **Megakaryoblasts**
   a. These large cells (25–40 μm in diameter) have a single large nucleus that may be indented or lobed and displays a fine chromatin network.
   b. Their basophilic, nongranular cytoplasm contains large mitochondria, many polysomes, some RER, and a large Golgi complex.
   c. Under the influence of the hormone **thrombopoietin**, megakaryoblasts divide endomitotically (i.e., no daughter cells are formed) and enlarge; the ploidy of the nucleus increases to as much as 64 N, giving rise to megakaryocytes.

t a b l e 10.6 Selected Characteristics of Neutrophil Precursor Cells

Characteristic	Myeloblast	Promyelocyte	Neutrophilic Myelocyte	Neutrophilic Metamyelocyte	Neutrophilic Stab Cell
Cell diameter (μm)	12–14	16–24	10–12	10–12	11–12
Nucleus shape	Large, round	Large, round	Flat (acentric)	Kidney (acentric)	Horseshoe
Color*	Reddish blue	Reddish blue	Blue to dark blue	Dark blue	Dark blue
Chromatin network	Very fine	Fine	Coarse	Very coarse	Very coarse
Number of nucleoli	2 or 3 (pale gray)	1 or 2 (pale gray)	Perhaps 1	None	None
Mitosis	Yes	Yes	Yes	No	No
Cytoplasmic appearance*	Blue clumps in pale blue background, cytoplasmic blebs at cell periphery	Bluish hue, no cytoplasmic blebs	Pale blue	Blue	Similar to mature neutrophils
Granules	None	Azurophilic	Azurophilic and specific	Azurophilic and specific	Azurophilic and specific

*Cells stained with Giemsa or Wright stain.

2. **Megakaryocytes**
   a. These extremely large cells (40–100 μm in diameter) have a single large **polypoid** nucleus that is highly indented (Figure 10.2).
   b. They possess a well-developed Golgi complex associated with the formation of α-granules, lysosomes, and dense bodies (δ-granules); they also contain many mitochondria and an extensive RER.
   c. Megakaryocytes lie just outside the sinusoids in the bone marrow and form **platelet demarcation channels**, which fragment into proplatelets (clusters of adhering platelets) or single platelets that are released into the sinusoidal lumen.

G. **Lymphocyte formation (lymphopoiesis)** begins with differentiation of **CFU-Ly (CLP)**, the lymphoid stem cell, into the **immunoincompetent** progenitor cells **CFU-LyB** and **CFU-LyT**. This step requires the presence of medium concentrations of **transcription factor PU.1** as well as intranuclear zinc finger transcription factors such as the **Ikaros family of transcription factors**. These zinc finger proteins have protruding hairpin-like extensions, maintained by zinc and iron ions that fit into grooves in the promoter or other regulatory regions of the DNA molecule and, thereby, activate or inhibit a particular gene. (It should be noted that zinc finger proteins bind not only to DNA but also to RNA, proteins, as well as to lipids.)

These **prelymphocytes** are processed and become mature immunocompetent cells.
1. **B lymphocyte (B-cell) maturation**
   a. Requires the presence of **Pax5** transcription factor.
   b. Pre-B lymphocytes acquire cell surface markers, including membrane-bound **antibodies**, which confer **immunocompetence**.
   c. In mammals, B-cell maturation occurs in the bone marrow, whereas in birds it occurs in the bursa of Fabricius (hence, **B** lymphocytes).
2. **T-lymphocyte (T-cell) maturation**
   a. Requires the presence of GATA-3 transcription factor.
   b. Progenitor T lymphocytes migrate to the **thymic cortex**, where they acquire cell surface markers, including **T-cell receptors,** which confer **immunocompetence**.
   c. Most of the newly formed T lymphocytes are destroyed in the cortex of the thymus and do not enter into circulation.
3. **Mature B and T lymphocytes** leave the bone marrow and thymus, respectively, and circulate to peripheral organs (e.g., the lymph nodes and spleen) to establish **clones** of immunocompetent lymphocytes (see Chapter 12).

VII. HEMOPOIETIC GROWTH FACTORS (CSFS)

A. **Hemopoiesis** is modulated by several **growth factors** and **cytokines**, including CSFs, stem cell factor (steel factor), interleukins, and macrophage-inhibiting protein-α (Table 10.7). **Stem cell factor** is probably the most important of the CSFs because it must be present to maintain a large enough population of PHSCs as well as multipotential hemopoietic stem cells and progenitor cells.

B. These factors may circulate in the bloodstream, acting as hormones, or they may act as local factors produced in the bone marrow that facilitate and stimulate formation of blood cells in their vicinity.

C. They act at low concentrations and bind to specific membrane receptors on single target cells.

D. Their various effects on target cells include control of mitotic rate, enhancement of cell survival, control of the number of times the cells divide before they differentiate, and promotion of cell differentiation.

E. **Hemopoietic stem cells** that do not contact growth factors, especially Stem Cell Factor, usually enter **apoptosis** and are eliminated by **macrophages**.

t a b l e 10.7	Hemopoietic Growth Factors	
Factors	**Principal Action of the Factor**	**Site of Origin of the Factor**
Stem cell factor	Facilitates hemopoiesis	Stromal cells of bone marrow
GM-CSF	Facilitates CFU-GM mitosis, differentiation, granulocyte activity	T cells, endothelial cells
G-CSF	Induces mitosis, differentiation of CFU-G; facilitates neutrophil activity	Macrophages, endothelial cells
M-CSF	Facilitates mitosis, differentiation of CFU-M	Macrophages, endothelial cells
IL-1 (IL-3, IL-6)	Facilitates proliferation of PHSC, CFU-S, CFU-Ly; suppresses erythroid precursors	Monocytes, macrophages, endothelial cells
IL-2	Promotes proliferation of activated T cells, B cells; facilitates NK cell differentiation	Activated T cells
IL-3	Same as IL-1; also facilitates proliferation of unipotential precursors except LyB and LyT	Activated T and B cells
IL-4	Promotes activation of T cells, B cells; facilitates development of mast cells, basophils	Activated T cells
IL-5	Facilitates proliferation of CFU-Eo; activates eosinophils	T cells
IL-6	Same as IL-1; also promotes differentiation of CTLs and B cells	Monocyte, fibroblasts
IL-7	Stimulates CFU-LyB and NK cell differentiation	Adventitial reticular cells?
IL-8	Promotes migration and degranulation of neutrophils	Leukocytes, endothelial cells, smooth muscle cells
IL-9	Promotes activation, proliferation of mast cells, modulates immunoglobulin E synthesis, stimulates proliferation of T helper cells	T helper cells
IL-10	Inhibits synthesis of cytokines by NK cells, macrophages, T cells; promotes CTL differentiation and B cell and mast cell proliferation	Macrophages, T cells
IL-12	Stimulates NK cells; promotes CTL and NK cell function	Macrophages
γ-Interferons	Activates monocytes, B cells; promotes CTL differentiation; enhances expression of class II human leukocyte antigen	T cells, NK cells
Erythropoietin	Promotes CFU-E differentiation, proliferation of burst-forming unit—erythroid	Endothelial cells of peritubular capillary network of kidney, hepatocytes
Thrombopoietin	Enhances mitosis, differentiation of CFU-Meg and megakaryoblasts	Hepatocytes and kidney cells

CFU, colony-forming unit; CSF, colony-stimulating factor; PHSC, pluripotential hemopoietic stem cell; CTL, cytotoxic lymphocyte; Eo, eosinophil; G, granulocyte; GM, granulocyte–monocyte; IL, interleukin; Ly, lymphocyte; M, monocyte; Meg, megakaryocyte; NK, natural killer; S, spleen.
Modified with permission from Gartner LP, Hiatt JL. *Color Textbook of Histology.* 2nd ed. Philadelphia, PA: Saunders; 2001.

Review Test

Directions: Each of the numbered items or incomplete statements in this section is followed by answers or completions of the statement. Select the ONE lettered answer that is BEST in each case.

1. Which of the following proteins associated with the erythrocyte plasma membrane is responsible for maintaining the cell's biconcave disk shape?

(A) HbA_1
(B) HbA_2
(C) Porphyrin
(D) Spectrin
(E) α-Actinin

2. Which of the following is an immunocompetent cell?

(A) Red blood cell
(B) Lymphocyte
(C) Platelet
(D) Neutrophil
(E) Basophil

3. Which of the following is derived from CFU-Meg (MKP cells)?

(A) Red blood cell
(B) Lymphocyte
(C) Platelet
(D) Neutrophil
(E) Basophil

4. Which of the following is derived from CFU-E?

(A) Red blood cell
(B) Lymphocyte
(C) Platelet
(D) Neutrophil
(E) Basophil

5. Which of the following is derived from CFU-GM?

(A) Red blood cell
(B) Lymphocyte
(C) Platelet
(D) Neutrophil
(E) Basophil

6. Which of the following is associated with demarcation channels?

(A) Red blood cell
(B) Lymphocyte
(C) Platelet
(D) Neutrophil
(E) Basophil

7. Which of the following is derived from myeloblasts?

(A) Red blood cell
(B) Lymphocyte
(C) Platelet
(D) Monocyte
(E) Basophil

8. Which one of the following cells is associated with antibody production?

(A) Red blood cell
(B) Lymphocyte
(C) Monocyte
(D) Neutrophil
(E) Basophil

9. Which of the following possesses specific and azurophilic granules?

(A) Red blood cell
(B) Lymphocyte
(C) Platelet
(D) Neutrophil
(E) Monocyte

10. Which of the following is derived from reticulocytes?

(A) Red blood cell
(B) Lymphocyte
(C) Platelet
(D) Neutrophil
(E) Basophil

11. A 4-year-old boy is taken by his parents to the pediatrician because of vomiting, headaches, and tenderness in the bones of his arms and legs. On palpation, the physician notes that many lymph nodes are enlarged, as is the liver. The pediatrician should order a complete blood count in order to determine whether or not the child may have

(A) chronic leukemia.
(B) infectious mononucleosis.
(C) von Willebrand disease.
(D) acute leukemia.
(E) pernicious anemia.

Answers and Explanations

1. **D.** Spectrin is associated with the erythrocyte cell membrane and assists in maintaining its biconcave disk shape (see Chapter 10 II B).

2. **B.** Lymphocytes are immunocompetent cells (see Chapter 10 VI G).

3. **C.** Platelets are derived from CFU-Meg (MKP cells) (see Chapter 10 VI F).

4. **A.** Red blood cells are derived from CFU-E (see Chapter 10 VI C).

5. **D.** Neutrophils are derived from CFU-GM (see Chapter 10 VI D).

6. **C.** Platelets are derived from megakaryocytes, and those cells possess demarcation channels (see Chapter 10 VI F).

7. **E.** Basophils are derived from myeloblasts (see Chapter 10 VI D).

8. **C.** Lymphocytes and plasma cells manufacture antibodies (see Chapter 10 VI G).

9. **D.** Neutrophils possess both azurophilic and specific granules (see Chapter 10 II B 2).

10. **A.** Red blood cells are derived from reticulocytes (see Table 10.5).

11. **D.** Acute leukemia is a disease of children with symptoms that include headaches; vomiting; swollen lymph nodes, liver, and spleen; and the sensation of tenderness in bones. Chronic leukemia is a disease that usually affects adults. von Willebrand disease is a coagulation disorder and does not have the same symptoms as acute leukemia. Infectious mononucleosis affects mostly young adults of high school and college age. Pernicious anemia is caused by vitamin B deficiency, and its symptoms do not resemble those of acute leukemia (see Chapter 10 II B 2 Clinical Considerations).

chapter 11

Circulatory System

I. OVERVIEW—BLOOD VASCULAR SYSTEM

The blood vascular system consists of the heart, arteries, veins, and capillaries. This system transports **oxygen and nutrients to tissues**, carries **carbon dioxide and waste products from the tissues**, and circulates **hormones** from the site of synthesis to their target cells.

A. The **heart** is a four-chambered pump composed of two **atria** and two **ventricles** and is surrounded by a fibroserous sac called the **pericardium**.

CLINICAL CONSIDERATIONS **Tetralogy of Fallot**

Tetralogy of Fallot is a **congenital malformation** consisting of a defective interventricular septum, hypertrophy of the right ventricle (due to a narrow pulmonary artery or valve), and transposed (dextroposed) aorta. It should be **repaired surgically** early in life, before the pulmonary constriction becomes exacerbated.

B. Atria are receiving chambers, whereas ventricles are discharging chambers. Moreover, the heart is divided functionally into the right heart (**pulmonary system**) and the left heart (**systemic system**). The right atrium receives venous blood from the body and discharges it into the right ventricle. From here the blood is pumped into the pulmonary trunk to be distributed to the lungs. Venous blood from the pulmonary system is received in the left atrium and then discharged into the left ventricle to be pumped out through the aorta into the systemic circulation.

The heart receives **sympathetic innervation** via upper thoracic levels of the spinal cord and **parasympathetic innervation** via vagus nerves, which **modulate the rate of the heartbeat** but do not initiate it. The heart (mostly the atria) also produces **atrial natriuretic peptide**, and **B-type natriuretic peptide**, hormones that increases secretion of sodium and water by the kidneys, inhibits renin release, and decreases blood pressure.

- Sympathetic innervation accelerates the heart rate, increases the force of the heartbeat, and dilates the coronary vessels.
- Parasympathetic innervation slows the heart rate, reduces the force of the heartbeat, and constricts the coronary vessels.

1. **Cardiac layers** (from internal to external)
   a. **Endocardium** lines the lumen of the heart and is composed of simple squamous epithelium (**endothelium**) and a thin layer of loose connective tissue. **Subendocardium**, a connective tissue layer that contains veins, nerves, and Purkinje fibers, underlies it.

    b. **Myocardium** consists of layers of striated **cardiac muscle cells** arranged in a spiral fashion about the heart's chambers and inserted into the fibrous skeleton. The myocardium contracts to propel blood into the arteries for distribution to the body.

    c. **Epicardium**, the outermost layer of the heart, constitutes the **visceral layer of the pericardium**. It is composed of simple squamous epithelium (**mesothelium**) on the external surface. Beneath the mesothelium lies fibroelastic connective tissue, containing nerves, the coronary vessels, and adipose tissue.

2. The **fibrous skeleton of the heart** consists of thick bundles of **collagen fibers** oriented in various directions and especially oriented to support the four valve rings of the heart valves. It also contains occasional foci of fibrocartilage.

3. **Heart valves**

    a. **Atrioventricular (AV)** valves are composed of a skeleton of fibrous connective tissue, arranged like an aponeurosis, and lined on both sides by endothelium. They are attached to the **annuli fibrosi** of the fibrous skeleton. The right AV valve is formed of three interlocking cusps **(tricuspid valve)**, whereas the left AV valve is formed of two interlocking cusps (**bicuspid or mitral valve**). These valves prevent regurgitation of ventricular blood into the atria.

    b. **Semilunar valves** in the pulmonary and aortic trunks are each composed of three cusps that approximate each other as they fill with arterial blood. They are lined with endothelium on both sides separated by sparse strands of connective tissue. These valves prevent regurgitation of pulmonary and aortic blood into the respective ventricles.

CLINICAL CONSIDERATIONS Rheumatic heart valve disease is a **sequel to childhood rheumatic fever** (subsequent to streptococcal infection), which causes scarring of the heart valves.

1. The disease is characterized by reduced elasticity of the heart valves, making them unable to close (**incompetence**) or unable open (**stenosis**) properly.

2. It most commonly affects the **mitral valve**, followed by the aortic valve.

---

4. The **impulse-generating and impulse-conducting system** of the heart comprises several specialized structures with coordinated functions that act to **initiate and regulate the heartbeat**.

    a. The **sinoatrial (SA) node**, the **pacemaker** of the heart, is composed of specialized cardiac cells located within the wall of the right atrium adjacent to the entry of the superior vena cava into the heart. It **generates impulses** that initiate contraction of atrial muscle cells; which are then conducted to the AV node.

    b. The **AV node** is located in the wall of the right atrium, adjacent to the tricuspid valve.

    c. The **AV bundle of His** is a band of conducting tissue radiating from the AV node into the interventricular septum, where it divides into two branches and continues as Purkinje fibers.

    d. **Purkinje fibers** are large, modified cardiac muscle cells (see Chapter 8 V B 9) that make contact with cardiac muscle cells at the apex of the heart via gap junctions, desmosomes, and fasciae adherentes.

    e. As indicated (in Section I B of the current chapter), the autonomic nervous system modulates the heart rate and stroke volume.

CLINICAL CONSIDERATIONS Cardiac arrest occurs when the heart ceases to beat, resulting in cessation of blood flow in the entire circulatory system. Cardiac death is imminenet unless cardiopulmonary resuscitation and defibrillation are conducted successfully and the electrical system of the heart is revived. Health conditions that may lead to cardiac arrest include, but are not limited to, tachycardia, fibrillation, and bradycardia.

table **11.1** Comparison of Tunicae in Different Types of Arteries

Tunica Components	Elastic Arteries	Muscular Arteries	Arterioles	Metarterioles
Intima				
Endothelium	+	+	+	+
Factor VIII in endothelium	+	+	+	−
Basal lamina	+	+	+	+
Subendothelial layer*	+	+	±	−
Internal elastic lamina	Incomplete	Thick, complete	Some elastic fibers	−
Media				
Fenestrated elastic membranes	40–70	−	−	−
Smooth muscle cells	Interspersed between elastic membranes	≤40 layers	1 or 2 layers	Discontinuous layer
External elastic lamina	Thin	Thick	−	−
Vasa vasorum	±	−	−	−
Adventitia				
Fibroelastic connective tissue	Thin layer	Thin layer	−	−
Loose connective tissue	−	−	+	±
Vasa vasorum	+	±	−	−
Lymphatic vessels	+	+	−	−
Nerve fibers	+	+	+	−

+, present and prominent; ±, present but not prominent; −, absent.
*In elastic arteries, the subendothelial layer is composed of loose connective tissue containing fibroblasts, collagen, and elastic fibers. In arterioles, this layer is less prominent; the connective tissue is sparse and contains a few reticular fibers.

C. **Arteries** conduct blood **away from the heart** to the organs and tissues. Arterial walls are composed of three layers (tunicae): the **tunica intima** (inner), **tunica media** (middle), and **tunica adventitia** (outer). Components of these layers and variations among types of arteries are summarized in Table 11.1.

1. **Types of arteries**
   a. **Elastic arteries (conducting arteries)** are large and include the **aorta** and its **major branches** (Figures 11.1 and 11.2).
      (1) Elastic arteries help **reduce changes in blood pressure** associated with the heartbeat.
      (2) Small vessels (**vasa vasorum**) and nerves are located in their tunicae adventitia and media. The vasa vasorum vascularizes the walls of the elastic arteries.
      (3) Thick, concentric sheaths of **elastic membranes**, known as **fenestrated membranes**, are located in the tunica media.
   b. **Muscular arteries** (distributing arteries) distribute blood to various organs.
      (1) They include most of the **named** arteries of the human body.
      (2) These medium-sized arteries are smaller than elastic arteries but larger than arterioles.
      (3) The tunica adventitia contains vasa vasorum.
      (4) The tunica media is thick, composed of layers of smooth muscle cells. Larger muscular arteries possess an **external elastic lamina** separating their boundary with the tunica adventitia (Figure 11.3).
      (5) The tunica intima is characterized by its endothelium and a prominent subendothelial **internal elastic lamina**.

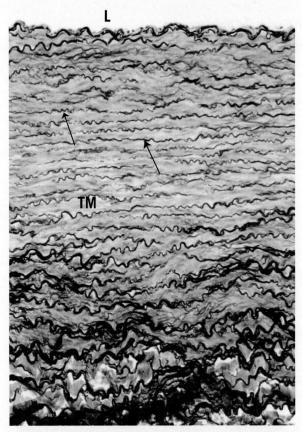

FIGURE 11.1. Light micrograph of the aorta (elastic stain) (×132). Observe the wavy elastic fibers (*arrows*) located in the tunica media (TM). Note the lumen (L) located at the top of the micrograph.

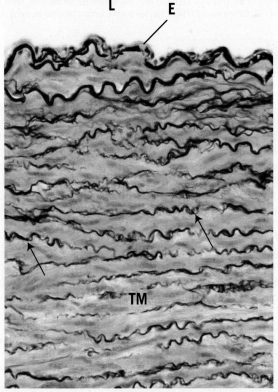

FIGURE 11.2. A light micrograph of the aorta (with elastic stain) at a higher magnification (×270). Observe the endothelial layer (E) adjacent to the lumen (L), Note that the tunica media (TM) contains an abundance of elastic fibers (*arrows*).

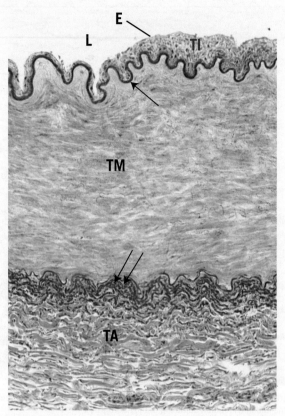

FIGURE 11.3. Light micrograph of an artery (×132). Observe the lumen (L), endothelial layer (E), internal elastic lamina (*single arrow*), tunica intima (TI), tunica media (TM), external elastic lamina (*double arrows*), and tunica adventitia (TA).

CLINICAL CONSIDERATIONS   Atherosclerosis

Atherosclerosis is the most frequent cause of morbidity of the vascular diseases. It is characterized by deposits of yellowish plaques (**atheromas**) in the intima of large and medium-sized arteries. The plaques may block blood flow to the region supplied by the affected artery. Continued deposits form plaques that reduce the lumina of the vessels, and the patient may feel referred pain and pressure. Sustained narrowing results in ischemia or complete blockage, which may be fatal if untreated. Major vessels affected by atherosclerosis include terminals of the coronary arteries, larger branches of the carotid arteries, cerebral arteries, large arteries of the lower extremities, renal arteries, and mesenteric arteries. Atherosclerosis of the cerebral arteries is the major cause of stroke (brain infarct). Other atheroscleroses affect the heart (see the section on ischemic heart disease), ischemic bowel disease, and renal arterial ischemia.

Ischemic (coronary) heart disease

Ischemic heart disease is usually caused by **coronary atherosclerosis,** which results in decreased blood flow to the myocardium. It may result (depending on its severity) in angina pectoris, myocardial infarction, chronic ischemic cardiopathy, or sudden cardiac death. Angioplasty is the current mode of treatment for partially clogged arteries, and bypass surgery is necessary for severely clogged arteries.

---

   c. **Arterioles** (10–100 μm in diameter) regulate blood pressure and are the terminal arterial vessels. They are the **smallest** arteries, with diameters of less than 0.1 mm and a narrow lumen; their luminal diameter usually equals the wall thickness.
      (1) The tunica adventitia is scant, whereas the tunica media consists of up to two layers of smooth muscle.
      (2) The tunica intima consists of an endothelium, basal lamina, and scant connective tissue.

d. Metarterioles (~8 μm in diameter) are narrow vessels arising from arterioles that give rise to **capillaries**.

(1) They are surrounded by incomplete rings of smooth muscle cells and possess individual smooth muscle cells (**precapillary sphincters**) that surround capillaries at their origin.

(2) Constriction of precapillary sphincters prevents blood from entering the capillary bed.

CLINICAL CONSIDERATIONS   **Arteriosclerosis**

Arteriosclerosis is characterized by rigidity and hyaline thickening of the blood vessel walls. It may involve the media of medium-sized arteries and eventual calcification in the media. Hyaline thickening usually attacks small arteries and arterioles in the kidneys and is usually associated with hypertension and diabetes mellitus.

---

2. **Vasoconstriction** primarily involves **arterioles** and reduces blood flow to a local region. Vasoconstriction is stimulated by **sympathetic nerve fibers** (see Chapter 9 IX B) via vasomotor nerves. These nerves do not synapse on the muscle cells of the tunica media; rather they discharge the neurotransmitter norepinephrine that diffuses throughout the muscle layer and induces contraction of cells via gap junctions that reduce luminal diameter.

3. **Vasodilation** is accomplished by **parasympathetic nerve fibers** as follows:

   a. Acetylcholine released from these nerve terminals stimulates the endothelium to release **nitric oxide**, previously known as endothelial-derived relaxing factor (EDRF).

   b. **Nitric oxide** diffuses to smooth muscle cells in the vessel wall and activates their cyclic guanosine monophosphate (cGMP) system, resulting in relaxation, which dilates the lumen.

CLINICAL CONSIDERATIONS   **Aneurysm is a ballooning out of an artery.**

1. An aneurysm occurs because of a weakness in the arterial or venous wall, which may result in rupture. Arterial aneurysms may result from age-related displacement of elastic fibers by collagen.

2. Aneurysms may be associated with **atherosclerosis** and **syphilis**. Atherosclerosis, especially of the abdominal aorta, may be due to genetic connective tissue disorders such as Marfan syndrome or Ehlers–Danlos syndrome (see Chapter 4, III A Clinical Considerations).

3. Dissecting aneurysms are most often located in the ascending aorta and are represented by a longitudinal tear in the wall characterized by tearing of the elastic and muscular tissues, resulting in rupture into the pericardial sac.

4. These conditions can be life-threatening because a weakness in an arterial wall may cause the artery to burst.

D. **Capillaries** are small vessels (about 8–10 μm in diameter and usually less than 1 mm long). Capillaries exhibit **selective permeability**, permitting the exchange of oxygen, carbon dioxide, metabolites, nutrients, metabolic wastes, signaling molecules, hormones, and other substances between the blood and tissues. They form **capillary beds** interposed between arterioles and venules.

1. **Capillary endothelial cells—General features.** Capillaries consist of a **single layer of endothelial cells** arranged as a continuum to form a cylinder, which is surrounded by a basal lamina and occasional **pericytes** (see Chapter 6 III A.2). Endothelial cells

   a. are nucleated, polygonal cells with an attenuated cytoplasm.

   b. possess a Golgi complex, ribosomes, mitochondria, and some rough endoplasmic reticulum (RER).

   c. contain intermediate filaments of **desmin**, **vimentin**, or both in the perinuclear zone; these filaments have a supportive function.

   d. are generally joined by **fasciae occludentes** (tight junctions); some desmosomes and gap junctions also are present. Characteristically, they contain pinocytotic vesicles.

   e. luminal diameter sometimes accommodates only one red blood cell at a time.

2. **Classification of capillaries.** There are three types of capillaries, depending on the structure of their endothelial cells and the continuity of the basal lamina (Figure 11.4).

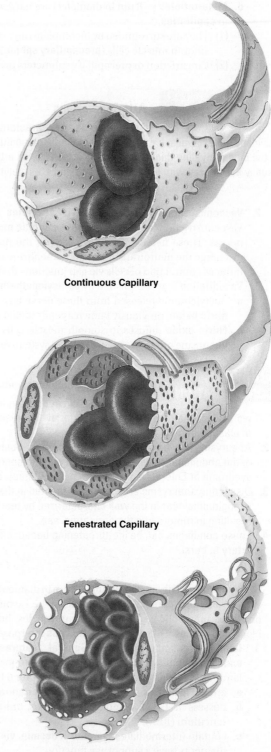

Continuous Capillary

Fenestrated Capillary

Capillaries consists of a simple squamous epithelium rolled into a narrow cylinder 8–10 μm in diameter. **Continuous (somatic) capillaries** have no fenestrae; material transverses the endothelial cell in either direction via **pinocytotic vesicles**. **Fenestrated (visceral) capillaries** are characterized by the presence of perforations, **fenestrae**, 60–80 μm in diameter, which may or may not be bridged by a diaphragm. **Sinusoidal capillaries** have a large lumen (30–40 μm in diameter), possess numerous fenestrae, have discontinuous basal lamina, and lack pinocytotic vesicles. Frequently, adjacent endothelial cells of sinusoidal capillaries overlap one another in an incomplete fashion.

Sinusoidal (Discontinuous) Capillary

FIGURE 11.4. The three types of capillaries. (Reprinted with permission from Gartner LP, Hiatt JL. *Color Atlas of Histology*. Baltimore, MD: Lippincott Williams & Wilkins; 2009:163.)

    a. Continuous (somatic) capillaries contain numerous **pinocytotic vesicles** except in the central nervous system (CNS), where they contain only a limited number of pinocytotic vesicles (a property that is partly responsible for the blood–brain barrier).

      (1) Continuous capillaries lack fenestrae and have a **continuous** basal lamina.

      (2) They are located in nervous tissue, muscle, connective tissue, exocrine glands, and the lungs.

    b. Fenestrated (visceral) capillaries are formed from endothelial cells that are perforated with **fenestrae**. These openings are 60 to 80 nm in diameter and are **bridged by a diaphragm** thinner than a cell membrane; in the renal glomerulus, the fenestrae are larger and lack a diaphragm.

      (1) Fenestrated capillaries have a **continuous** basal lamina and few pinocytotic vesicles.

      (2) They are located in endocrine glands, the intestine, the pancreas, and the glomeruli of kidneys.

    c. Sinusoidal capillaries (sinusoids) possess many large **fenestrae that lack diaphragms**.

      (1) Sinusoidal capillaries are 30 to 40 µm in diameter, much larger than continuous and fenestrated capillaries.

      (2) Sinusoidal capillaries have a **discontinuous** basal lamina and lack pinocytotic vesicles.

      (3) Gaps may be present at the cell junctions, permitting leakage between endothelial cells.

      (4) They are located in the liver, spleen, bone marrow, lymph nodes, and adrenal cortex.

3. Permeability of capillaries is dependent on the morphology of their endothelial cells and on the size, charge, and shape of the traversing molecules. Permeability is altered during the inflammatory response by **histamine** and **bradykinin**.

    a. Some substances **diffuse**, whereas others are **actively transported** across the plasma membrane of capillary endothelial cells.

    b. Other substances move across capillary walls via **small pores** (intercellular junctions) or **large pores** (fenestrae and pinocytotic vesicles).

    c. Leukocytes leave the bloodstream to enter the tissue spaces by penetrating intercellular junctions. This process is called **diapedesis**.

4. Metabolic functions of capillaries are carried out by the **endothelial cells**, and include the following (see Table 11.2):

    a. Conversion of inactive angiotensin I to active angiotensin II (especially in the lung). This powerful vasoconstrictor also stimulates secretion of aldosterone, a hormone that promotes water retention.

    b. Deactivation of various pharmacologically active substances (e.g., bradykinin, serotonin, thrombin, norepinephrine, prostaglandins).

    c. Breakdown of lipoproteins to yield triglycerides and cholesterol.

    d. Release of prostacyclin, a potent vasodilator and inhibitor of intravascular platelet aggregation.

    e. Release of the relaxing factor **NO** (**nitric oxide**) and contraction factor (**endothelin 1**).

    f. Regulation of transendothelial migration of inflammatory cells (**neutrophils**).

    g. Release of tissue factors responsible for blood coagulation.

5. Blood flow to capillary beds occurs either from **metarterioles** (with precapillary sphincters) or from **terminal arterioles** (Figure 11.5).

    a. Central channels are vessels that traverse a capillary bed and connect arterioles to small venules. Their proximal portion is the **metarteriole** (possessing precapillary sphincters), and their distal portion is the **thoroughfare channel** (with no precapillary sphincter) (see Figure 11.5).

    b. Metarterioles supply blood to the capillary bed, whereas thoroughfare channels receive blood from capillary beds.

6. Arteriovenous shunt (bypassing a capillary bed)

    a. Contraction of precapillary sphincters forces the blood flow from the **metarteriole** directly into the **thoroughfare channel**, thus bypassing the capillary bed and draining into a postcapillary venule.

    b. AV anastomoses are small vessels that directly connect arterioles to venules, bypassing the capillary bed. They function in **thermoregulation**, especially in the skin where they are abundant. These anastomoses also control blood pressure and flow.

table **11.2**   Endothelial Cell Functions

Function	Principal Locations	Mode of Action	Notations
Permeability	Capillaries and postcapillary venules	Paracellular; Transcellular	Between cells; Caveolae, VVO*, diapedesis
Hemostasis promotion	Throughout the vascular system	Release of tissue factor, von Willebrand factor, plasminogen-activator inhibitor, and protease activated receptors	Weibel–Palade bodies house both von Willebrand Factor and tissue factor. If the integrity of the vascular endothelium is compromised, these factors are released in order to form a blood clot and stop the escape of blood from the vessel
Hemostasis inhibition	Throughout the vascular system	Endothelial cells secrete and/or express:Tissue pathway factor inhibitor; thrombomodulin; heparin; plasminogen activator; prostacyclin; nitric oxide; and endothelial protein C receptor	These anticoagulants are always present in the normal, intact endothelium and prevent coagulation to ensure that blood remains in a fluid state
Vasomotor tone	Arterioles	*Vasodilatation*: nitric oxide (NO†), prostacyclin *Vasoconstriction*: endothelins 1, 2, and 3; prostaglandins; thromboxane A$_2$; and angiotensin II	Vasodilator and vasoconstrictor molecules are released in response to local or systemic factors; angiotensin II is produced by the conversion of angiotensin I by the endothelial cell membrane-bound ACE
Thermoregulation	Microcirculation in the dermis and bronchial tree	The close proximity of capillary beds to the surface of the skin and the luminal bronchial surface permits heat exchange with the external environment	Vasoconstriction reduces blood flow into the capillary beds, thus conserving body heat. Vasodilatation increases blood flow into capillary beds, thus releasing body heat
Leukocyte trafficking	Postcapillary (high endothelial venules [HEVs])	L-selectins, chemokine receptor 7, and lymphocyte-associated antigens of lymphocytes interact with peripheral node addressin, chemokine ligand 21, and intercellular adhesion molecules of endothelial cells of HEVs which facilitate the migration of lymphocytes into the stroma of secondary lymphoid organs	Similar method permits the migration of other leukocytes out of postcapillary venules (non-HEVs) during the inflammatory process
Angiogenesis	Throughout the vascular system	Vascular endothelial growth factors released by endothelial cells and angiogenic factors released by tumor cells prompt other endothelial cells as well as pericytes to proliferate and form endothelial tubes that will eventually develop their own tunicae media and adventitia	Repairs vascular damage during wound healing as well as providing for vascularization of growing tumors
Angiotensin II formation	Mostly in lung capillary beds	ACE converts angiotensin I to the potent vascular smooth muscle contractant angiotensin II	Angiotensin II elevates blood pressure, thereby increasing glomerular filtration rate and facilitates additional resorption of sodium from the ultrafiltrate

ACE, angiotensin-converting enzyme.
*VVO—Vesicular–vacuolar organelles are believed to be aggregates of fused caveoli.
†Nitric oxide (NO) was known as endothelial-derived relaxing factor (EDRF); according to some authors, prostacyclin is also considered to be EDRF.

E. **Veins** conduct blood away from the organs and tissues and return it **to the heart**. Veins contain about 70% of the body's total blood volume at any given time. Their walls are composed of three layers: the **tunica intima** (inner), **tunica media** (middle), and **tunica adventitia** (outer), the thickest and most prominent. Vasa vasorum are more numerous in veins than in arteries. A distinct internal elastic lamina is also absent in veins. The components of these layers and the variations among different types of veins are summarized in Table 11.3.

1. **Comparison with arteries.** Veins have thinner walls and larger, more irregular lumina than the companion arteries. They may have valves in their lumina that prevent retrograde flow of the blood (Figure 11.6).

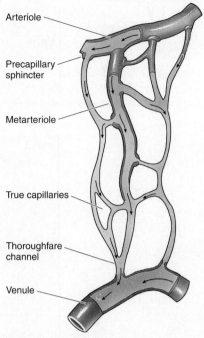

FIGURE 11.5. Blood flow to capillary beds. Some capillary beds, such as those of the skin, can be bypassed under certain circumstances. One method of controlling blood flow is the use of **central channels** that convey blood from an arteriole to a venule. The proximal half of the central channel is a **metarteriole**, a vessel with an incomplete smooth muscle coat. Flow of blood into each capillary that arises from the metarteriole is controlled by a smooth muscle cell, the **precapillary sphincter**. The distal half of the central channel is the **thoroughfare channel**, which has no smooth muscle cells and which accepts blood from the capillary bed. If the capillary bed is to be bypassed, the precapillary sphincters contract, preventing blood flow into the capillary bed, and the blood goes directly into the venule. (Reprinted with permission from Gartner LP, Hiatt JL. *Color Atlas of Histology.* 5th ed. Baltimore, MD: Lippincott Williams & Wilkins; 2009:163.)

2. **Types of veins**
   a. **Large veins** include the vena cava and pulmonary veins. These veins possess **cardiac muscle** in the tunica adventitia for a short distance as they enter the heart. This layer also contains vasa vasorum and nerves.

table **11.3** Comparison of Tunicae in Different Types of Veins

Tunica Components	Large Veins	Medium and Small Veins	Venules
Intima			
Endothelium	+	+	+
Basal lamina	+	+	+
Valves	In some	In some	−
Subendothelial layer	+	+	−
Media			
Connective tissue	+	Reticular, elastic fibers	±
Smooth muscle cells	+	+	±
Adventitia			
Smooth muscle cells	Longitudinal bundles	−	−
Collagen layers with fibroblasts	+	+	+

+, present and prominent; ±, present but not prominent; −, absent.

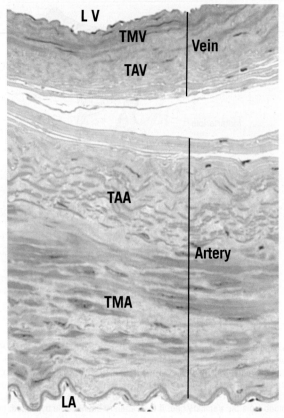

FIGURE 11.6. Light micrograph of an artery and vein (×270). Vein—lumen (LV), tunica media (TMV), and tunica adventitia (TAV). Artery—tunica adventitia (TAA), tunica media (TMA), and lumen (LA).

b. **Small and medium-sized veins** include the external jugular vein. These veins have a diameter of 1 to 9 mm.
c. **Venules** have a diameter of 0.2 to 1 mm and are involved in **exchange of metabolites** with tissues and in **diapedesis** (exiting of blood cells through vessel walls).

CLINICAL CONSIDERATIONS   **Varicose veins** are abnormally tortuous **dilated veins**, usually of the **leg**.
1. They are caused by a decline in muscle tone, degenerative alteration of the vessel wall, and valvular incompetence. They generally occur in older people, being most prevalent in women. Pregnant women are also susceptible to varicose veins.
2. When they occur in the region of the anorectal junction, they are known as **hemorrhoids**.

F. Specialized sensory mechanisms within arteries include three types of sensors: the **carotid sinus**, the **carotid body**, and the **aortic bodies**.
1. **Carotid sinus** is a **baroreceptor** in the wall of the internal carotid artery just as it begins at the common carotid artery. Sensory endings of the glossopharyngeal nerve embedded with the wall of the artery are sensitive to changes in pressure that distend the vessel, thus initiating a signal to the vasomotor center of the brain. The resultant response triggers adjustments to the tension on the arterial wall via the smooth muscles of the tunica media, effecting changes in blood pressure.
2. **Carotid body** is a **chemoreceptor** at the bifurcation of the common carotid artery. Specialized nerve endings of the vagus and glossopharyngeal cranial nerves are sensitive to oxygen and carbon dioxide levels as well as H^+ concentration. Glomus (type 1) cells and sheath (type 2)

cells, which envelop the glomus cells, constitute the parenchyma. Nerve endings lose their Schwann cells upon entering the parenchyma, becoming covered instead by sheath cells. Impulses are shuttled to the brain by these two cranial nerves for processing.

3. **Aortic bodies** are located in the wall of the arch of the aorta at the junction of the common carotid and subclavian arteries. Their structure and function are similar to those of the carotid body.

4. **Hormonal control of low blood pressure starts with the kidney:**
   a. **Kidney produces renin**
   b. Renin cleaves angiotensinogen circulating in the blood, forming angiotensin I, a mild vasoconstrictor.
   c. **Angiotensin I is converted into angiotensin II** by angiotensin-converting enzyme (ACE), located on the luminal plasmalemmas of capillary endothelia (especially capillaries of the lungs).
   d. Angiotensin II, a potent vasoconstrictor, causes the walls of arterioles to contract, which raises blood pressure.
   e. Antidiuretic hormone, or vasopressin, secreted by the pituitary gland, is another potent vasoconstrictor employed after severe hemorrhage.

II. OVERVIEW—LYMPHATIC VASCULAR SYSTEM

This system consists of peripheral lymphatic capillaries, lymphatic vessels of gradually increasing size, and lymphatic ducts. The lymphatic vascular system **collects excess tissue fluid (lymph) and returns it to the venous portion of the cardiovascular system**. It drains most tissues with the exception of the nervous system and bone marrow.

A. Lymphatic capillaries are thin-walled vessels that begin as **blind-ended channels** (e.g., **lacteals**) adjacent to capillary beds where they collect lymph.
   1. They are composed of a single layer of **attenuated endothelial cells** that lack fenestrae and fasciae occludentes. They possess a sparse basal lamina.
   2. Lymph enters these leaky capillaries via spaces between overlapping endothelial cells.
   3. Small lymphatic anchoring filaments between the surrounding connective tissue and the abluminal plasma membrane assist in maintaining luminal patency in these delicate vessels.

B. Large lymphatic vessels possess valves and are similar in structure to small veins, except that they have larger lumina and thinner walls.
   1. Lymph nodes that filter the lymph are interposed along their routes.
   2. These vessels converge to form the **thoracic duct** and **right lymphatic duct**. The thoracic duct empties into the venous system at the junction of the left internal jugular vein with the subclavian vein, whereas the right lymphatic duct empties into the venous system at a similar location on the right side of the neck.

CLINICAL CONSIDERATIONS   **Edema** is a pathologic process resulting in an **increased volume of tissue fluid**.

Edema may be caused by venous obstruction or decreased venous blood flow (as in congestive heart failure), increased capillary permeability (due to injury), starvation, excessive release of histamine, and obstruction of lymphatic vessels. It is common during pregnancy and in older persons. Edema that is responsive to localized pressure (i.e., depressions persist after release of pressure) is called **pitting edema**. Edema can be a symptom of a serious underlying disorder, including heart disease; liver disease; or diseases of the thyroid, lymphatic system, or the kidneys, with serious consequences.

Review Test

Directions: Each of the numbered items or incomplete statements in this section is followed by answers or completions of the statement. Select the ONE lettered answer that is BEST in each case.

1. The epicardium is one of the three layers of the heart. It is
(A) continuous with the endocardium.
(B) also known as the visceral pericardium.
(C) composed of modified cardiac muscle cells.
(D) capable of increasing intraventricular pressure.
(E) capable of decreasing the rate of contraction.

2. The atrial muscle of the heart produces a hormone that
(A) decreases blood pressure.
(B) increases blood pressure.
(C) causes vasoconstriction.
(D) facilitates the release of renin.
(E) facilitates sodium resorption in the kidneys.

3. The generation of impulses in the normal heart is the responsibility of which of the following structures?
(A) Atrioventricular (AV) node
(B) AV bundle of His
(C) Sympathetic nerves
(D) Sinoatrial (SA) node
(E) Purkinje fibers

4. Metarterioles, vessels interposed between arterioles and capillary beds,
(A) function to control blood flow into arterioles.
(B) possess a complete layer of smooth muscle cells in their tunica media.
(C) possess precapillary sphincters.
(D) receive blood from thoroughfare channels.
(E) possess valves to regulate the direction of blood flow.

5. Which of the following statements concerning innervation of blood vessels is true?
(A) Vasoconstriction is controlled by parasympathetic nerve fibers.
(B) Acetylcholine acts directly on smooth muscle cells.
(C) Acetylcholine acts directly on endothelial cells.
(D) Vasodilation is controlled by sympathetic nerve fibers.
(E) Nitric oxide acts as a vasoconstrictor.

6. Which of the following characteristics distinguishes somatic capillaries from visceral capillaries?
(A) Presence or absence of fenestrae
(B) Size of the lumen
(C) Thickness of the vessel wall
(D) Presence or absence of pericytes
(E) Thickness of the basal lamina

7. The blood–brain barrier is thought to exist because capillaries in the central nervous system have which of the following characteristics?
(A) Discontinuous basal lamina
(B) Fenestrae with diaphragms
(C) Fenestrae without diaphragms
(D) A few pinocytic vesicles
(E) No basement membrane

8. Which of the following statements about healthy, intact capillaries is true?
(A) They control blood pressure.
(B) They are lined by a simple columnar epithelium.
(C) They have a smooth muscle coat.
(D) They inhibit clot formation.
(E) Satellite cells share their basal lamina.

9. A patient complains of shortness of breath even after only mild exercise. She states that she has had this condition for 2 years but recently has noticed that it has become more pronounced. Her medical history indicates that she had rheumatic fever when she was a child. Auscultation indicates an enlarged heart. What may the physician expect to find with other diagnostic tests?

(A) Mitral valve stenosis
(B) Tetralogy of Fallot
(C) Pulmonary artery aneurysm
(D) Coronary heart disease
(E) Ischemic heart disease

10. Diagnostic tests for ischemic heart disease usually reveal

(A) malformed heart valves.
(B) atherosclerosis of coronary arteries.
(C) irregular heartbeat.
(D) faulty SA valve.
(E) arteriosclerosis of coronary arteries.

11. Vasa vasorum function in a way that is similar to

(A) AV valves.
(B) semilunar valves.
(C) coronary arteries.
(D) elastic arteries.
(E) metarterioles.

12. Which one of the following possesses a distinct internal elastic lamina?

(A) Capillary
(B) Metarteriole
(C) Arteriole
(D) Muscular artery
(E) Vein

13. Ischemic heart disease is the usual sequel to

(A) arteriosclerosis.
(B) abdominal aortic aneurysm.
(C) rheumatic fever.
(D) varicose veins.
(E) atherosclerosis.

Answers and Explanations

1. **B.** The pericardium is a fibroserous sac that encloses the heart. The innermost layer of the pericardium, the epicardium, is also known as the visceral pericardium (see Chapter 11 I A 1).

2. **A.** Atrial natriuretic peptide, which decreases blood pressure, is produced mainly by cardiac muscle cells of the right atrium. It inhibits the release of renin and causes the kidneys to decrease the resorption of sodium and water (see Chapter 11 I A 1 b).

3. **D.** Impulses are generated in the sinoatrial node, which is the pacemaker of the heart. They are then conducted to the AV node. The bundle of His and Purkinje fibers conduct impulses from the AV node to the cardiac muscle cells of the ventricles. Sympathetic nerves can increase the rate of the heartbeat but do not originate it (see Chapter 11 I A 4 a).

4. **C.** The proximal portion of a central channel is known as a metarteriole, whereas its distal portion is the thoroughfare channel. Blood from metarterioles may enter the capillary bed if their precapillary sphincters are relaxed. If the precapillary sphincters of metarterioles are constricted, blood bypasses the capillary bed and flows directly into thoroughfare channels and from there into a venule (see Chapter 11 I B 1 d).

5. **C.** Acetylcholine stimulates the endothelial cells of a vessel to release nitric oxide (EDRF), which causes relaxation of smooth muscle cells. Thus, acetylcholine does not act directly on smooth muscle cells (see Chapter 11 I B 2).

6. **A.** Somatic (continuous) capillaries lack fenestrae, whereas visceral (fenestrated) capillaries are characterized by their presence. Both types of capillary possess a continuous basal lamina and are surrounded by occasional pericytes (see Chapter 11 I C 2).

7. **D.** Capillaries in the CNS are of the continuous type and thus lack fenestrae but have a continuous basal lamina. In contrast to continuous capillaries in other parts of the body, they contain only a few pinocytic vesicles; this characteristic is thought to be partly responsible for the blood–brain barrier (see Chapter 11 I C 2).

8. **D.** The smooth endothelial lining of intact, healthy capillaries inhibits clot formation. Capillaries do not control blood pressure (see Chapter 11 I C 2).

9. **A.** A person who has had rheumatic fever as a child may develop heart valve disease later in life. Although the mitral valve is the one most commonly affected, the other valves may also be involved. The mitral valve becomes inflamed, fibrotic, and eventually incompetent or stenotic. This condition leads to respiratory hypertension and edema, which restricts respiratory function. The key is a history of rheumatic fever, because those individuals are predisposed to developing heart valve diseases (see Chapter 11 I A 3 Clinical Considerations).

10. **B.** Diagnostic tests for ischemic heart disease reveal atherosclerosis of the coronary vessels. Over time, excessive plaque composed of cholesterol and fats is layered beneath the intima of these vessels, thus restricting blood flow to the myocardium of the heart, leading to angina pectoris, an infarction, or perhaps sudden death (see Chapter 11 I B 1 Clinical Considerations).

11. **C.** Vasa vasorum are the small blood vessels that serve the walls of elastic and muscular arteries with oxygen and nutrients just as the coronary arteries provide for the walls of the heart (see Chapter 11 I B 1).

12. **D.** The muscular artery possesses a distinct internal elastic lamina. Elastic arteries possess an incomplete internal elastic lamina, whereas capillaries, arterioles, metarterioles, and veins do not possess an internal elastic lamina (see Table 11.1 and Chapter 11 I D).

13. **E.** Ischemic heart disease is usually caused by coronary atherosclerosis, resulting in decreased blood flow to the myocardium. It may develop into angina pectoris, myocardial infarction, chronic ischemic cardiopathy, or sudden cardiac death. On the other hand, arteriosclerosis (hardening of the arteries) usually attacks renal arteries and is related to hypertension and diabetes mellitus (see Chapter 11 I B Clinical Considerations).

I. OVERVIEW—THE LYMPHOID (IMMUNE) SYSTEM

A. The lymphoid system consists of **capsulated lymphoid tissues** (thymus, spleen, tonsils, and lymph nodes); **diffuse lymphoid tissue**; and lymphoid cells, primarily **T lymphocytes** (T cells), **B lymphocytes** (B cells), and **macrophages.** Capsulated lymphoid organs are of two types, **primary lymphoid organs** that "educate" lymphocytes so that they become immunocompetent cells; these are the **bone marrow** (discussed in Chapter 10 Section IV) and the **thymus** (discussed in this chapter, Section VI B). **Secondary lymphoid organs** sequester immunogens and allow immunocompetent cells and antigen-presenting cells (APCs) to interact with the immunogens and with each other to initiate an immune reaction and eliminate the antigenic attack. The **diffuse lymphoid tissue, lymph nodes, spleen,** and **tonsils** are the secondary lymphoid organs and are discussed in Section VI of this chapter.

B. The **immune system** has two components: the innate immune system (nonspecific) and the adaptive immune system (specific).

  1. The **innate immune system** has no immunological memory; it acts rapidly, but in a nonspecific manner. Its chief constituents are complement proteins, toll-like receptors (TLRs), mast cells (see Chapter 6 III A 4), eosinophils (see Chapter 10 Table 10.2), neutrophils (see Chapter 10 Table 10.2), macrophages (see Chapter 6 III B 1), and natural killer (NK) cells (see Section II D).

     a. **Complement proteins** are blood-borne proteins (C1–C9) that function in nonspecific host defense and initiate the inflammatory process.

     b. **TLRs** in humans are a family of 10 receptors that are integral proteins located either in the cell membranes or in the membranes of endosomes of specific cells of the innate immune system.

        (1) It is believed that in order to perform their function, they have to pair up with their counterpart, usually the same TLR (forming homodimers); however, TLR2 can form dimers with TLR1 and TLR6 (forming heterodimers).

        (2) TLRs have key functions in the recognition of repeating molecular patterns that exist in pathogens, known as **pathogen-associated molecular patterns** (**PAMPs**).

        (3) Each TLR, or TLR pair, recognizes PAMPs that are specific to them (Table 12.1).

        (4) TLRs 1, 2, 4, 5, 6, and 10 are integral proteins of the cell membrane and recognize molecular patterns belonging to bacteria, protozoa, and fungi, whereas TLRs 3, 7, 8, and 9 are integral proteins of endosomal membranes and recognize molecular patterns belonging to nucleic acids of viruses (and some other microorganisms).

        (5) For instance, TLR4 recognizes lipopolysaccharides of gram-negative bacteria, and TLR2 recognizes peptidoglycan of gram-positive bacteria. Once these receptors bind to their ligand, they cause the release of **tumor necrosis factor** α (**TNF-α**), **interleukins 1 and 12 (IL-1 and IL-12)**, and other systemic inflammation-inducing **cytokines.**

t a b l e **12.1**	Toll-like Receptors, Their Location, and Function	
Receptor	**Location**	**Function**
TLR1	Cell membrane of macrophages, neutrophils, B lymphocytes, and dendritic cells	In conjunction with TLR2, it binds to triacylated lipopeptides as well as to peptidoglycans of gram-positive bacteria. Peptidoglycan coats of gram-negative bacteria are much thinner; therefore, the reactivity is much less pronounced.
TLR2	Cell membranes of T reg cells, B lymphocytes, dendritic cells, and macrophages	Binds to lipoteichoic acid of gram-positive bacteria as well as various lipopeptides and lipoproteins of various bacteria, and to zymosan of fungi. In conjunction with TLR6, it binds to diacylated lipopeptides. See its binding abilities in conjunction with TLR1 in the row above.
TLR3	Endosomes of macrophages and dendritic cells	Binds to double-stranded viral RNA.
TLR4	Cell membranes of macrophages, dendritic cells, neutrophils, and endothelial cells	Binds to the endotoxin LPS of gram-negative bacteria but requires the homodimers state along with the presence of MD2 in order to recognize LPS.
TLR5	Cell membranes of macrophages, dendritic cells, and intestinal epithelial cells	Binds to the protein flagellin of bacterial flagella.
TLR6	Cell membranes of macrophages, mast cells, and B lymphocytes	Binds to lipopeptides of the bacteria-like organism, *Mycoplasma*. In conjunction with TLR2, it binds to diacylated lipopeptides.
TLR7	Endosomes of specialized dendritic cells* and B lymphocytes	Binds to single-stranded viral RNA.
TLR8	Endosomes of macrophages, dendritic cells, type I pneumocytes, and mast cells	Binds to single-stranded viral RNA.
TLR9	Endosomes of macrophages, specialized dendritic cells*	Binds to bacterial and viral DNA.
TLR10	Cell membranes of macrophages and dendritic cells	Possibly binds to profilin-like proteins of the parasite *Toxoplasma gondii*.

LPS, lipopolysaccharide; MD2, myeloid differentiation factor 2.
*Specialized dendritic cells are plasmacytoid dendritic cells that constitute only ½% of mononuclear cells of the peripheral circulation. When activated, they release the antiviral agents IFN-α and IFN-β, and type I interferons.

(6) Activation of TLRs also facilitates the induction of an adaptive immune response such as the recruitment of NK cells, macrophages, neutrophils, and dendritic cells to the region.

(7) Many TLRs, including TLR4 and TLR2 as well as TNF-α and IL-1, activate the **NF-κB pathway (nuclear factor kappa-light chain enhancer of activated B cells)**.

    (a) **NF-κB** is a family of five proteins that form dimers with each other (homodimers or heterodimers) that are closely bound and thereby kept in the inactive state by inhibitory proteins known as **IκB**.

    (b) When TLR2 or TLR4 or TNF-α or IL-1 binds its ligands, it **activates a kinase** that phosphorylates IκB and releases NF-κB. The phosphorylated IκB becomes ubiquinated and is sent to **proteasomes** for destruction.

    (c) The released **NF-κB** is translocated into the **nucleus** where, in conjunction with a coactivator protein, it finds its target gene and **initiates its transcription**. These protein products of these genes activate **innate immune responses** and **inflammatory responses**.

2. The **adaptive immune system** is evolutionarily more recent than the innate immune system. It possesses four characteristics: ability to distinguish self from nonself, memory, specificity, and diversity. The cells of the adaptive immune system, namely T lymphocytes, B lymphocytes, and APCs, communicate with one another by the use of signaling molecules (**cytokines**) and cell surface markers (e.g., cluster of differentiation proteins), thus relaying information to each other in response to antigenic invasion.

C. The immune system functions primarily to defend the organism by mounting **humoral immune responses** against foreign substances (**antigens**) and **cell-mediated immune responses** against microorganisms, tumor and transplanted cells, and virus-infected cells.

Individuals may suffer from **congenital immunodeficiency disorders**, usually a recessive X-linked genetic defect that affects males to a much greater extent than females. The most common symptoms are recurrent respiratory infections that have a tendency to progress to pneumonia. Additional indicators are multiple skin and oral infections, such as yeast infections of the mouth (thrush) or of the vagina. In some cases, such as **X-linked agammaglobulinemia**, B lymphocytes do not develop, resulting in scarcity of plasma cells and consequently lack of immunoglobulin production.

II. CELLS OF THE IMMUNE SYSTEM

A. Overview—Cells of the immune system: T lymphocytes, B lymphocytes, and APCs

  1. Cells of the immune system include **clones of T lymphocytes (T cells)** and **B lymphocytes (B cells)**. A clone is a small number of **identical** cells that can recognize and respond to a single or a small group of related antigenic determinants known as epitopes.

  a. An **epitope** is that small portion of an antigen to which an **antibody (immunoglobulin)** binds. A single antigen may have a number of epitopes, each different, recognized by different antibodies each of which is specific to each of those epitopes.

  b. The region of the antibody that binds to an epitope is known as a **paratope**.

  c. It is important to realize that, instead of recognizing antigens, antibodies recognize those portions of antigens that act as epitopes.

  Exposure to antigen and one or more **cytokines** induce **activation** of **resting T** and **B cells**, leading to their proliferation and differentiation into **effector cells** (Figure 12.1). Both B cells and T cells arise in the bone marrow, T cells leave the bone marrow to mature in the thymus, whereas B cells remain in and mature in the bone marrow.

  2. APCs (e.g., macrophages, lymphoid dendritic cells, Langerhans cells, follicular dendritic cells, M cells, and B cells), **mast cells**, and **granulocytes** are also cells of the immune system (see Chapter 6 III A and B).[1]

B. T lymphocytes

  1. Overview—T lymphocytes

  a. T lymphocytes include several functionally distinct subtypes and are responsible for **cell-mediated immune responses.** They assist B cells in developing humoral responses to **thymic-dependent antigens.**

  b. T-cell receptors (TCRs) are heterodimers, that is, they are composed of two dissimilar protein chains: α and β or γ and δ. TCRs are present only on the surfaces of T lymphocytes and are always associated with a CD3 molecule; although they belong to the Ig (immunoglobulin) superfamily unlike Igs, they are not secreted. TCRs recognize only **protein** antigens.

    (1) γ/δ **T cells** are more uniform, are much fewer in number, do not form memory T cells, and are usually located in the intestinal mucosa; they react to antigens that are indicative of microbial assault.

    (2) α/β **T cells** constitute the bulk of the T-cell population, form memory T cells, and, although they react slower than γ/δ T cells, they are responsible for most T-cell responses.

  c. It is important to realize that T cells do not recognize antigens; instead they recognize only **epitopes** that are bound to **major histocompatibility complex (MHC) molecules** on the surface of **APCs**. Since T cells require that the epitopes be presented in conjunction with MHC molecules, they are said to be **MHC restricted** (see Section III of this chapter).

  2. Maturation of α/β T cells, γ/δ T cells, and NKT cells occurs in the thymus. Only α/β **T cells** spend a considerable time in the thymus and they go through a series of steps in their "education" to become immunocompetent cells. Although γ/δ **T cells and NKT cells** also

---

[1] Although B cells can presents epitopes to T cells and are thus antigen-presenting cells, their role in this function is probably limited to the secondary (anamnestic) immune response rather than the primary immune response.

Antigen-dependent cross-linking of the surface antibodies activates the B cell, which places the epitope–MHC II complex on the external aspect of its plasmalemma.

The TCR and CD4 molecules of the T$_H$2 cell recognize the B cell's MHC II–epitope complex. In addition, binding of the B cell's CD40 molecule to the T$_H$2 cell's CD40 receptor induces the B cell to proliferate and the T$_H$2 cell to release of IL-4, IL-5, and IL-6.

IL-4, IL-5, and IL-6 induce the activation of B cells and their differentiation into B memory and plasma cells.

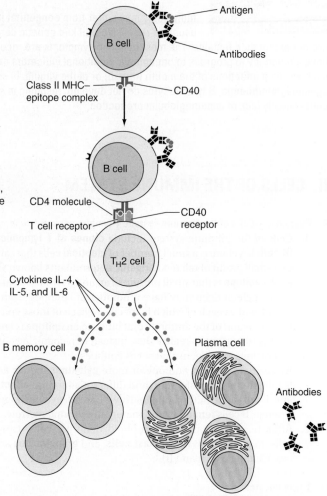

A

FIGURE 12.1. Schematic overview of the interactions among the various cells of the immune system. **A.** Thymic-dependent antigen-induced B memory and plasma cell formation.

spend some time in the thymus, their "education" to become immunocompetent cells is very sparse. This textbook will describe the maturation only of α/β T cells, and that involves the following events:

a. Immunoincompetent progenitor T lymphocytes migrate from the bone marrow to enter the thymus at the corticomedullary junction and migrate to the **outer region of the thymic cortex**. Once in the thymus, they are also referred to as **thymocytes.** These thymocytes have neither **CD4** nor **CD8** (**c**luster of **d**ifferentiation) surface **markers** and, therefore, are known as **double negative T cells.** However, thymocyte plasmalemma possesses **Notch-1 receptors** that permit these cells to respond to cytokines released by epithelial reticular cells to become T cells.

b. Within the **outer thymic cortex**, thymocytes undergo **gene rearrangements** and begin to express antigen-specific TCRs, which are integral membrane proteins. Because they express both CD4 and CD8 surface markers, they are known as **double positive T cells**. These cells are now **immunocompetent.**

c. Double positive T cells that do not recognize **self-MHC–epitope complex molecules** offered to them by **epithelial reticular cells** of the thymic cortex are forced into apoptosis, because they failed to recognize the body's own MHC molecules and the body's own epitopes. Double positive T cells that were able to recognize the self-MHC–epitope complex are

The TCR and CD4 molecule of the T$_H$1 cell binds to the epitope and the MHC II of the APC, respectively. The binding induces the APC to express B7 molecules on its plasmalemma, which then binds to the CD28 molecule of the T$_H$1 cell, inducing that cell to release IL-2.

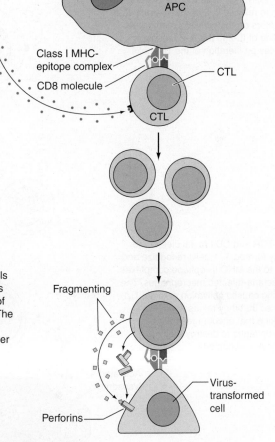

The same APC expresses the MHC I-epitope complex, which is recognized by the CD8 molecule and the TCR of the CTL. In addition, the CD28 molecule of the CTL binds with the B7 molecule on the APC plasmalemma. These interactions induce the expression of IL-2 receptors on the CTL plasma membrane. Binding of IL-2 (released by the T$_H$1 cell) to the IL-2 receptors of the CTL induces that cell to proliferate.

The plasmalemma of virally transformed cells expresses MHC I-epitope complex, which is recognized by the CD8 molecule and TCR of the newly formed cytotoxic T lymphocytes. The binding of the CTL induces these cells to secrete perforins and fragmentins. The former assemble to form pores in the plasma membrane of the transformed cell, and framentin drives the transformed cell into apoptosis.

B

FIGURE 12.1. (*Continued*) **B.** Cytotoxic T lymphocyte activation and cell killing.

permitted to enter the medulla of the thymus. It is interesting to note that 90% of the double positive T cells die in the cortex.

   d. Still in the **thymic cortex**
      (1) double positive T cells contact epithelial reticular cells that bear **MHC I–epitope complexes** stop expressing CD4 markers and become **single positive T cells** that express only **CD8 markers**.
      (2) double positive T cells contact epithelial reticular cells that bear **MHC II–epitope complexes** stop expressing CD8 markers and become **single positive T cells** that express only **CD4 markers**.
      (3) Those **single positive T cells** that remain alive enter the **medulla of the thymus** as full-fledged immunocompetent, but **naïve, T cells**.

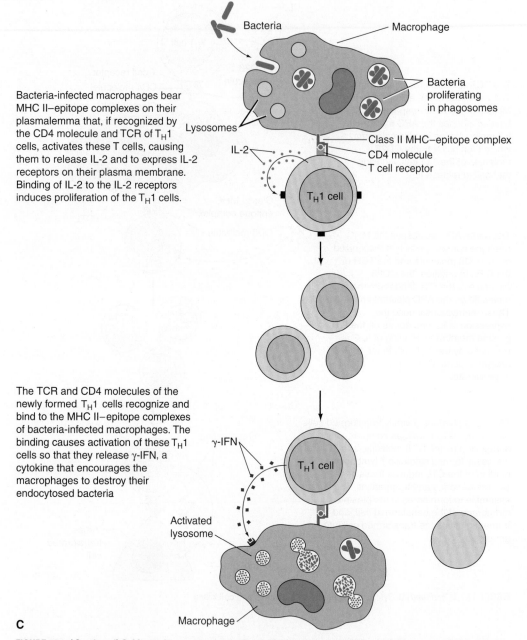

Bacteria-infected macrophages bear MHC II–epitope complexes on their plasmalemma that, if recognized by the CD4 molecule and TCR of T$_H$1 cells, activates these T cells, causing them to release IL-2 and to express IL-2 receptors on their plasma membrane. Binding of IL-2 to the IL-2 receptors induces proliferation of the T$_H$1 cells.

The TCR and CD4 molecules of the newly formed T$_H$1 cells recognize and bind to the MHC II–epitope complexes of bacteria-infected macrophages. The binding causes activation of these T$_H$1 cells so that they release γ-IFN, a cytokine that encourages the macrophages to destroy their endocytosed bacteria

C

FIGURE 12.1. (*Continued*) **C.** Macrophage activation by T$_H$1 cells. IL, interleukin; MHC, major histocompatibility complex; TCR, T-cell receptor; APC, antigen-presenting cell; CTL, cytotoxic T lymphocyte; IFN, interferon. (Adapted with permission from Gartner LP, Hiatt JL. *Color Textbook of Histology.* 2nd ed. Philadelphia, PA: WB Saunders; 2001:282–284.)

    e. The final step in the maturation of T cells occurs in the **medulla of the thymus**, where there is another test: **medullary epithelial reticular cells** present self-epitopes on MHC I and MHC II molecules to single positive T cells, and those T cells whose TCRs bind to the MHC–epitope complex are also forced into apoptosis to prevent a possible **autoimmune response**. These epithelial reticular cells also express the transcription factor **AIRE** (**a**uto**i**mmune **re**gulator), which assists in the recognition of certain tissue-specific antigens such as **insulin** and **filaggrin** (protein in the stratum corneum of skin) (see Chapter 14 Section II B 2 c), and force T cells that would be triggered by these proteins to initiate an immune response into apoptosis.

  f. The T cells that survive this final test are permitted to leave the thymic medulla to be distributed by the circulatory system to various regions of the body.

  g. The entire process of T cell development is directed by a variety of **growth factors** and **signaling molecules** released by the various types of **epithelial reticular cells** of the thymus.

3. T lymphocyte subtypes. There are three types of T cells: naïve, memory, and effector T cells. Some have a number of subtypes.

  a. Naïve T cells are immunologically competent cells that have not as yet been activated (i.e., they have not come into contact with their designated antigen outside the thymic cortex), but possess CD45RA surface markers. Once activated, they undergo cell division and form both memory T cells and effector T cells.

  b. Memory T cells, derived from naïve T cells, possess CD45R0 surface molecules. There are two classes of these cells, central memory T cells (CR7+) and effector memory T cells (CR7–).

   (1) Central memory T cells (**TCMs**) reside in the paracortex of lymph nodes. If they interact with an epitope that they recognize when APCs present it to them, they cause the APC to release IL-12, which induces TCMs to undergo cell division, and the newly formed cells differentiate into effector T memory cells.

   (2) Effector T memory cells migrate to inflammatory sites, where they undergo cell division and form **effector T cells.**

  c. Effector T cells are derived from effector T memory cells and are capable of initiating an immune response. The subtypes of effector T cells are T helper cells, cytotoxic T lymphocytes (CTLs, T killer cells), and regulatory T cells (T reg cells).

   (1) T helper cells (T_H0, T_H1, T_H2, T17, and $T_H\alpha\beta$) are **CD4+** cells. After activation, these cells synthesize and release numerous growth factors known as **cytokines (lymphokines).** **T_H0 cells** differentiate into the other four types of T helper cells.

     (a) T_H1 cells regulate responses against viral or bacterial invasions and instruct macrophages in killing bacteria.

     (b) T_H2 cells regulate humoral responses against parasitic or mucosal attacks by stimulating B cells to produce antibodies.

     (c) T17 cells manufacture and release IL-17, which recruits neutrophils and enhances their bactericidal activities.

     (d) $T_H\alpha\beta$ cells are activated by IL-10 as well as interferon α or β (INF-α or INF-β) to act against viruses.

     (e) The cytokines **IL-4, IL-5,** and **IL-6** released by T_H2 cells induce B cells to proliferate and mature and thus respond to an antigenic stimulus, whereas **IL-10** inhibits the formation of T_H1 cells, **IL-9** enhances the proliferation of T_H2 cells as well as mast cell responses, and IL-13 retards T_H1 cell development and induces the development of B cells.

     (f) Other cytokines produced by T_H1 cells, such as IL-2, IFN-γ, and others, **modulate the immune response** in diverse ways (Table 12.2). Macrophages synthesize and release IL-12, which restricts the development of T_H2 cells and encourages the formation of T_H1 cells.

CLINICAL CONSIDERATIONS **Acquired immunodeficiency syndrome (AIDS)** is caused by infection with **human immunodeficiency virus,** which preferentially invades T_H cells, causing a severe depression in their number and thus **suppressing both cell-mediated and humoral immune responses.**

1. AIDS is characterized by **secondary infections** by opportunistic microorganisms that cause pneumonia, toxoplasmosis, candidiasis, and other diseases.

2. It is also characterized by the development of certain malignancies, such as **Kaposi sarcoma** and **non-Hodgkin lymphoma.**

| t a b l e   **12.2** | Biological Activities of Selected Cytokines in the Immune Response* | | |

Cytokine	Secreted by	Target Cell	Action
IL-1a, IL-1b	Macrophages and epithelial cells	T cells, macrophages	Activates both T lymphocytes and macrophages
IL-2	T_H1 cells	Activated T cells, B cells	Induces mitosis of activated T and B cells
IL-4	T_H2 cells	B cells	Induces mitosis of B cells, their transformation into plasma cells; promotes isotype switching from IgM to IgG and IgE
IL-5	T_H2 cells	B cells	Induces mitosis, maturation of B cells; promotes isotype switching from IgM to IgE
IL-6	Antigen-presenting cells and T_H2 cells	T cells, activated B cells	Activates T cells, induces maturation of B cells to IgG-forming plasma cells
IL-10	T_H2 cells	T_H1 cells	Inhibits formation of T_H1 cells; retards their ability to manufacture cytokines
IL-12	B cells, macrophages	NK cells, T cells	Activates NK cells, facilitates formation of T_H1-like cells
IL-18	Macrophages	T_H1 cells and NK cells	Acts on T_H1 cells to produce IFN-γ and enhances NK cell activity
IL-23	Macrophages	CD8+ T cells	decreases the motility of CD8+ T cells
TNF-α	Macrophage	Macrophages	Macrophages self-activate to manufacture, release IL-12
	T_H1 cells	Activated macrophages	Promotes production of oxygen radicals facilitating bacterial killing within endosomes of activated macrophages
INF-α	Virally attacked cells	NK cells, macrophages	Activates macrophages, NK cells
INF-β	Virally attacked cells	NK cells, macrophages	Activates macrophages, NK cells
IFN-γ	T_H1 cells	Macrophages, T cells	Activates cytotoxic T cells to kill altered and/ or foreign cells; promotes phagocytosis by macrophages

Ig, immunoglobulin; IL, interleukin; INF, interferon; NK, natural killer; T_H, T helper; TNF, tumor necrosis factor.
*See Chapter 10 for discussion of cytokines involved in hemopoiesis.

(2) **T cytotoxic cells** are **CD8+** cells. After priming by an antigenic stimulus via an APC, T cells are induced by **IL-2** to proliferate, forming new **CTLs**, which mediate (via **perforins** and **granzymes**) **apoptosis** of foreign cells as well as virally altered self-cells (Figure 12.1).

(3) **T reg cells** (previously called T suppressor cells) are **CD4+** cells. T reg cells are of two types, natural and inducible.
   (a) **Natural T reg cells** (**nT reg cells**) originate in the thymus, possess, in addition to the CD4 marker, **CD25** and **Foxp3** markers (**forkhead family transcription factor box p3**), and suppress the immune response in a non–antigen-specific manner. Naïve T cells are converted to natural T reg cells by dendritic cells of the thymus under the influence of the cytokine **thymic stromal lymphopoietin (TSLP)**. Interestingly, among the richest sources of TSLP are the cells of **Hassall corpuscles** of the thymus, which has been implicated in inducing nT reg cell formation.
   (b) **Inducible T reg cells** (also known as **T_H3 cells**) originate outside the thymus from naïve T cells. They inhibit the formation of T_H1 cells, thus suppressing the immune response.

(4) **Natural T killer cells** are similar to NK cells except that they have to go to the thymus to become immunologically competent. They are unusual in that they recognize **lipid antigens** that are presented to them by APCs in conjunction with a CD1 molecule. Natural T killer cells manufacture and secrete IL-4, IL-10, and INF-γ, and sport a limited range of TCRs on their plasma membranes.

C. B lymphocytes
  1. **Overview—B lymphocytes**
     a. B lymphocytes originate and mature into **immunocompetent** cells within the bone marrow. They are responsible for the **humoral immune response.** These cells go through a series of developmental steps going from pre-B cells through immature and finally **transitional B cells**, where they express different light and heavy chains of immunoglobulins on their cell membranes. Transitional B cells travel to the spleen where they either **die** or **undergo final maturation** and become mature B cells.
     b. **Mature B cells** express immunoglobulins IgD and the monomeric form of IgM on the external aspect of their plasma membranes (known as **surface immunoglobulins [sIgs]**); all of the immunoglobulin molecules on a particular B cell recognize and bind to the **same antigenic determinant** (epitope). There are several types of B cells, but B-2 B cells and B-1 B cells are the most predominant forms.
        (1) **B-2 B cells** are the "conventional" B cells *and will be referred to as "B cells"* in this textbook; they are the most numerous and are present throughout the body; they must interact with T cells to propagate (in the bone marrow) and to become activated; they recognize an immense number of **epitopes**; and they are able to switch isotypes (i.e., switch in the synthesis of antibody types) and establish **memory B cells**. They are considered to be firmly related to the adaptive immune system.
        (2) **B-1 B cells** are much fewer in number than B cells and are usually limited to the gastrointestinal and respiratory systems; they very seldom require T-cell interaction; they do not have to regenerate in the bone marrow but proliferate peripherally; they target **carbohydrates** rather than proteins; they very seldom switch isotypes; and they do not establish memory B-1 B cells. They cross over between the innate and adaptive immune systems.
     c. CD40 molecules are present on the plasmalemmae of B cells. They interact with CD40 receptors on T_H2 cells, causing release of cytokines that
        (1) facilitate proliferation and transformation of B cells into B memory and plasma cells and
        (2) inhibit T_H1 cell proliferation.
     d. The specific cytokines that are released by T helper cells depend on the **invading pathogen.**
        (1) IL-4 and IL-5 are released by T helper cells in response to parasitic worms causing B cells to switch to IgE formation.
        (2) IL-6 and IFN-γ are released by T helper cells in response to bacteria and viruses in the connective tissue, causing B cells to switch to IgG formation.
        (3) Transforming growth factor β (TGF-β) is released by T helper cells in response to the presence of bacteria and viruses on mucosal surfaces causing B cells to switch to IgA formation.
     e. B lymphocytes can present epitopes complexed with class II human leukocyte antigen (HLA) to T_H1 cells; therefore, they are considered to be **APCs**.
     f. When activated, B lymphocytes release **IL-12** to induce T_H1 cell formation and NK cell activation.
     g. During a humoral immune response to an antigenic challenge, B lymphocytes proliferate and differentiate to form plasma cells and B memory cells (Figure 12.1A).
  2. **Plasma cells** lack surface antibody and actively synthesize and secrete **antibody specific against the challenging antigen.**
  3. **B memory cells** are **long-lived committed immunocompetent cells** that are formed during proliferation in response to an antigenic challenge. They do not react against the antigen but remain in the circulation or in specific regions of the lymphoid system. Since they increase the size of the original clone, they **provide a faster and greater secondary response (anamnestic response)** against a future challenge by the same antigen.
  4. There are also two groups of B cells in the spleen: the more populous follicular B cells and fewer marginal zone B cells.
     a. **Follicular B cells** are more populous and are located in the primary and secondary follicles of the spleen (see VI C 3 of this chapter); they sport IgM, IgD, and CD21 surface markers; and

they are T cell dependent for immune function. They are believed to be in the final stage of their maturation into fully functioning mature B cells.
   b. **Marginal zone B cells** are fewer in number than follicular B cells; are located in the marginal zone of the spleen (see VI C 3 of this chapter); they sport IgM, CD1, CD9, and CD21 on their plasmalemmae; they are T cell independent for their immune functions. They react primarily to self-antigens and bacterial invasion.

CLINICAL CONSIDERATIONS **Common variable immunodeficiency** is a disease of the young, developing in patients who are between 10 and 20 years of age. Although these patients have normal B-cell population, they do not manufacture enough immunoglobulins, with the consequence of being prone to recurrent respiratory infections and the development of autoimmune disorders such as rheumatoid arthritis, thyroiditis, and Addison disease. Affected individuals frequently suffer from gastrointestinal disorders, such as diarrhea and insufficient absorption of nutrients from the alimentary canal.

Hodgkin disease is a malignant **neoplastic transformation of lymphocytes.**

1. It occurs mostly in young men. It is characterized by the presence of **Reed Sternberg cells**, which are giant cells with two large, vacuolated nuclei, each with a dense nucleolus.
2. Signs and symptoms include painless progressive **enlargement of the lymph nodes, spleen**, and **liver**; anemia; fever; weakness; anorexia; and weight loss.

D. **NK cells** belong to a category of **null cells**, a small group of peripheral-blood lymphocytes that **lack the surface determinants** that are characteristic of T and B lymphocytes. However, they do possess two specific receptors: **killer activation receptors** that respond to stress molecules and **killer inhibition receptors** that respond to MHC Class I molecules. It is these receptors that aid them in the recognition of virally altered cells and tumor cells that have to be forced into apoptosis.
   1. As soon as they are formed, NK cells are immunocompetent. They do not have to enter the thymic environment.
   2. Not only are NK cells not MHC restricted but they also exhibit an apparently **nonspecific cytotoxicity** against tumor cells and virus-infected cells. The mechanism by which NK cells recognize these target cells is not yet understood.
   3. NK cells can also kill specific target cells that have antibodies bound to their surface antigens in a process known as **antibody-dependent cell-mediated cytotoxicity (ADCC)**; macrophages, neutrophils, and eosinophils also exhibit ADCC.
   4. NK cells use **perforins** and **granzymes** to drive the virally altered cells or tumor cells into **apoptosis.**

E. **Macrophages** function both as **APCs** and as **cytotoxic effector cells** in ADCC.
   1. When acting as APCs, macrophages phagocytose antigens, fragment them into small antigenic components, known as **epitopes**, and present them to T cells.
   2. Macrophages produce and release **IL-1**, which helps activate T_H cells and self-activate macrophages. Moreover, they produce **TNF-α**, which also self-activates macrophages and induces the release of IL-12; in conjunction with **IFN-γ** facilitates killing of endocytosed bacteria (Table 12.2). In addition, macrophages secrete **prostaglandin E_2 (PGE$_2$)**, which decreases certain immune responses, **IL-6**, which activates T cells and stimulates B cells to differentiate into plasma cells, **IL-12**, which activates T_H1 cells to proliferate and activates NK cells, **IL-18**, which acts on T_H1 cells to produce IFN-γ and also enhances NK cell activity, and **IL-23**, which decreases the motility of CD8+ T cells. It should be noted that **IL-1**, **IL-6**, **and TNF-α** act together to induce an **inflammatory process.**

III. ANTIGEN PRESENTATION AND THE ROLE OF MHC MOLECULES

A. MHC

1. The MHC (major histocompatibility complex) is a large genetic complex with many loci that encode two main classes of integral membrane molecules: **class I molecules (MHC I)**, which are expressed by nearly all **nucleated cells**, and **class II molecules (MHC II)**, which are expressed by the various cells that function as **APCs.**

2. In humans, the MHC is referred to as the **HLA complex (human lymphocyte antigen).** Therefore, MHC I is class I HLA, and MHC II is class II HLA. As described below, MHC I molecules bind epitopes derived from **endogenous proteins**, whereas MHC II molecules bind epitopes derived from **exogenous proteins.** Both types of MHC molecules present their epitopes to T cells.

B. Immunogens are molecules that are capable of **inducing an immune response.** All immunogens are **antigens**, that is, molecules whose **epitopes** can react with an **antibody** or a **TCR (T cell receptor).** Most, but not all, antigens are immunogens.

1. **Exogenous immunogens** are derived from proteins that were endocytosed or phagocytosed by APCs and degraded intracellularly, yielding antigenic peptides containing an epitope that enter the *trans*-Golgi network (TGN).

2. In the TGN, the complex is sorted into specialized antigenic peptides (containing an epitope) that associate with **class II HLA molecules** (MHC II molecules).

   a. These epitopes are relatively long, composed of 13 to 25 amino acids.

   b. Class II HLA molecules are synthesized on the rough endoplasmic reticulum (RER) and are loaded within the RER cisternae with a protein known as **CLIP** (**cl**ass II–associated **i**nvariant **p**rotein).

   c. The class II HLA–CLIP complex enters the Golgi apparatus, where it is delivered to MIIC vesicles (**MHC class II compartment vesicles** that already contain epitopes derived from exogenous immunogens), where the CLIP is exchanged for the epitope.

   d. The epitope–class II HLA complexes are transported to and displayed on the cell surface, where they are **presented** to T cells.

3. **Endogenous immunogens** are derived from proteins that were produced **within** host cells (these may be **viral proteins** synthesized in virus-infected cells or **tumor proteins** synthesized in cancerous cells).

   a. **Class I HLA molecules** (MHC I molecules), synthesized on the RER surface, enter the RER cisternae.

   b. Endogenous immunogens are degraded by organelles of the host cells, known as **proteasomes**, into short polypeptide fragments. These fragments are antigenic peptides (8–12 amino acids in length) known as **epitopes.**

   c. The epitopes are transported by **TAP1** and **TAP2** (**tra**nsporter **p**roteins 1 and 2) into the RER cisternae.

   d. Within the RER cisternae, the epitopes derived from endogenous immunogens are loaded on the **class I HLA.**

   e. The peptide–class I HLA complexes are transported to the Golgi complex for sorting and eventual delivery within clathrin-coated vesicles to the cell surface, where they are presented to T cells.

C. MHC (HLA) restriction—T lymphocytes. Each subtype of T lymphocytes (except T memory cells) recognizes only epitopes that are associated with either MHC I or MHC II (class I or class II HLA) molecules as follows:

1. T_H1 and T_H2 cells (CD4+ cells) recognize MHC II (class II HLA) molecules.

2. Cytotoxic T cells (CD8+ cells) recognize MHC I (class I HLA) molecules.

3. T memory cells (CD45R0 cells) recognize both MHC I and MHC II (class I and class II HLA) molecules.

IV. IMMUNOGLOBULINS

Immunoglobulins are glycoproteins that are synthesized and secreted by **plasma cells.** They constitute the active agents of the humoral immune response and have **specific antibody activity** against one antigen or a few closely related antigens. Immunoglobulins bind antigens to form antigen–antibody complexes, which are cleared from the body by various means, some of which involve the **complement system**, whereas others involve **eosinophils.**

A. Structure—Immunoglobulins
1. **Immunoglobulins** are composed of monomers containing two **heavy chains** and two **light chains.**
2. Each immunoglobulin possesses a **constant region** that is identical in all immunoglobulin molecules of the same isotype.
3. Each immunoglobulin also possesses a **variable region** that differs in the antibody molecules that recognize different antigens. Thus, the **variable regions determine the specificity** of an antibody molecule (i.e., its ability to bind to a particular antigenic determinant). Large antigens may have multiple antigenic determinants, which induce production of antibodies with different specificities.

B. Immunoglobulin classes (Table 12.3)
1. Human serum contains five classes (**isotypes**) of immunoglobulins, which differ in the amino acid composition of their **heavy-chain constant regions.**

table **12.3**   Immunoglobulin (Ig) Isotypes and Their Characteristics

Class	Type of Ig	Cytokines Required for Isotype Switch	Fraction of All Igs (%) and Half-Life (Days) in Serum	Binding to Cells	Biological Characteristics
IgA	Secretory antibody	TGF-β	10–15% 6 days	Forms temporary attachment to epithelial cells as it is being secreted	Secreted as dimers into saliva, tears, bile, lumen of gut, and milk (providing passive immunity for infants); dimers protected by their secretory component. IgA provides protection against pathogens and invading antigens.
IgD	Reaginic antibody		0.2% 3–8 days	B-cell plasmalemma	Allows B cells to recognize antigens and elicits an immune response by inducing B-cell transformation into plasma cells.
IgE	Reaginic antibody	IL-4 and IL-5	Much less than 1% 2–5 days	Plasmalemmae of mast cells and basophils	Antigenic binding to IgE located on mast cell and basophil plasma membranes, induces these cells to release their pharmacological agents inducing an instantaneous hypersensitivity response.
IgG	Serum immunoglobulin	IFN-γ, IL4, and IL-6	65–75% 23 days	Neutrophils and macrophages	IgG can penetrate the placental barrier, thereby providing the fetus with passive immunity. IgG binds to antigenic sites on invading pathogens, opsonizing them facilitating phagocytosis by macrophages and neutrophils. IgG induces NK cells, thus initiating ADCC.
IgM	First to be formed in immune response		8–10% 5–10 days	IgM is a pentamer; however, its monomeric form binds to B cells.	Pentameric IgM activates the complement system. The principal place of formation of IgM is the spleen.

IFN, interferon; IL, interleukin; NK, natural killer; ADCC, antibody-dependent cell-mediated cytotoxicity.

2. The different isotypes exhibit functional differences.
    a. **IgA** is secretory immunoglobulin that is released, in the form of dimers, into tears, bile, saliva, milk, and as part of the nasal discharge to protect the body (and the nursing infant) from pathogenic microorganisms and invading antigens. It is protected from digestive enzymes by its **secretory component** synthesized by epithelial cells and hepatocytes.
    b. **IgD** and **IgE** are reaginic antibodies; IgE binds to IgE receptors of mast cells and basophils and prompts the release of pharmacologic agents from these cells to initiate an **immediate hypersensitivity response.** IgD binds to B-cell plasma membranes and permits these cells to recognize antigens and thus initiate a response against antigenic challenges by prompting B cells to differentiate into antibody-secreting **plasma cells.**
    c. **IgG**, the most abundant serum immunoglobulin, crosses the placental barrier to shield the fetus—a process known as **passive immunity.** It attaches to antigenic sites on invading microorganisms, thus opsonizing these pathogens, making them available for phagocytosis by macrophages and neutrophils. These antibodies activate NK cells, thus initiating **ADCC.**
    d. **IgM** forms pentamers and is the first isotype to be formed in an immune response. It activates the **complement system.** Its monomeric form binds to the B-cell plasma membrane.

V. DIFFUSE LYMPHOID TISSUE

Diffuse lymphoid tissue is considered to be a secondary lymphoid tissue. It is especially prominent in the mucosae of the gastrointestinal and respiratory systems. It is organized as nonencapsulated clusters of lymphoid cells or as lymphoid (lymphatic) nodules. Diffuse lymphoid tissue is collectively called **mucosa-associated lymphoid tissue (MALT).**

A. **MALT** consists of two major types: **bronchus-associated lymphoid tissue (BALT)** and **gut-associated lymphoid tissue (GALT).** Both types possess lymphoid nodules that are isolated from one another, except in the case of Peyer patches.

B. **Peyer patches** are aggregates of lymphoid nodules found in the **ileum.** They are components of the GALT.

C. **Lymphoid (lymphatic) nodules** are transitory dense spherical **accumulations of lymphocytes** (mostly B cells). The dark, peripheral region of nodules (**corona**) is composed mainly of small, newly formed lymphocytes. Lymphoid nodules of the GALT are isolated from the lumina of their respective tracts by **microfold (M) cells**, which transfer antigens from the lumen and present them (**without** processing them into epitopes) to lymphocytes and macrophages lying in deep invaginations of their basal cell surfaces. From here, an appropriate immune response is mounted by lymphoid tissue in the underlying lamina propria.
    1. **Secondary nodules,** formed in response to an antigenic challenge, have a lightly staining central area called the **germinal center**, which is composed of B lymphocytes (**lymphoblasts [centroblasts]** as well as **centrocytes**). A darker region, known as the **mantle (corona)**, is composed of resting B cells that are being displaced from the germinal center by the newly formed B cells. In addition to centroblasts and centrocytes, the germinal center houses B memory cells, plasma cells, migrating dendritic cells, follicular dendritic cells, macrophages, and reticular cells.
        a. **Centroblasts** do not display surface immunoglobulins (sIgs), whereas centrocytes have expressed sIgs.
        b. **Centrocytes** that express sIgs against self are forced into apoptosis.
        c. Surviving centrocytes become **B memory cells** or **plasma cells.**
        d. **Migrating dendritic cells,** derived from the bone marrow, are located in various regions of the body, and when they encounter an antigen, they travel to a nearby lymphoid nodule or lymph node to precipitate an immune reaction.

e. **Follicular dendritic cells** are resident cells of lymph nodes or lymphoid nodules and challenge the sIgs of newly formed centrocytes and force those centrocytes that do not possess the proper sIgs into apoptosis. **Macrophages** phagocytose the remnants of apoptotic cells.

f. **Reticular cells** are fibroblast-like cells that manufacture reticular fibers (type III collagen) to form the supporting skeleton of the lymphoid nodule and lymph node.

2. **Primary nodules** lack germinal centers and are composed of resting B memory cells, plasma cells, migrating dendritic cells, follicular dendritic cells, macrophages, and reticular cells.

VI. LYMPHOID ORGANS

A. **Lymph nodes**

1. **Overview—Lymph nodes are secondary lymphoid organs.**

   a. A lymph node is a small, ovoid to kidney-shaped structure with a capsule that sends **trabeculae** into the substance of the node (Figure 12.2).

   b. The **convex** surface of a lymph node receives afferent lymphatic vessels, whereas the **concave** surface (the **hilum**) is the site where arterioles enter and venules and efferent lymphatic vessels exit.

   c. Lymph nodes possess a **stroma** composed of **stromal cells** and a supportive framework rich in **reticular fibers.**

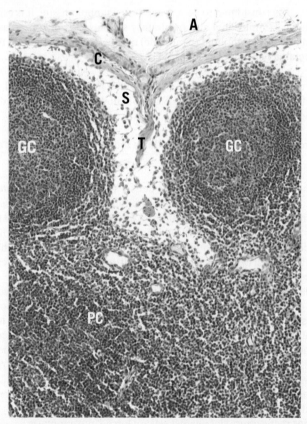

FIGURE 12.2. This photomicrograph of a human lymph node demonstrates that the capsule (C) of the node is surrounded by adipose tissue (A). The capsule sends trabeculae (T) into the substance of the node. Note the presence of the subcapsular and paratrabecular sinusoids (S) as well as the germinal centers (GC) of the lymphoid nodules. The paracortex (PC) is evident between the cortex and the medulla (×132).

d. Function. Lymph nodes filter lymph, maintain and produce T and B cells, and possess memory cells (especially T memory cells). Antigens delivered to lymph nodes by APCs are recognized by T cells, and an immune response is initiated. Additionally, some of the **stromal cells** and some of the **dendritic cells** of lymph nodes express the transcription factor **AIRE** (**a**uto**i**mmune **re**gulator), which selectively induces anti-self-T cells that escaped destruction in the thymus to go into apoptosis.

2. **Structure—Lymph nodes.** Lymph nodes are divided into three regions: the outermost **cortex**, the middle **paracortex**, and the innermost **medulla** (Figure 12.2). Stromal cells of these regions release a variety of **chemotactic chemokines lymphocytes (CCLs)** that attract lymphocytes. Depending on the CCL released, B cells or T cells are attracted to a particular region of the lymph node. In order to attract both B cells and T cells, CCLs are conveyed to the luminal endothelial cell membranes of postcapillary venules, the region where lymphocytes leave the circulatory system to enter the substance of the lymph node. Once in the lymph node stroma, both B cells and T cells are segregated within the cortex of the lymph node by those CCLs to which each responds.

   a. The **cortex of lymph nodes**

      (1) lies deep to the capsule, from which it is separated by a subcapsular sinus.

      (2) is incompletely subdivided into compartments by connective tissue septa derived from the capsule.

      (3) contains lymphoid nodules and sinusoids.

         (a) Lymphoid nodules are composed mainly of B cells but also of some T cells, follicular dendritic cells, macrophages, and reticular cells. They may possess a germinal center and then they are known as secondary lymphatic nodules.

         (b) Sinusoids are endothelium-lined lymphatic spaces that extend along the capsule and trabeculae and are known as **subcapsular** and **cortical sinusoids**, respectively.

   b. The **paracortex of the lymph node** is located between the cortex and the medulla.

      (1) It is composed of a non-nodular arrangement of **mostly T lymphocytes** (the thymus-dependent area of the lymph node) and **dendritic cells**.

      (2) The paracortex is the region where circulating lymphocytes gain access to lymph nodes via **postcapillary (high endothelial) venules (HEVs)**.

   c. The **medulla of a lymph node** lies deep to the paracortex and cortex, except at the region of the hilum. It is composed of medullary sinusoids and medullary cords.

      (1) Medullary sinusoids are endothelium-lined spaces supported by reticular fibers and reticular cells. They frequently contain macrophages and receive lymph from the cortical sinuses.

      (2) Medullary cords are composed of lymphocytes and plasma cells.

B. **The thymus is a primary lymphoid organ.**

   1. **Overview—Thymus**

      a. The thymus is a bilobed structure located in the neck. It is derived from both **endoderm** (**epithelial reticular cells**), derived from the third pharyngeal pouch of the embryo, and **mesoderm (lymphocytes [thymocytes])**. The development of the epithelial reticular cells of the thymus (especially in the medulla) is dependent on the formation and release of **lymphotoxins**, members of the tumor necrosis factor family of cytokines. In the absence of these proteins the thymus does not develop or function properly. The thymus begins to involute near the time of puberty.

      b. A connective tissue **capsule** surrounds the thymus. The septa of this capsule divide the parenchyma into incomplete lobules, each of which contains a **cortical** and **medullary region** (Figure 12.3). The thymus does not possess lymphoid nodules.

   2. **Structure—Thymus**

      a. **The thymic cortex** is supplied by arterioles in the septa; these arterioles provide capillary loops that enter the substance of the cortex. The cortex is the region in which **T-cell maturation** occurs.

         (1) Epithelial reticular cells (Figure 12.3)

            (a) There are six types of epithelial reticular cells (see Table 12.4). They are pale cells (derived, during embryogenesis, from the third and perhaps fourth pharyngeal pouches) and have a large ovoid lightly staining nucleus that often displays a nucleolus.

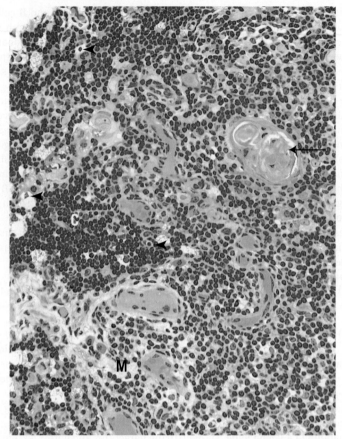

FIGURE 12.3. This low-power photomicrograph of the monkey thymus displays the dense cortex (C) and the lighter medulla (M). Note the numerous epithelial reticular cells (*arrowheads*) that are quite evident in the cortex as well as the thymic (Hassall) corpuscles (*arrow*) in the medulla (×132).

t a b l e 12.4 Reticular Epithelial Cells of the Thymus

Type	Location	Function
Cortex		
I	Junction of the capsule and the cortex as well as surrounding the trabeculae that partially separates thymic lobules from each other	Forms a barrier between the thymic parenchyma and the rest of the body; it also assists in the formation of the blood–thymus barrier by surrounding blood vessels in the thymic cortex
II	Stellate-shaped cells in the cortex where the processes of adjacent cells form desmosomes with each other	The processes surround and form compartments isolating maturing T cells. They express MHC I and MHC II and self-antigen molecules and present them to maturing T cells
III	On the cortical aspect of the corticomedullary junction	They form the boundary between the cortex and the medulla. They express MHC I and MHC II and self-antigen molecules and present them to maturing T cells
Medulla		
IV	On the medullary aspect of the corticomedullary junction	They and type III cells isolate the cortex from the medulla
V	Throughout the medulla	Form the cytoarchitectural framework of the medulla and form compartments for T cells
VI	Medulla	Form Hassall corpuscles, which are believed to be responsible for deletion of T-cell clones that would recognize and attack self-proteins. Manufacture and release thymic stromal lymphopoietin that aids in the formation of natural T reg cells

(b) They possess **long processes** that surround the thymic cortex, isolating it from both the connective tissue septa and the medulla. These processes, which are filled with bundles of **tonofilaments**, form desmosomal contacts with each other.

(c) They manufacture **thymosin**, **serum thymic factor**, **thymopoietin**, and **thymic stromal lymphopoietin**, hormones that function in the transformation of immature T lymphocytes into immunocompetent T cells.

(2) Thymocytes

(a) Thymocyte plasmalemma possesses Notch-1 receptors that permit these cells to respond to cytokines released by epithelial reticular cells to become T cells. Once committed to the T-cell lineage, they are known as **immature T lymphocytes** and are noted to be present within the thymic cortex in different stages of differentiation.

(b) Thymocytes are surrounded by processes of epithelial reticular cells, which help segregate thymocytes from antigens during their maturation.

(c) They migrate toward the medulla as they mature. Most T cells die in the cortex, and the dead cells are phagocytosed by macrophages.

(d) Surviving T cells are naïve. They leave the thymus and are distributed to secondary lymphoid organs by the vascular system.

(3) Blood–thymus barrier

(a) This barrier exists in the **cortex only**, making it an immunologically protected region.

(b) It ensures that antigens escaping from the bloodstream do not reach developing T cells in the thymic cortex.

(c) It consists of the following layers: **endothelium** of the thymic capillaries and the associated basal lamina, **perivascular connective tissue** and **cells** (e.g., pericytes and macrophages), and **type I epithelial reticular cells** and their basal laminae.

b. Thymic medulla

(1) The thymic medulla is continuous between adjacent lobules and contains large numbers of **epithelial reticular cells** and **mature T cells**, which are loosely packed, causing the medulla to stain lighter than the cortex (Figure 12.3).

(2) It also contains whorl-like accretions of type VI epithelial reticular cells called **Hassall corpuscles** (**thymic corpuscles**). These structures display various stages of keratinization and increase in number with age. It has been shown that these epithelial reticular cells manufacture **TSLP (thymic stromal lymphopoietin)**, a cytokine that facilitates dendritic cell maturation which, in turn, elicit the transformation of naïve T cells into natural T reg cells.

(3) Mature T cells exit the thymus via venules and efferent lymphatic vessels from the thymic medulla. The T cells then migrate to secondary lymphoid structures.

(4) Hormones acting on the thymus

(a) Thymosin, thymopoietin, thymulin (thymic factor), somatotropin, thymic stromal lymphopoietin, and thymic humoral factor promote the formation of immunocompetent T cells.

(b) Thyroxin encourages thymulin production by epithelial reticular cells.

(c) Adrenocorticosteroids depress T-cell formation in the thymus.

CLINICAL CONSIDERATIONS **DiGeorge syndrome**, also called **congenital thymic aplasia**, is characterized by the congenital absence of the thymus and parathyroid glands, resulting from abnormal development of the third and fourth pharyngeal pouches.

1. This syndrome is associated with **abnormal cell-mediated immunity** but relatively normal humoral immunity.
2. It usually results in **death** from **tetany** or uncontrollable **infection**.

C. Spleen

1. Overview—Spleen

a. A simple squamous epithelium (peritoneum) covers the dense irregular collagenous connective tissue **capsule** of the spleen, which sends **trabeculae** into the substance of the spleen to form a supportive framework (Figure 12.4).

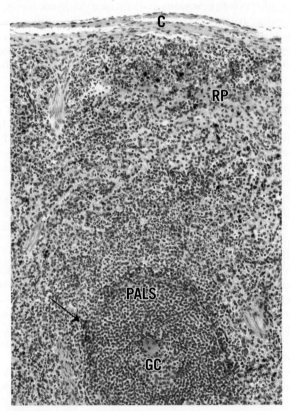

FIGURE 12.4. This low-power photomicrograph displays the smooth capsule (C) of a human spleen. Observe that the spleen is not divided into a cortex and a medulla; instead, it has red pulp (RP) and white pulp. Note the presence of a lymphoid nodule with a germinal center (GC) composed of B lymphocytes. The lymphoid nodule is invested by the T-cell–rich region of the spleen, known as the periarterial lymphatic sheath (PALS). The *arrow* points to the marginal zone located between the white pulp and the RP (×132).

    b. The spleen is similar to lymph nodes in that it possesses a hilum, but differs from both the thymus and the lymph nodes in that it **lacks a cortex and medulla.** It further differs from lymph nodes because it has no **afferent lymphatic vessels.**

    c. The spleen is divided into **red pulp** and **white pulp**; the latter contains lymphoid elements. These two regions are separated from each other by the **marginal zone** (Figure 12.4).

    d. Function—Spleen. The spleen filters blood, phagocytoses damaged and aged erythrocytes, and is a site of proliferation of B and T lymphocytes and the production of antibodies by plasma cells. In some animals, such as the dog but not in humans, it stores red blood cells.

2. Vascularization of the spleen is derived from the **splenic artery**, which enters the hilum and gives rise to trabecular arteries.

    a. Trabecular arteries leave the trabeculae, become invested by a **periarterial lymphatic sheath** (**PALS**, described later), and are known as central arteries.

    b. Central arteries branch but maintain their lymphatic sheath until they leave the white pulp to form several straight penicillar arteries.

    c. Penicillar arteries enter the red pulp. They have three regions: pulp arterioles, macrophage-sheathed arterioles, and **terminal arterial capillaries.** These last named vessels either drain directly into the splenic sinusoids (**closed circulation**) or terminate as open-ended vessels within the splenic cords of the red pulp (**open circulation**).

    d. Splenic sinusoids are drained by pulp veins, which are tributaries of the trabecular veins; these in turn drain into the splenic vein, which exits the spleen at the hilum.

3. Structure—Spleen

    a. White pulp of the spleen includes **all** of the organ's lymphoid tissue (diffuse and nodular), such as **lymphoid nodules** (mostly B cells) and **PALS** (mostly T cells) around the central arteries. It also contains macrophages and other APCs.

b. The **marginal zone (MZ) of the spleen**

(1) is a **sinusoidal region** between the red and white pulps at the periphery of the PALS (Figure 12.4).

(2) receives blood from capillary loops derived from the central artery and is thus the **first site where blood contacts the splenic parenchyma.**

(3) is richly supplied by avidly phagocytic macrophages and other APCs. There are two types of macrophages in the marginal zone: the **MZ macrophages** and the **MZ metallophilic macrophages.**

(a) MZ macrophages express molecules on their surface that recognize pathogens such as bacteria, viruses, and yeasts.

(b) MZ metallophilic macrophages express molecules that bind to cell-bound oligosaccharide ligands; these macrophages also interact with **marginal zone B cells** (see Section II C 4 b in this chapter), promoting them to migrate to the white pulp of the spleen and present blood-borne antigens to T cells.

(4) The **MZ** is the region where circulating T and B lymphocytes **enter the spleen** before becoming segregated to their specific locations within the organ and where **interdigitating dendritic cells** are able to display their MHC–epitope complex for recognition by T cells.

(5) Stromal cells of the MZ release a variety of **CCLs (chemotactic chemokines lymphocytes)** that attract lymphocytes. Depending on the CCL released, B cells or T cells are attracted to a particular region of the spleen. In order to attract both B cells and T cells to the MZ, CCLs are conveyed to the luminal endothelial cell membranes of MZ sinusoids. Once in the spleen parenchyma, both B cells and T cells are segregated within the white pulp of the spleen by those CCLs to which each responds.

c. Red pulp of the spleen (Figure 12.4) is composed of an interconnected network of sinusoids supported by a loose type of reticular tissue (**splenic cords**).

(1) Sinusoids

(a) are lined by long fusiform endothelial cells separated by relatively large blood-containing intercellular spaces.

(b) have a discontinuous basal lamina underlying the endothelium and circumferentially arranged ribs of reticular fibrils.

(2) Splenic cords (cords of Billroth) contain plasma cells, stellate reticular cells, blood cells, and macrophages enmeshed within the spaces of the reticular fiber network. Processes of the macrophages enter the lumina of the sinusoids through the spaces between the endothelial cells.

D. **Tonsils** are **aggregates of lymphoid tissue**, which sometimes lack a capsule. All tonsils are in the upper section of the digestive tract, lying beneath but in contact with the epithelium. B and T cells in the three sets of tonsils are localized in different regions of any particular tonsil. The mechanism of distribution is similar to that which occurs in lymph nodes and the spleen, and depends on the various **chemotactic chemokines for lymphocytes** (**CCLs**) secreted by stromal cells. Tonsils assist in combating antigens entering via the nasal and oral epithelia.

1. Palatine tonsils

a. possess **crypts**, deep invaginations of the stratified squamous epithelium covering of the tonsils, frequently containing debris;

b. possess primary and secondary (with germinal centers) lymphoid nodules;

c. are separated from subjacent structures by a connective tissue **capsule.**

2. The **pharyngeal tonsil** is a **single** tonsil in the posterior wall of the nasopharynx.

a. It is covered by a pseudostratified ciliated columnar epithelium.

b. Instead of crypts, it has longitudinal pleats (infoldings).

c. Possesses primary and secondary (with germinal centers) lymphoid nodules.

3. Lingual tonsil

a. is on the dorsum of the posterior third of the tongue and is covered by a stratified squamous nonkeratinized epithelium.

b. possesses deep **crypts**, which frequently contain debris. Ducts of the posterior mucous glands of the tongue often open into the base of these crypts.

c. possesses primary and secondary (with germinal centers) lymphoid nodules.

Review Test

Directions: Each of the numbered items or incomplete statements in this section is followed by answers or completions of the statement. Select the ONE lettered answer that is BEST in each case.

1. Which of the following statements concerning T helper cells is true?

(A) They possess membrane-bound antibodies.
(B) They can recognize and interact with antigens in the blood.
(C) They produce numerous cytokines.
(D) They function only in cell-mediated immunity.
(E) Their activation depends on interferon-γ.

2. Which of the following statements concerning T cytotoxic (T_C) cells is true?

(A) They assist macrophages in killing microorganisms.
(B) They possess antibodies on their surfaces.
(C) They possess CD8 surface markers.
(D) They possess CD28 surface markers.
(E) They secrete interferon-γ.

3. Which of the following cell types is thought to function in suppressing the immune response?

(A) Inducible T reg cells
(B) B cells
(C) T memory cells
(D) T_H cells
(E) Mast cells

4. Which of the following statements concerning interferon-γ is true?

(A) It is produced by T memory cells.
(B) It is produced by T reg cells.
(C) It activates macrophages.
(D) It inhibits macrophages.
(E) It induces viral proliferation.

5. A patient who was given penicillin had an adverse reaction to the antibiotic. Although the reaction was due to the actions of mast cells, the response occurred because mast cells have IgE receptors in their cell membranes. Which of the following cells produced the IgE decorating the plasma cell's surface?

(A) T memory cells
(B) B memory cells
(C) T helper cells
(D) Plasma cells
(E) T cytotoxic cells

6. Which of the following statements concerning the thymus is true?

(A) Lymphoid nodules form much of the thymic cortex.
(B) Epithelial reticular cells form Hassall corpuscles.
(C) T cells migrate into the medulla, where they become immunologically competent.
(D) Most T cells that enter the thymus are killed in the medulla.
(E) Macrophages are essential components of the blood–thymus barrier.

7. Which of the following statements concerning Hassall corpuscles is true?

(A) They are located in the thymic cortex of young individuals.
(B) They are located in the thymic cortex of old individuals.
(C) They are derived from mesoderm.
(D) They are located in the thymic medulla.
(E) They are derived from T memory cells.

8. After their maturation in the thymus and release into the circulation, T lymphocytes migrate preferentially to which of the following sites?

(A) Paracortex of lymph nodes
(B) Cortical lymphoid nodules of lymph nodes
(C) Hilum of lymph nodes
(D) Lymphoid nodules of the tonsils
(E) Lymphoid nodules of the spleen

9. In which of the following sites do lymphocytes become immunocompetent?

(A) Germinal center of secondary lymphoid nodules
(B) White pulp of the spleen
(C) Thymic cortex
(D) Red pulp of the spleen
(E) Paracortex of lymph nodes

10. Which of the following statements about IgG is true?

(A) It is located in the serum and on the membrane of B cells.
(B) It can cross the placental barrier.
(C) It is involved in allergic reactions.
(D) It exists as a pentamer.
(E) It binds to antigens on the body surface and in the lumen of the gastrointestinal tract.

Answers and Explanations

1. **C.** T helper cells produce a number of cytokines that affect other cells involved in both the cell-mediated and humoral immune responses. T helper cells possess antigen-specific TCRs (not antibodies) on their membranes. These cells recognize and interact with antigenic determinants that are associated with class II HLA molecules on the surface of APCs. IL-1 is necessary for activation of T helper cells (see Chapter 12 II B 3 c).

2. **C.** T cytotoxic cells are CD8+ cells. CD28 molecules are present on T_H1 cells. IFN-γ is released by T_H1 cells, which also assist macrophages in killing microorganisms (see Chapter 12 II B 3 c).

3. **A.** The immune response is decreased by inducible T reg cells. They suppress the formation of T_H1 cells, thereby suppressing the immune response (see Chapter 12 II B 3 c).

4. **C.** Interferon-γ activates macrophages, NK cells, and T cytotoxic cells, enhancing their phagocytic or cytotoxic activity or both (see Chapter 12 II E 2).

5. **D.** Individuals allergic to penicillin produce IgE antibodies. The cells that manufacture IgE are plasma cells. After an antigenic challenge, proliferation and differentiation of B cells give rise to plasma cells and B memory cells (see Chapter 12 II C 2).

6. **B.** Epithelial reticular cells of the medulla congregate to form Hassall (thymic) corpuscles (see Chapter 12 VI B 2 b).

7. **D.** Hassall corpuscles are concentric accretions of epithelial reticular cells (derived from endoderm) found only in the medulla of the thymus (see Chapter 12 VI B 2 b).

8. **A.** T lymphocytes are preferentially located in the paracortex of lymph nodes, whereas B lymphocytes are found in lymphoid nodules located in lymph nodes, tonsils, and the spleen (see Chapter 12 VI A 2 a).

9. **C.** T lymphocytes mature and become immunocompetent in the cortex of the thymus, whereas B lymphocytes do so in the bone marrow. After an antigenic challenge, lymphocytes proliferate and differentiate in various lymphoid tissues (see Chapter 12 II B 2 and II C 1).

10. **B.** IgG is the most abundant immunoglobulin isotype in the serum. It can cross the placental barrier but does not bind to the B-cell plasma membrane. It exists as a monomer, functions to activate complement, and acts as an opsonin (see Chapter 12 IV B 2).

13 Endocrine System

I. OVERVIEW—THE ENDOCRINE SYSTEM

A. The endocrine system is composed of several **ductless glands, clusters of cells** within certain organs, and isolated single **endocrine cells**, known as the diffuse neuroendocrine system (DNES) cells, located in the epithelial lining of the respiratory and gastrointestinal systems (discussed in chapters 15 and 16, respectively).

B. Glands of the endocrine system include the **pituitary gland** (and a region of the brain known as the **hypothalamus**), as well as the **thyroid, parathyroid, adrenal**, and **pineal** glands. Additional components of the endocrine system, such as the Islets of Langerhans, adipose tissue, female gonads, and male gonads, are discussed in the pertinent chapters.

C. **Function.** The endocrine system secretes hormones into nearby capillaries and interacts with the nervous system to modulate and control the body's metabolic activities.

II. HORMONES

Hormones are **chemical messengers** that are carried via the bloodstream to distant **target cells**. They include low-molecular-weight **water-soluble** proteins, polypeptides, and amino acids (e.g., insulin, glucagon, follicle-stimulating hormone [FSH]) and **lipid-soluble** substances, principally the **steroid hormones** (e.g., progesterone, estradiol, and testosterone).

A. **Water-soluble hormones** interact with specific cell surface receptors on target cells, which communicate a message that generates a biological response by the cell.
   1. **G protein–linked receptors** are used by some hormones (e.g., epinephrine, thyroid-stimulating hormone [TSH], serotonin). Binding of the hormone to the G protein–linked receptor leads to the production of a second messenger that evokes a target-cell response.
   2. **Catalytic receptors** are used by insulin and growth hormone. Binding of the hormone to the catalytic receptor activates protein kinases that phosphorylate target proteins.

B. **Lipid-soluble hormones** diffuse across the plasma membrane of target cells and bind to specific receptors in the cytosol or in the nucleus, forming hormone–receptor complexes that regulate transcription of deoxyribonucleic acid (DNA).

III. OVERVIEW—PITUITARY GLAND (HYPOPHYSIS) AND HYPOTHALAMUS

The **pituitary gland** lies below the hypothalamus in a bony housing known as the **hypophyseal fossa**, a depression in the **sella turcica** of the sphenoid bone located in the base of the middle cranial fossa of the skull.

The **hypothalamus** is a region of the diencephalon of the brain; it possesses nuclei that are structurally and functionally linked to the pituitary gland. The structural link is via a series of axons whose cell bodies are located in the **supraoptic** and **paraventricular** nuclei of the hypothalamus. These axons form the **hypothalamo-hypophyseal tract** and terminate in the pars nervosa of the pituitary gland, where they store and, when needed, release their hormones. The functional connection is via **releasing hormones** that are synthesized in the **arcuate, paraventricular** (and **medial paraventricular**), **periventricular, ventromedial**, and **dorsal nuclei** of the hypothalamus. These hormones are released by the neurons located in these nuclei, enter a capillary bed, and make their way, via the **hypophyseal portal system** to a second capillary bed in the anterior lobe of the pituitary gland, leave the capillary bed, and bind to their respective target cells in the anterior pituitary.

The **pituitary gland** is a relatively small gland, weighing only about 0.6 g in men and 1.2 g in women who are pregnant or who have given birth to two or more children. The pituitary is divided into two major subdivisions, the **adenohypophysis** and the **neurohypophysis** (Figure 13.1). Each subdivision is derived from a distinct embryonic analog, which is reflected in its unique cellular constituents and functions.

A. The adenohypophysis is also called the **anterior pituitary gland** (Figures 13.1 and 13.2). It originates from an ectodermal diverticulum of the stomodeum **(Rathke pouch)**. The adenohypophysis is subdivided into the **pars distalis, pars intermedia**, and **pars tuberalis**.

1. The **pars distalis** is supported by a connective tissue capsule and framework. It consists of irregular cords composed of two types of parenchymal cells, **chromophils** and **chromophobes**, lying adjacent to **fenestrated** capillaries.

   a. **Chromophils** (Figures 13.1 and 13.3)

      (1) Overview. **Chromophils** are parenchymal cells that stain intensely because of their hormone-containing secretory granules. They synthesize, store, and release several hormones. They are regulated by specific **stimulatory** and **inhibitory hormones** produced by neurons, referred to as **neurosecretory cells**, in the **hypothalamus**. These hormones are conveyed to the pars distalis via a system of portal blood vessels originating in the **median eminence**.

      (2) Types. Chromophils are classified into two types, acidophils and basophils, depending on the dyes they bind using special histological stains. With hematoxylin–eosin stain, the distinction between the two cell types is much less obvious.

         (a) **Acidophils** (Tables 13.1 and 13.2) bind acidic dyes and often stain **orange** or **red**. They are small cells of two subtypes: somatotrophs and mammotrophs.

            1. **Somatotrophs** constitute about 50% of the chromophils and produce **somatotropin (growth hormone)**. They are stimulated by **somatotropin-releasing hormone** and are inhibited by **somatostatin**.

            2. **Mammotrophs** (**lactotrophs**) constitute about 10% of the chromophil population, except in multiparous women, where they may be as high as 30%. Mammotrophs produce **prolactin**, which is stored in small secretory granules. They are stimulated by **prolactin-releasing hormone** and **thyrotropin-releasing hormone (TRH)** and are inhibited by **dopamine** (until re-identified that it was designated as **prolactin-inhibiting hormone**).

         (b) **Basophils** (Tables 13.1 and 13.2) bind basic dyes and typically stain **blue**. They include three subtypes: corticotrophs, thyrotrophs, and gonadotrophs.

            1. **Corticotrophs** constitute about 10% of the chromophil population. They produce **pro-opiomelanocortin (POMC)** whose by-products are **adrenocorticotropic hormone (ACTH)**, **melanocyte-stimulating hormone (MSH)**, and **lipotropic**

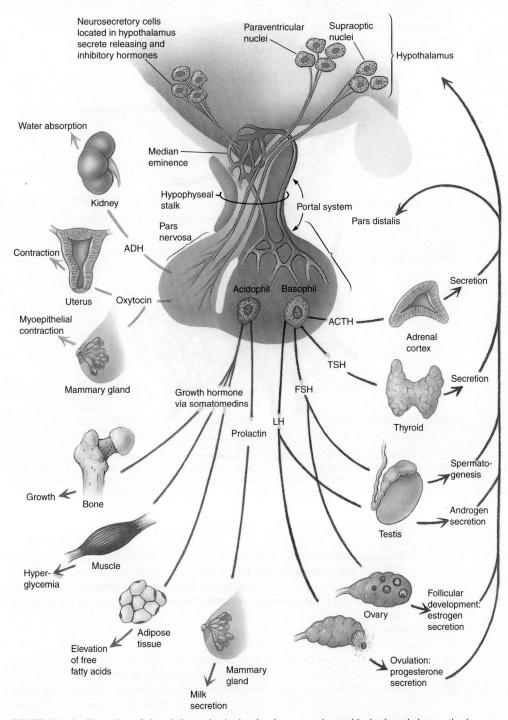

FIGURE 13.1. An illustration of the pituitary gland, showing its connections with the hypothalamus, the hormones it releases, and the effects of these hormones on organs and tissues of the body. ADH, antidiuretic hormone; ACTH, adrenocorticotropic hormone; TSH, thyroid-stimulating hormone; FSH, follicle-stimulating hormone; LH, luteinizing hormone. (From Gartner LP, Hiatt JL. *Color Atlas of Histology.* 5th ed. Baltimore, MD: Lippincott William & Wilkins; 2009:206.)

hormone **(LTH)**, a precursor of β-endorphin. They are stimulated by **corticotropin-releasing hormone**.

2. **Thyrotrophs** constitute about 5% of the chromophil population, produce **TSH**, and are stimulated by **TRH**.

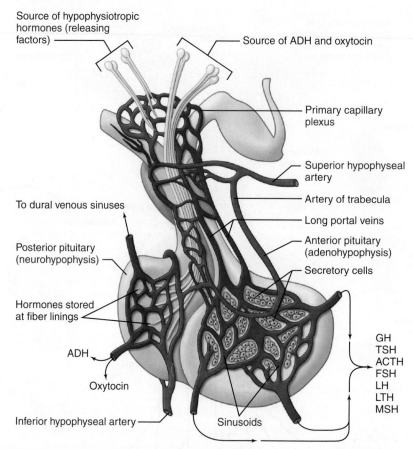

Source of hypophysiotropic hormones (releasing factors)

Source of ADH and oxytocin

Primary capillary plexus

Superior hypophyseal artery

Artery of trabecula

Long portal veins

Anterior pituitary (adenohypophysis)

Secretory cells

To dural venous sinuses

Posterior pituitary (neurohypophysis)

Hormones stored at fiber linings

ADH

Oxytocin

Inferior hypophyseal artery

Sinusoids

GH
TSH
ACTH
FSH
LH
LTH
MSH

FIGURE 13.2. A diagram of the pituitary gland showing its connections to the hypothalamus, sites of hormone synthesis and storage, and vascularization. The adenohypophysis is shown at the right and consists of the pars distalis, pars tuberalis, and pars intermedia (not shown). The neurohypophysis consists of the infundibulum (stalk) and pars nervosa. Various releasing and inhibiting hormones stored in the median eminence are transferred, via the hypophyseal portal system, to the pars distalis. ADH, antidiuretic hormone; GH, growth hormone; TSH, thyroid-stimulating hormone; ACTH, adrenocorticotropic hormone; FSH, follicle-stimulating hormone; LH, luteinizing hormone. (Reprinted with permission from Morton P, Fontaine D. *Critical Care Nursing.* 10th ed. Philadelphia, PA: Wolters Kluwer Health/Lippincott Williams & Wilkins; 2012:959.)

   3. Gonadotrophs constitute about 10% of the chromophil population. They produce **FSH** and **luteinizing hormone (LH)** in both sexes, although in men, the latter is sometimes referred to as **interstitial cell–stimulating hormone**. Gonadotrophs are stimulated by **gonadotropin-releasing hormone**, also known as LH-releasing hormone.

 b. Chromophobes (Figure 13.3)
   (1) are parenchymal cells that stain poorly.
   (2) appear as small cells under the light microscope; the cells lack (or have only a few) secretory granules and are arranged close to one another in clusters.
   (3) sometimes resemble degranulated chromophils in the electron microscope, suggesting that they may represent different stages in the life cycle of various acidophil and basophil populations.
   (4) may also represent undifferentiated cells that are capable of differentiating into various types of chromophils.
 c. Folliculostellate cells
   (1) are numerous in the pars distalis and lie between the chromophils and chromophobes.
   (2) possess long processes that form gap junctions with processes of other folliculostellate cells.
   (3) produce many peptides that are thought to regulate the production of pars distalis hormones via a paracrine effect.

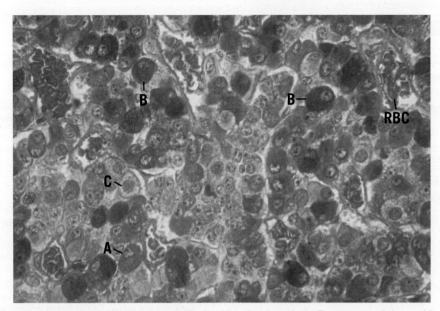

FIGURE 13.3. A light micrograph of cells in the pars distalis of the adenohypophysis. The two types of chromophil cells are easily identified using the trichrome stain. Basophils (B) stain blue, and acidophils (A) stain red. Chromophobes (C) are smaller and show little affinity for the stain. Many erythrocytes (red blood cells [RBCs]) are present in the capillaries (×300).

2. The **pars intermedia** lies between the pars distalis and pars nervosa.
   a. It contains many **colloid-containing cysts (Rathke cysts)** that are lined by cuboidal cells.
   b. It also possesses **basophilic cells**, which sometimes extend into the pars nervosa. These cells secrete the **prohormone POMC**, which is cleaved to form **ACTH, lipotropin,** and **MSH.** In humans, MSH acts to induce melanocytes to produce melanin and may act in various ways to modulate inflammatory responses throughout the body, and it may play a role in controlling stores of body fat.
3. The **pars tuberalis** surrounds the cranial part of the infundibulum (hypophyseal stalk).
   a. It is composed of cuboidal **basophilic cells**, arranged in cords along an abundant capillary network.
   b. Its cells may secrete FSH and LH, but this has not been confirmed.

CLINICAL CONSIDERATIONS **Pituitary adenomas** are **common tumors** of the anterior pituitary.

1. They enlarge and often suppress secretions by the remaining pars distalis cells.
2. These tumors frequently destroy surrounding bone and neural tissues and are treated by surgical removal.

B. **The neurohypophysis** (Figures 13.1 and 13.2; Table 13.1) is also called the **posterior pituitary gland.** It originates from an evagination of the hypothalamus and is divided into the **infundibulum,** which is continuous with the hypothalamus, and the **pars nervosa,** or main body of the neurohypophysis.
   1. **Hypothalamo-hypophyseal tract**
      a. contains the unmyelinated axons of **neurosecretory cells** whose cell bodies are located in the **supraoptic** and **paraventricular nuclei** of the hypothalamus.
      b. transports **oxytocin** and **antidiuretic hormone (ADH; vasopressin)**, each bound to **neurophysin** (a binding protein specific for each hormone) to the pars nervosa (see Table 13.2). Oxytocin binds to neurophysin I, whereas ADH binds to neurophysin II. Additionally, acetylcholine and adenosine triphosphate (ATP) are transported to the pars nervosa by the axons that compose the hypothalamo-hypophyseal tract.

table **13.1**	Physiological Effects of Pituitary Hormones	
Cell	**Hormone**	**Major Function**
Hormones released by the pars distalis		
Acidophils		
Somatotrophs	Somatotropin (growth hormone)	Increases metabolism in most cells; indirectly stimulates epiphyseal plate, growth of long bones via production of insulin-like growth factors I, II
Mammotrophs (Lactotrophs)	Prolactin	Development of mammary gland during pregnancy, milk synthesis during lactation
Basophils		
Corticotrophs	POMC whose by-products are ACTH, MSH, and lipotropin	ACTH stimulates glucocorticoid secretion by zona fasciculata cells of adrenal cortex; MSH stimulates melanocytes to manufacture melanin pigments; Lipotropin also stimulates melanocytes to manufacture melanin, but also mobilizes lipids by inducing lipolysis and the formation of steroids.
Gonadotrophs	FSH	Stimulates growth of secondary ovarian follicles, estrogen secretion in women; stimulates spermatogenesis via production of androgen-binding protein in Sertoli cells in men
	LH or interstitial cell–stimulating hormone	Ovulation, formation of corpus luteum, and progesterone secretion in women; testosterone synthesis by Leydig cells of testis in men
Thyrotrophs	TSH	Stimulates synthesis and release of T_3, T_4 by follicular cells
Hormones released by the pars nervosa		
Neurosecretory cells of hypothalamus (primarily in the paraventricular nucleus)	Oxytocin	Induces contraction of smooth muscle in wall of uterus at parturition and in myoepithelial cells of mammary gland during nursing
Neurosecretory cells of hypothalamus (primarily in the supraoptic nucleus)	ADH	Renders kidney collecting tubules permeable to water, which is resorbed to produce a concentrated urine; constricts smooth muscle in wall of arterioles

POMC, pro-opiomelanocortin; ACTH, adrenocorticotropic hormone; MSH, melanocyte-stimulating hormone; FSH, follicle-stimulating hormone; LH, luteinizing hormone; TSH, thyroid-stimulating hormone; ADH, antidiuretic hormone.

2. **Pars nervosa**
   a. contains the distal ends of the hypothalamo-hypophyseal axons and is the site where the neurosecretory granules in these axons are stored in accumulations known as **Herring bodies**.
   b. releases oxytocin and ADH into fenestrated capillaries in response to nerve stimulation.
3. **Pituicytes**
   a. occupy approximately 25% of the volume of the pars nervosa.
   b. are glial-like cells that support axons in this region.
   c. possess numerous cytoplasmic processes and contain lipid droplets, intermediate filaments, and pigments.

CLINICAL CONSIDERATIONS   **Diabetes Insipidus**

Diabetes insipidus results from inadequate amounts of ADH; it is discussed in Chapter 18 V C Clinical Considerations.

C. **Vascularization of the pituitary gland**
   1. **Arterial supply** is from two pairs of blood vessels derived from the internal carotid artery.
      a. The right and left **superior** hypophyseal arteries serve the pars tuberalis, infundibulum, and median eminence.
      b. The right and left **inferior** hypophyseal arteries serve mostly the pars nervosa.

t a b l e **13.2**	Hormones of the Hypothalamus	
Hormone	Nucleus	Primary Functions
Oxytocin	Primarily the paraventricular nucleus	Induces contraction of smooth muscle in wall of uterus at parturition and in myoepithelial cells of mammary gland during nursing
ADH; vasopressin	Primarily the supraoptic nucleus	Renders kidney collecting tubules permeable to water, which is resorbed to produce a concentrated urine; constricts smooth muscle in wall of arterioles
CRH	Arcuate, medial paraventricular, and periventricular nuclei	Induces the release of POMC by the corticotrophs of the anterior pituitary
Dopamine	Arcuate nucleus	Inhibits prolactin release by mammotrophs (lactotrophs) of the anterior pituitary
GnRH	Arcuate, dorsal, paraventricular, and ventromedial nuclei	Induces the release of LH and FSH by gonadotrophs of the anterior pituitary
Somatostatin	Arcuate nucleus	Inhibits somatotropin release by the somatotrophs of the anterior pituitary
Somatotropin-releasing factor (SRH) (also known as growth hormone–releasing factor, GHRH)	Arcuate nucleus	Induces the release of somatotropin (growth hormone) by the somatotrophs of the anterior pituitary
TRH	Dorsal, paraventricular, and ventromedial nuclei	Induces the release of TSH by the thyrotrophs as well as prolactin by the mammotrophs (lactotrophs) of the anterior pituitary

ADH, antidiuretic hormone; CRH, corticotropin-releasing hormone; POMC, pro-opiomelanocortin; GnRH, gonadotropin-releasing hormone; LH, luteinizing hormone; FSH, follicle-stimulating hormone; SRH, somatotropin-releasing hormone; GHRH, growth hormone–releasing hormone; TRH, thyrotropin-releasing hormone; TSH, thyroid-stimulating hormone.

2. **Hypophyseal portal system** (Figures 13.1 and 13.2)
   a. The **primary capillary plexus** consists of fenestrated capillaries coming off the superior hypophyseal arteries.
      (1) This plexus is located in the **median eminence**, where stored hypothalamic neurosecretory hormones enter the blood.
      (2) It is drained by **hypophyseal portal veins**, which descend through the infundibulum into the adenohypophysis.
   b. The **secondary capillary plexus** consists of **fenestrated** capillaries derived from the hypophyseal portal veins. This plexus is located in the **pars distalis**, where neurosecretory hormones leave the blood to stimulate or inhibit the parenchymal cells.

CLINICAL CONSIDERATION

Sheehan Syndrome

Sheehan syndrome is necrosis of the anterior pituitary gland due to a sudden reduction in blood pressure of the newborn as a result of postpartum hemorrhage. The bulk of the anterior pituitary becomes necrotic and only the peripheral parenchymal cells remain healthy and viable. The functionality of the adenohypophysis depends on the severity of the necrotic event; the wider the parenchymal destruction, the less function remains. Interestingly, the neurohypophysis is usually unaffected because it has a different blood supply.

Hemosiderosis

Patients afflicted with **hemochromatosis (iron overload)**, whether as a function of heredity or acquired due to multiple transfusions, present with iron deposits in the pituitary gland, especially in the gonadotrophs. This condition is known as **hemosiderosis** and is fortunately treatable either by phlebotomy or by chelating the iron with one of the available chelating agents in the pharmaceutical armamentarium.

D. **Regulation of the pars distalis** (Figures 13.1 and 13.2)
   1. Neurosecretory cells in the hypothalamus synthesize specific hormones that enter the hypophyseal portal system and stimulate or inhibit the parenchymal cells of the pars distalis (see Table 13.2).
   2. The hypothalamic neurosecretory cells in turn are regulated by the level of hormones in the blood (**negative feedback**) or by other physiological (or psychological) factors.
   3. Some hormones (e.g., thyroid hormones, cortisol) exert negative feedback on the pars distalis directly.

IV. OVERVIEW—THYROID GLAND (Figure 13.4)

The thyroid gland is composed of two lobes connected by an **isthmus**. It is surrounded by a dense irregular collagenous connective tissue capsule, in which (posteriorly) the **parathyroid glands** are embedded. The thyroid gland is subdivided by capsular septa into lobules containing **follicles**. These septa also serve as conduits for blood vessels, lymphatic vessels, and nerves.

A. **Thyroid follicles** are spherical structures filled with **colloid**, a viscous gel consisting mostly of **iodinated thyroglobulin** (Figure 13.5)
   1. Surrounding the colloid within each follicle is a single layer of epithelial cells, called **follicular cells**. In addition, one or more **parafollicular cells** occasionally lie sandwiched between the follicular cells. Both of these parenchymal cell types rest upon the basal lamina surrounding the follicle, which separates them from the abundant network of **fenestrated capillaries** in the connective tissue.
   2. **Function.** Thyroid follicles synthesize, store, and release thyroid hormones.

B. **Follicular cells** (Figure 13.6)
   1. **Structure**
      a. Follicular cells are normally cuboidal, but they become columnar when stimulated and squamous when inactive.
      b. They possess a distended rough endoplasmic reticulum (RER) with many ribosome-free regions, a supranuclear Golgi complex, many lysosomes, and rod-shaped mitochondria.
      c. Follicular cells also contain many small **apical vesicles**, which are involved in the transport and release of thyroglobulin and enzymes into the colloid.
      d. They possess short, blunt microvilli that extend into the colloid.
   2. **Synthesis and release of the thyroid hormones thyroxine (T_4) and triiodothyronine (T_3)** occur by the sequence of events illustrated in Figure 13.7. These processes are evoked by **TSH**, which binds to G protein–linked receptors on the basal surface of follicular cells.

CLINICAL CONSIDERATIONS — Graves disease is characterized by a diffuse **enlargement of the thyroid gland** and **protrusion of the eyeballs** (exophthalmic goiter).

1. This disease is associated with the presence of columnar-shaped thyroid follicular cells, excessive production of thyroid hormones, and decreased amounts of follicular colloid.
2. It is caused by the binding of autoimmune immunoglobulin G (IgG) antibodies to TSH receptors, which stimulates the thyroid follicular cells. Additionally, inflammatory cells, such as T cells, neutrophils, and macrophages, invade the connective tissues of the retro-orbital region and release cytokines that activate fibroblasts not only to increase their production of proteoglycans but also to differentiate into fat cells. Since proteoglycans readily attract Na^+ ions which attract water molecules, the connective tissue volume increases; moreover, the additional number of fat cells also acts to increase the volume of the retro-orbital connective tissue, putting increased pressure on the back of the eyeball, pushing it forward, resulting in protrusion of the eye.

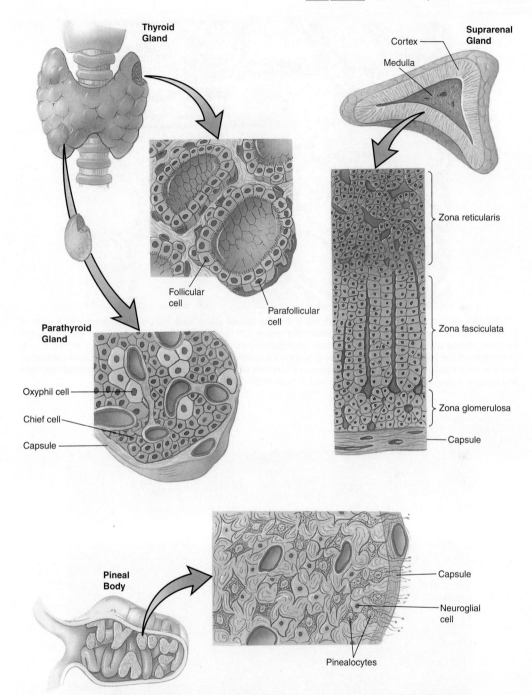

FIGURE 13.4. A diagram showing features of the thyroid, parathyroid, adrenal, and pineal glands. (From Gartner LP, Hiatt JL. *Color Atlas of Histology.* 5th ed. Baltimore, MD: Lippincott William & Wilkins; 2009:207.)

C. **Parafollicular cells** are also called **clear (C) cells** because they stain less intensely than thyroid follicular cells (Figures 13.5 and 13.8).

   1. Parafollicular cells are present singly or in small clusters of cells between the follicular cells and basal lamina.

   2. These cells belong to the population of **DNES cells**, previously known as **a**mine **p**recursor **u**ptake and **d**ecarboxylation (**APUD**) cells, or enteroendocrine cells.

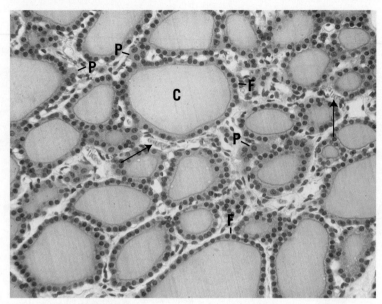

FIGURE 13.5. A light micrograph showing follicles within the thyroid gland. Each follicle is surrounded by a layer of follicular cells (F) and contains a central colloid-filled region (C). The follicular cells synthesize and secrete thyroid hormones bound within a large protein molecule, thyroglobulin, which makes up most of the colloid. A second type of endocrine cell, the parafollicular cell (P), is also present in the thyroid gland. It has no contact with the colloid and is often found in small clusters at or near the basal surfaces of the follicular cells. The parafollicular cell synthesizes calcitonin and releases it into the rich network of capillaries (*arrows*) existing between the follicles (×150).

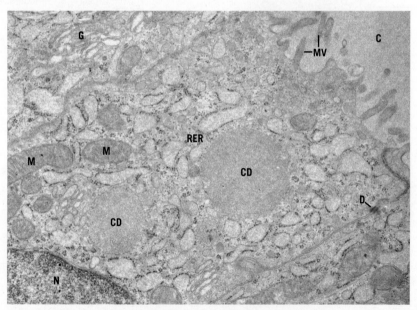

FIGURE 13.6. Electron micrograph of thyroid follicular cells. Two large colloid droplets (CD), a distended rough endoplasmic reticulum (RER) with many ribosome-free regions, and a Golgi apparatus (G) are observed. Microvilli (MV) extend into the lumen of a follicle-containing colloid (C). Also present are mitochondria (M), a nucleus (N), and a desmosome (D) (×7,500).

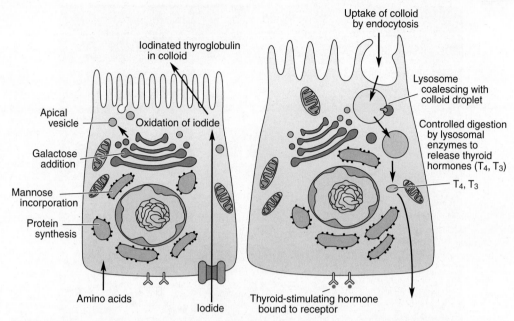

FIGURE 13.7. Synthesis and release of T_4 and T_3 by follicular cells of the thyroid gland. **A.** Thyroglobulin is synthesized like other secretory proteins. Circulating iodide (I^-) is actively transported into the cytosol via sodium-iodide symporters, so that the iodide concentration in the follicular cells becomes 20 to 30 times greater than it is in the blood. Iodide leaves the follicular cell to enter the colloid via **pendrin**, an iodide–chlorine transporter. At the same time, noniodinated **thyroglobulin**, packaged with the enzyme **thyroid peroxidase** is also being released into the colloid. At the colloid follicular cell interface, thyroid peroxidase oxidizes the iodide to form iodine (I) and iodinates tyrosine residues on the thyroglobulin molecule, forming monoiodotyrosine and diiodotyrosine residues; therefore, iodination occurs mostly at the apical plasma membrane. A rearrangement, by oxidative coupling, of the neighboring iodinated tyrosine residues of thyroglobulin in the colloid produces **triiodotyrosine (T_3)** and **tetraiodotyrosine (T_4, thyroxine)**. **B.** Binding of thyroid-stimulating hormone to receptors on the basal surface stimulates follicular cells to become columnar and to form apical pseudopods, which engulf colloid by endocytosis. After the colloid droplets fuse with lysosomes, controlled hydrolysis of iodinated thyroglobulin liberates T_3 and T_4 into the cytosol. These hormones move basally and are released basally to enter the bloodstream and lymphatic vessels, where they bind with the carrier protein, thyroxine-binding globulin, that ferries the hormones to their target cells. (Adapted with permission from Junqueira LC, Carneiro J, Kelley RO. *Basic Histology.* 9th ed. Stamford, CT: Appleton & Lange; 1998:403, and from Fawcett DW. *Bloom and Fawcett: A Textbook of Histology.* 12th ed. New York, NY: Chapman & Hall; 1994:496.)

3. They possess elongated mitochondria, substantial amounts of RER, a well-developed Golgi complex, and many membrane-bound dense secretory granules.

4. They synthesize and release **calcitonin**, a polypeptide hormone, in response to high blood calcium levels.

D. Physiological effects of thyroid hormones

1. T_4 and T_3 act on a variety of target cells. These hormones **increase the basal metabolic rate** and thus promote heat production. They have broad effects on gene expression and the induction of protein synthesis. T_4 has a much longer half-life (approximately 6 days vs. less than a day) but is much less active than T_3. Both hormones have to enter the nucleus to perform their function.

2. **Calcitonin** functions primarily to lower blood calcium levels by inhibiting bone resorption by osteoclasts.

CLINICAL CONSIDERATIONS   **Simple goiter (enlargement of the thyroid gland)** is caused by insufficient iodine (<10 µg/day) in the diet.

1. It is usually not associated with either hyperthyroidism or hypothyroidism.

2. Simple goiter is treated by administration of dietary iodine.

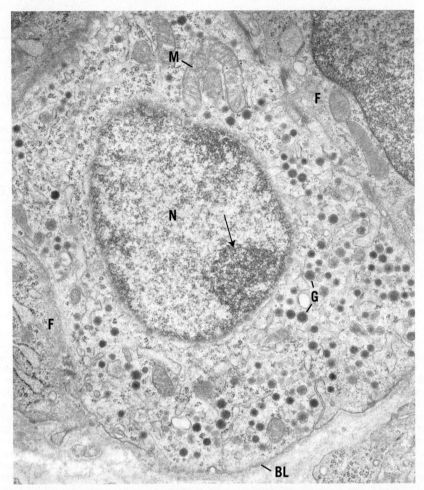

FIGURE 13.8. Electron micrograph of a parafollicular cell (clear cell, C cell) in the thyroid gland. This cell lies between the follicular cells (F) within the basal lamina (BL) enveloping the follicle. Its nucleus (N) displays a nucleolus (*arrow*), and its cytoplasm possesses elongated mitochondria (M). In response to high levels of calcium in the blood, the parafollicular cell releases the hormone calcitonin by exocytosis of the dense granules (G) in its cytoplasm. The calcitonin enters nearby fenestrated capillaries and lowers blood calcium levels by inhibiting osteoclast bone resorption throughout the body (×7,000).

V. PARATHYROID GLANDS (Figure 13.4)

A. **Overview**
 1. The parathyroid glands are four small glands that lie on the posterior surface of the thyroid gland, embedded in its connective tissue capsule.
 2. They have a parenchyma composed of two types of cells, **chief cells** and **oxyphil cells**.
 3. They are supported by septa from the capsule, which penetrate each gland and also convey blood vessels (Figure 13.4) into its interior.
 4. They become infiltrated with fat cells in older persons, and the number of oxyphil cells also increases.

B. **Chief cells** are small basophilic cells arranged in clusters (Figure 13.9).

 1. Chief cells form anastomosing cords, surrounded by a rich, fenestrated capillary network.
 2. These cells possess a central nucleus, a well-developed Golgi complex, abundant RER, small mitochondria, glycogen, and secretory granules of variable size.

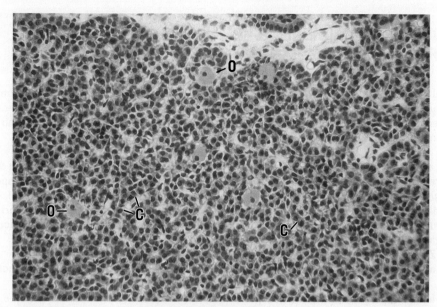

FIGURE 13.9. A light micrograph of the parathyroid gland. Chief cells (C) are small basophilic cells arranged in cords along capillaries. They synthesize and secrete parathyroid hormone that raises blood calcium levels primarily by mobilizing calcium from the bone. Oxyphil cells (O) are also present in the parathyroid gland. They are acidophilic, much larger than the chief cells, and few in number, but they increase in number with age. Oxyphils contain many large elongated mitochondria, but the function of these cells is not known (×150).

3. **Function.** They synthesize and secrete **parathyroid hormone** (**PTH**, or **parathormone**), which raises blood calcium levels. High blood calcium levels **inhibit** the production of PTH. The hormone acts on osteoclasts (see Chapter 7 II C 4 and II J) and also induces the decrease in calcium excretion by the thick ascending limb of Henle loop.

4. **Mechanism.** The cell membrane of chief cells possesses a transmembrane Ca^{2+} receptor (**CaSR**) that binds calcium ions. In the presence of calcium ions, CaSR activates G proteins that shut off the release of parathormone, whereas if calcium ions do not bind to CaSR, the inhibitory activity of the G protein is suppressed and the chief cell releases parathormone.

C. **Oxyphil cells** are large, eosinophilic cells that are present singly or in small clusters within the parenchyma of the gland (Figure 13.9).

1. Oxyphil cells possess many large, elongated mitochondria, a poorly developed Golgi complex, and only a limited amount of RER.

2. Their function is not known.

D. **PTH** functions primarily to **increase blood calcium levels** by indirectly stimulating osteoclasts to resorb bone. In concert with calcitonin, the hormone produced and released by the C cells of the thyroid gland, PTH provides a dual mechanism for regulating blood calcium levels. A near absence of PTH (hypoparathyroidism) may be caused by accidental surgical removal of the parathyroid glands, which leads to **tetany**, characterized by hyperexcitability and spastic skeletal muscle contractions throughout the body.

CLINICAL CONSIDERATIONS

Hyperparathyroidism is overactivity of the parathyroid glands, resulting in excess secretion of PTH and consequent bone resorption (see Chapter 7 II J 1).

1. Hyperparathyroidism is associated with **high blood calcium levels**, which may lead to deposition of calcium salts in the kidneys and the walls of blood vessels.

2. It may be caused by a benign tumor of the parathyroid glands.

VI. OVERVIEW—ADRENAL (SUPRARENAL) GLANDS (Figure 13.4)

Adrenal glands lie embedded in fat at the superior pole of each kidney. They are derived from two embryonic sources: the ectodermal neural crest, which gives rise to the **adrenal medulla**, and the mesoderm, which gives rise to the **adrenal cortex**. The adrenal glands are invested by their own collagenous capsule.

A. **The adrenal cortex** (Table 13.3) contains parenchymal cells that synthesize and secrete but **do not store** various steroid hormones. The production of steroid hormones is dependent on a specific protein, **steroidogenic acute regulatory protein (StAR)** that facilitates the transport of cholesterol across the outer membranes of mitochondria. The adrenal cortex is divided into three concentric histologically recognizable regions: the **zona glomerulosa, zona fasciculata, and zona reticularis** (Figure 13.10).

1. **Zona glomerulosa**
   a. synthesizes and secretes **mineralocorticoids**, mostly **aldosterone** and some **deoxycorticosterone**. Hormone production is stimulated by angiotensin II and ACTH.
   b. is composed of small cells arranged in arch-like cords and clusters. These cells have a few small lipid droplets, an extensive network of smooth endoplasmic reticulum (SER), and mitochondria with **shelf-like cristae**.

2. **Zona fasciculata**
   a. synthesizes and secretes **glucocorticoids**, namely **cortisol and corticosterone**. Hormone production is stimulated by ACTH (Figure 13.11).
   b. is composed of columns of cells and **sinusoidal capillaries** oriented perpendicularly to the capsule.
   c. cells contain many lipid droplets and (in tissue sections) appear so vacuolated that they are called **spongiocytes** (Figure 13.12). These cells also possess spherical mitochondria with **tubular** and **vesicular cristae**, SER, RER, lysosomes, and **lipofuscin pigment granules**.

3. **Zona reticularis**
   a. synthesizes and secretes **weak androgens** (mostly **dehydroepiandrosterone** and some **androstenedione**) and perhaps small amounts of glucocorticoids. Hormone production is stimulated by ACTH.
   b. is composed of cells, arranged in anastomosing cords. Many large **lipofuscin pigment granules** are common in these cells (Figure 13.12) and are believed to represent lipid-containing residues of lysosomal digestion.

table 13.3   Adrenal Gland Cells and Hormones

Cell	Hormone	Function
Adrenal cortex		
Zona glomerulosa	Mineralocorticoids (mostly aldosterone)	Regulate electrolyte, water balance via effect on cells of renal tubules
Zona fasciculata	Glucocorticoids (cortisol, corticosterone)	Regulate carbohydrate metabolism by promoting gluconeogenesis; promote breakdown of proteins, fat; anti-inflammatory properties; suppress immune response
Zona reticularis	Weak androgens (dehydroepiandrosterone, androstenedione)	Promote masculine characteristics
Adrenal medulla		
Chromaffin cells	Epinephrine	Fight-or-flight response; increases heart rate and force of contraction; relaxes bronchiolar smooth muscle; promotes glycogenolysis and lipolysis
	Norepinephrine	Little effect on cardiac output, rarely used clinically

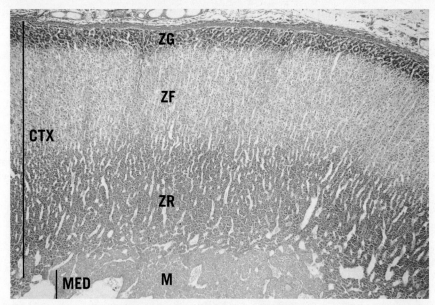

FIGURE 13.10. A light micrograph of the adrenal gland showing the different regions of the cortex (CTX) and a portion of the medulla (MED). Cells in the outermost zona glomerulosa (ZG) are arranged in clusters and secrete mineralocorticoids; cells in the middle zona fasciculata (ZF) are arranged in cords between sinusoidal capillaries and secrete glucocorticoids and a small amount of androgens; and cells of the innermost zona reticularis (ZR) are arranged in anastomosing cords and secrete androgens and small amounts of glucocorticoids. Cells in the adrenal medulla (M), called chromaffin cells, synthesize, store, and secrete epinephrine and norepinephrine (×16).

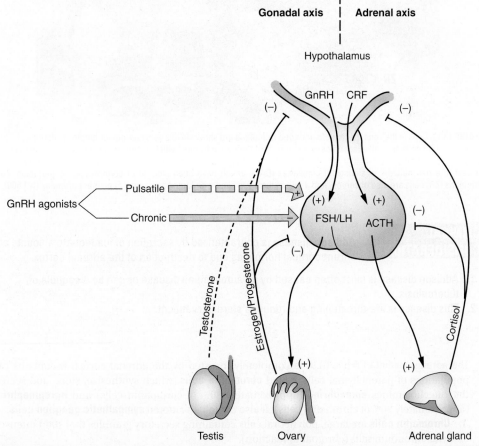

FIGURE 13.11. Regulation of glucocorticoid secretion by the adrenal cortex via stimulation by corticotropin-releasing hormone and adrenocorticotropic hormone (ACTH) and the negative feedback of cortisol at both the pituitary and the hypothalamic levels. GnRH, gonadotropin-releasing hormone; CRF, corticotropin-releasing factor; FSH, follicle-stimulating hormone; LH, luteinizing hormone. (Reprinted with permission from Rosenfeld G, Loose D. *BRS Pharmacology*. 5th ed. Baltimore, MD: Wolters Kluwer Health/Lippincott Williams & Wilkins; 2009:218.)

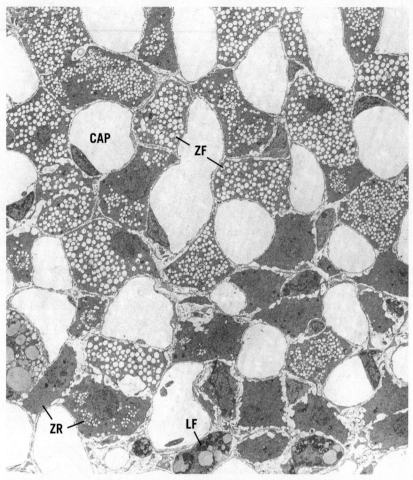

FIGURE 13.12. Cells of the zona fasciculata and zona reticularis are shown in this very low-power electron micrograph. Zona fasciculata (ZF) cells are called spongiocytes because of their appearance, which is caused by the extraction of the many lipid droplets in their cytoplasm that have been removed through the process of fixation and dehydration. The spongiocytes lie next to a rich network of sinusoidal capillaries (CAP), which have been cleared of erythrocytes by perfusion. Zona reticularis (ZR) cells are also observed, and a few of them are filled with large lipofuscin (LF) pigment granules (×1,500).

| CLINICAL CONSIDERATIONS | **Addison disease** is characterized by secretion of inadequate amounts of adrenocortical hormones due to destruction of the adrenal cortex. |

1. Addison disease is most often caused by an autoimmune disease or can be a sequela of tuberculosis.
2. This disease is life-threatening and requires steroid treatment.

B. **The adrenal medulla** (Table 13.3) is completely invested by the adrenal cortex. It contains two populations of parenchymal cells, called **chromaffin cells**, which synthesize, store, and secrete the catecholamines **epinephrine** (approximately 80% of chromaffin cells) and **norepinephrine** (approximately 20% of chromaffin cells). It also contains scattered **sympathetic ganglion cells**.
   1. **Chromaffin cells** are large, polyhedral cells containing secretory granules that stain intensely with chromium salts (chromaffin reaction).
      a. Chromaffin cells are arranged in short, irregular cords surrounded by an extensive capillary network.

    b. They are innervated by **preganglionic sympathetic (cholinergic) fibers**, making these cells analogous in function to postganglionic sympathetic neurons.

    c. They possess a well-developed Golgi complex, isolated regions of RER, and numerous mitochondria.

    d. They also contain large numbers of membrane-bound granules containing one of the catecholamines, ATP, enkephalins, and **chromogranins**, which may function as binding proteins for epinephrine and norepinephrine.

  2. **Catecholamine release** occurs in response to intense emotional stimuli and is mediated by the preganglionic sympathetic fibers that innervate the chromaffin cells.

CLINICAL CONSIDERATIONS   A **pheochromocytoma** is a tumor arising in catecholamine-secreting chromaffin cells of the adrenal medulla. The tumor is rare; it is found in both sexes, and 90% of the time it is benign. However, its secretion of excessive amounts of epinephrine and norepinephrine leads to **hypertension** (episodic or sustained), although the patient may remain asymptomatic. Increased levels of catecholamines and their metabolites in the urine are diagnostic of pheochromocytoma. If the tumor is detected early and is surgically removed, the hypertension is correctable, but if not, prolonged and sustained hypertension may prove fatal.

C. **Blood supply to the adrenal glands** is derived from the superior, middle, and inferior adrenal arteries, which form three groups of vessels: to the capsule, to parenchymal cells of the cortex, and directly to the medulla.

  1. **Cortical blood supply**

    a. A **fenestrated** capillary network bathes cells of the zona glomerulosa.

    b. **Straight, discontinuous, fenestrated** capillaries supply the zona fasciculata and zona reticularis.

  2. **Medullary blood supply**

    a. **Venous blood** rich in hormones reaches the medulla via the discontinuous fenestrated capillaries that pass through the cortex.

    b. **Arterial blood** from direct branches of capsular arteries forms an extensive fenestrated capillary network among the chromaffin cells of the medulla.

    c. **Medullary veins** join to form the suprarenal vein, which exits the gland.

VII. PINEAL GLAND (PINEAL BODY, EPIPHYSIS)

A. **Overview** (Figure 13.4)

  1. The pineal gland **projects from the roof of the diencephalon**.

  2. Its secretions vary with the light and dark cycles of the day, thereby regulating the individual's circadian rhythm. Although the pineal gland is buried deep within the head, it receives information about the light and dark conditions from special ganglion cells in the retina of the eye. These ganglion cells send their information about the presence of daylight via the retinohypothalamic tract that projects to the suprachiasmatic nucleus of the hypothalamus, from where information reaches the superior cervical sympathetic ganglion whose postganglionic sympathetic fibers reach the pineal gland by riding on the tunica adventitia of blood vessels that supply the pineal.

  3. This gland has a capsule formed of the **pia mater**, from which septa (containing blood vessels and unmyelinated nerve fibers) extend to subdivide it into incomplete lobules.

  4. It is composed primarily of pinealocytes, which constitute approximately 95% of the cells, and neuroglial cells (interstitial cells), which constitute about 5% of the cells.

  5. It also contains calcified concretions **(brain sand)** in its interstitium. The function of these concretions is unknown, but they increase during short light cycles and decrease during periods of darkness.

B. **Pinealocytes** are pale-staining cells with numerous long processes that end in dilations near capillaries.

 1. Pinealocytes contain many secretory granules, microtubules, microfilaments, and unusual structures called **synaptic ribbons**.

 2. These cells synthesize and immediately secrete **melatonin** but almost only at night. During the day, melatonin synthesis is mostly inhibited.

 3. Pinealocytes may also produce **arginine vasotocin**, a peptide that appears to be an antagonist of LH and FSH; they also secrete small quantities of serotonin, histamine, and dopamine. Most of the serotonin manufactured by the pinealocytes is converted to melatonin in a two-step reaction, the first of which is catalyzed by the enzyme **N-acetyltransferase**. It is the activity of this particular enzyme that is inhibited during daylight conditions, thus preventing the formation of melatonin during daylight.

C. **Neuroglial (interstitial) cells** resemble astrocytes, with elongated processes and a small, dense nucleus. They contain microtubules and many microfilaments and intermediate filaments.

CLINICAL CONSIDERATIONS Melatonin is used to treat jet lag and seasonal affective disorder (SAD), an emotional response to shorter daylight hours during the winter.

Review Test

Directions: Each of the numbered items or incomplete statements in this section is followed by answers or completions of the statement. Select the ONE lettered answer that is BEST in each case.

1. Protein hormones act initially on target cells by

(A) attaching to receptors on the nuclear membrane.
(B) attaching to receptors in the nucleolus.
(C) diffusing through the plasma membrane.
(D) attaching to receptors on the plasma membrane.
(E) attaching to receptors on the rough endoplasmic reticulum membrane.

2. Which of the following statements concerning adrenal parenchymal cells is true?

(A) Those of the zona fasciculata produce androgens.
(B) Those of the adrenal medulla produce epinephrine and norepinephrine.
(C) Those of the zona glomerulosa produce glucocorticoids.
(D) Those of the cortex contain numerous secretory granules.
(E) Those of the zona reticularis produce mineralocorticoids.

3. Characteristics of pinealocytes include which one of the following?

(A) They produce melatonin.
(B) They resemble astrocytes.
(C) They contain calcified concretions of unknown function.
(D) They act as postganglionic sympathetic cells.
(E) They are unaffected by dark and light cycles.

4. Prolactin is synthesized and secreted by which of the following cells?

(A) Acidophils in the pars distalis
(B) Basophils in the pars tuberalis
(C) Somatotrophs in the pars distalis
(D) Basophils in the pars intermedia
(E) Gonadotrophs in the pars distalis

5. ACTH is produced by which of the following cells?

(A) Chromophobes in the pars distalis
(B) Neurosecretory cells in the median eminence
(C) Basophils in the pars distalis
(D) Neurons of the paraventricular nucleus in the hypothalamus
(E) Basophils in the pars intermedia

6. The histological appearance of a thyroid gland being stimulated by TSH would show which of the following?

(A) Decreased numbers of follicular cells
(B) Increased numbers of parafollicular cells
(C) Column-shaped follicular cells
(D) An abundance of colloid in the lumen of the follicle
(E) Decreased numbers of parafollicular capillaries

7. A 40-year-old woman is diagnosed with Graves disease. Which of the following characteristics would be associated with her condition?

(A) Inadequate levels of iodine in her diet
(B) Weight gain
(C) Flattened thyroid follicular cells
(D) Excessive production of thyroid hormones
(E) Increased amounts of follicular colloid

8. Which one of the following hormones lowers blood calcium levels by inhibiting bone resorption?

(A) Calcitonin
(B) Epinephrine
(C) Parathyroid hormone
(D) Prolactin
(E) T_3

9. A 51-year-old man underwent surgery for removal of a carcinoma on his trachea. After surgery, he suffered excessive nervousness, muscle cramps, and spasmodic skeletal muscle contractions in his arms, legs, and feet. Laboratory tests revealed markedly low levels of calcium in his blood. Treatment with intravenous calcium and vitamin D led to recovery in a few weeks. Which one of the following conditions is responsible for these symptoms in this patient following surgery?

(A) Hypothyroidism
(B) Hyperthyroidism
(C) Hypoparathyroidism
(D) Graves disease
(E) Hyperparathyroidism

10. Which one of the following hormones plays a role in regulating body temperature by promoting heat production?

(A) Calcitonin
(B) Epinephrine
(C) Parathyroid hormone
(D) Prolactin
(E) Triiodothyronine (T_3)

Answers and Explanations

1. **D.** Protein hormones initiate their action by binding externally to transmembrane receptor proteins in the target-cell plasma membrane. Receptors for some hormones (e.g., TSH, serotonin, epinephrine) are linked to G proteins; other receptors, including those for insulin and growth hormone, have protein kinase activity (see Chapter 13 II A).

2. **B.** Chromaffin cells in the adrenal medulla synthesize and store epinephrine and norepinephrine in secretory granules, which also contain ATP, chromogranins, and enkephalins. The cortical parenchymal cells of the zona fasciculata produce glucocorticoids, and those of the zona glomerulosa produce mineralocorticoids. The cortical parenchymal cells do not store their secretory products and thus do not contain secretory granules (see Chapter 13 VI).

3. **A.** Pinealocytes, the parenchymal cells of the pineal gland, produce melatonin at night and serotonin during the day. The pineal gland also contains neuroglial cells that resemble astrocytes, and its interstitium has calcified concretions called brain sand (see Chapter 13 VII).

4. **A.** Prolactin is produced by mammotrophs, one of the two types of acidophils located in the pars distalis of the pituitary gland. As their name implies, these cells produce a hormone that regulates the development of the mammary gland during pregnancy and lactation (see Chapter 13 III A).

5. **C.** ACTH is produced by corticotrophs, a type of basophil, present in the pars distalis of the pituitary gland (see Chapter 13 III A).

6. **C.** Stimulation of the thyroid gland by TSH causes the follicular cells to become more active and column shaped. They form apical pseudopods and engulf colloid, which is removed from the lumen of the follicle by endocytosis and broken down by controlled lysosomal hydrolysis to yield the thyroid hormones T_3 and T_4. Parafollicular cells and capillaries do not contain receptors for TSH (see Chapter 13 IV).

7. **D.** Graves disease (exophthalmic goiter) results in an enlarged thyroid gland due to stimulation of the follicular cells to produce an excessive amount of thyroid hormones by binding of autoimmune antibodies to TSH receptors. Follicular cells actively remove colloid from the lumen of the follicles. Heat intolerance and weight loss are common, but the disease is not caused by iodine deficiency (see Chapter 13 IV B Clinical Considerations).

8. **A.** Calcitonin lowers blood calcium levels and thus has an effect antagonistic to that of parathyroid hormone. It is produced by parafollicular cells of the thyroid gland (see Chapter 13 IV D).

9. **C.** Upon removal of the carcinoma from his neck, the parathyroid glands were also removed or damaged, causing hypoparathyroidism (a lack of parathyroid hormone that increases blood calcium). Treatment with calcium (and vitamin D, which aids in its absorption) corrected these symptoms. The marked neuromuscular irritability in the absence of calcium reveals its importance in regulating skeletal muscle contraction (see Chapter 13 V D).

10. **E.** Triiodothyronine (T_3) and thyroxine (T_4) both increase the basal metabolic rate, which affects heat production and body temperature. These thyroid hormones also have many other effects (see Chapter 13 IV D).

chapter 14

Skin

I. OVERVIEW—THE SKIN

A. The skin is the heaviest organ, about 16% of the total body weight.

B. It is composed of two layers, the **epidermis** and the **dermis**, which interdigitate to form an irregular contour.

C. A deeper superficial fascial layer, the **hypodermis**, lies under the skin. This layer, which is not considered part of the skin, consists of loose connective tissue that binds skin loosely to the subjacent tissue.

D. The skin contains several epidermal derivatives (sweat glands, hair follicles, sebaceous glands, nails, and the mammary glands, discussed in Chapter 19). The skin along with its derivatives is called the **integument**.

E. Function. The skin protects the body against injury, desiccation, and infection; regulates body temperature; absorbs ultraviolet (UV) radiation, which is necessary for synthesis of vitamin D; and contains receptors for touch, temperature, and pain stimuli from the external environment. Additionally, skin acts as an excretory organ via sebaceous, sweat, and apocrine glands.

II. EPIDERMIS

A. Overview—Epidermis
   1. The epidermis is the **superficial layer** of the skin. Primarily of **ectodermal origin**, it is classified as **stratified squamous keratinized epithelium**. The epidermis is composed predominantly of **keratinocytes** and three other types of cells: **melanocytes, Langerhans cells**, and **Merkel cells**.
   2. The epidermis is constantly being regenerated. **Regeneration**, which occurs approximately every 30 days, is carried out by the mitotic activity of keratinocytes, which normally divide at night.
   3. The epidermis has deep downgrowths called **epidermal ridges** that **interdigitate** with projections of the dermis (**dermal ridges**), resulting in a highly irregular interface. Each dermal ridge is often further subdivided into two secondary dermal ridges by a narrow downgrowth of the epidermis, called an **interpapillary peg**. Where the epidermis overlies the dermal ridges,

surface ridges are produced. On the fingertips, these surface ridges are visible as **fingerprints**, whose configuration is genetically determined and thus unique to each individual.

4. Interestingly, it has been suggested that keratinocytes may participate in immune reactions because they manufacture and release various signaling molecules, such as interleukins, interferons, tumor necrosis factors, and colony-stimulating factors that stimulate the immune system.

B. **Layers of the epidermis** (Figure 14.1, Table 14.1)

1. The **stratum basale (stratum germinativum)** is the **deepest layer** of the epidermis and is composed mostly of keratinocytes that are cuboidal to columnar in shape. These **mitotically active** cells are attached directly to the basal lamina of the basement membrane by **hemidesmosomes** (see Chapter 5 III B) and to each other by desmosomes. These cells manufacture and house **keratins 5 and 14**. The stratum basale also contains **melanocytes** and **Merkel cells**.

2. The **stratum spinosum** consists of a few layers of polyhedral keratinocytes (**prickle cells**). Their extensions, termed "intercellular bridges" by early histologists, are now known to terminate in **desmosomes** (see Chapter 5 II A 3). Keratinocytes and their nuclei become larger and flatter a characteristic of squamous cells. This layer also contains **Langerhans cells**.

    a. Keratinocytes in the deeper aspects of the stratum spinosum are also **mitotically active**.

    b. The **malpighian layer** (stratum malpighii) consists of the stratum spinosum and stratum basale. Nearly all of the mitotic activity in the epidermis occurs in this region, and cell division occurs at night. It is believed that interleukin-1 and epidermal growth factor facilitate, whereas transforming growth factor suppresses the mitotic activity of these cells.

    c. In the superficial regions of the stratum spinosum, keratinocytes:

        (1) Contain **membrane-coating granules (Odland bodies, lamellar bodies)**, whose contents are rich in lipids, especially glycosphingolipids, ceramides, and phospholipids. The lipid contents of some of these granules are released into the intercellular spaces in the form of lipid-containing sheets that are **impermeable to water** and **many foreign substances**.

        (2) Form the **intermediate filaments keratins 1** and **10**, replacing the keratin types located in the cells of the stratum basale. These new keratins form *thin* bundles of intermediate filaments, known as **tonofilaments**.

        (3) Form **keratohyalin granules**, that is, non-membrane-bound structures, whose main components are the proteins **filaggrin** and **tricohyalin**. The keratohyalin granules envelop the thin bundles of tonofilaments and cause them to become cross-linked, thereby forming *thick* bundles of **tonofibrils**.

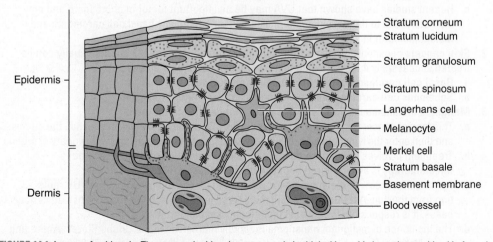

FIGURE 14.1. Layers of epidermis. The stratum lucidum is present only in thick skin and is best observed in skin from the palms of the hands and the soles of the feet. Melanocytes lie between keratinocytes in the stratum basale. (Adapted with permission from Ham AH, Cormack DH. *Histology.* 8th ed. Philadelphia, PA: Lippincott; 1979:625.)

table **14.1** Histological Features of Skin

Divisions	Layers	Characteristics
Epidermis*	Stratum corneum	The most superficial layer of epidermis Many flattened dead "cells" called squames, packed with keratin filaments Surface cells are sloughed
	Stratum lucidum	Indistinct homogeneous layer of keratinocytes; present only in thick skin Cells lack nuclei and organelles Cytoplasm is packed with keratin filaments and eleidin
	Stratum granulosum	Flattened nucleated keratinocytes arranged in 3–5 layers Cells contain many coarse keratohyalin granules associated with tonofilaments Membrane-coating (waterproofing) granules occasionally present Present only in thick skin
	Stratum spinosum	Several layers of keratinocytes, called prickle cells because they appear spiny Desmosomes, associated with tonofilaments, connect cells between processes (intercellular bridges) Keratinocytes contain membrane-coating (waterproofing) granules Keratinocytes are mitotically active, especially in deeper layers Langerhans cells are also present in this layer
	Stratum basale (stratum germinativum)	Deepest layer of epidermis, composed of a single layer of tall cuboidal keratinocytes Keratinocytes are mitotically active Melanocytes and Merkel cells are also present in this layer
Dermis†	Papillary layer	Superficial thin layer of connective tissue that interdigitates with epidermal ridges of the epidermis Forms dermal papillae where Meissner corpuscles and capillary loops may be found Contains delicate collagen (type I and type III) fibers Contains anchoring fibrils (type VII collagen), microfibrils (fibrillin), and elastic fibers
	Reticular layer	Extensive part of the dermis, lying deep to the papillary layer Contains thick bundles of collagen (type I) fibers and elastic fibers Arteries, veins, and lymphatics are present Location of sweat glands and their ducts, Pacinian corpuscles, and nerves In thin skin, contains hair follicles, sebaceous glands, and arrector pili muscles

*Stratified squamous keratinized epithelium.
†Dense, irregular connective tissue.

CLINICAL CONSIDERATIONS

1. **UV radiation and skin damage**
   a. Exposure of unprotected skin to UV light can cause harmful effects to the cells, even in the absence of sunburn.
   b. Sunscreen with a sun protection factor (SPF) rating of 15 or higher may protect against UVB wavelengths, but offers no protection against the longer UVA wavelengths.
   c. Recent studies have shown that UVA may be an important factor in photoaging and may ultimately lead to the development of skin cancer (especially basal cell carcinoma and melanoma) later in life.

2. **Skin cancers** commonly originate from cells in the epidermis. These cancers usually can be treated successfully if they are diagnosed early and surgically removed.
   a. **Basal cell carcinoma** arises from basal keratinocytes.
   b. **Squamous cell carcinoma** arises from cells of the stratum spinosum.

3. **Malignant melanoma** is a form of skin cancer that can be life-threatening.
   a. This form of cancer originates from **melanocytes** that divide, transform, and invade the dermis and then enter the lymphatic and circulatory systems, **metastasizing** to a wide variety of organs.
   b. Treatment involves **surgical removal** of the skin lesion and regional lymph nodes. **Chemotherapy** is also required because of the extensive metastases.
   c. Approximately 86% of melanomas are believed to be caused by exposure to UV radiation from the sun. Although malignant melanoma accounts for less than 5% of skin cancer cases, it is responsible for the vast majority of skin cancer deaths.
   d. The incidence of malignant melanoma is rapidly increasing in the United States. According to the National Cancer Institute in the year 2014, there will be more than 76,000 new cases of malignant melanoma, resulting in more than 9,000 fatalities in the United States.

3. The **stratum granulosum** is the most superficial layer of the epidermis, in which it comprises three to five layers of flattened keratinocytes that contain even more and bigger accumulations of **keratohyalin granules, thick bundles of keratin filaments (tonofibrils)**, and **membrane-coating granules**.

   a. **Keratohyalin granules** stain intensely with basophilic stains, thus are very pronounced in histological sections.

   b. The cytoplasmic aspect of the plasma membrane of keratinocytes in the stratum granulosum is reinforced by an electron-dense layer 10 to 12 nm thick.

   c. Cells in the superficial layers of the stratum granulosum form **tight junctions** with one another and with the cells of the stratum lucidum in thick skin and with cells of the stratum corneum in thin skin. These tight junctions are rich in the membrane protein **claudin**.

   d. The lipid contents of the membrane-coating granules are released into the extracellular space to form a water-impermeable barrier, preventing nutrients from reaching the superficial-most layer of cells of the stratum granulosum and those of the strata lucidum and corneum. Therefore, those cells undergo apoptosis, their organelles die, and the cells become **keratohyalin-tonofibril-filled** "hulls." The impermeable layer also prevents aqueous fluid from entering the epidermal layers from the external environment.

4. The **stratum lucidum** is a clear, homogeneous layer just superficial to the stratum granulosum; it is often difficult to distinguish in histological sections. It is found only in **palmar** and **plantar skin**. This layer consists of keratinocytes that **have neither nuclei** nor organelles, but contain an abundance of tonofibrils embedded in keratohyalin, frequently referred to as **eleidin**.

5. The **stratum corneum** is the most **superficial layer** of the epidermis (Figure 14.2). It may consist of as many as 15 to 20 layers of flattened, nonnucleated dead "cells" filled with **keratohyalin-keratin complex**. These **nonviable scale-like** structures are called **squames** (or horny cells), and have the shape of a 14-sided polygon.

   a. The keratohyalin–keratin complex lines the plasma membrane of the stratum corneum cell and is further strengthened by three proteins **involucrin**, **small proline-rich protein**, and **loricrin**, thereby establishing a thickened **cornified cell envelope**.

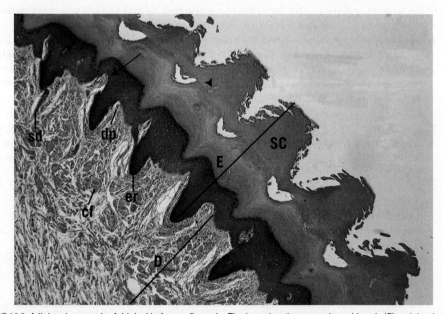

FIGURE 14.2. A light micrograph of thick skin from a fingertip. The boundary between the epidermis (E) and the dermis (D) is markedly irregular due to epidermal downgrowths, called epidermal ridges (er), which interdigitate with dermal ridges, called dermal papillae (dp). The epidermis (E) over the fingertips is very thick due to its stratum corneum (SC), which forms surface ridges that are visible as fingerprints. Sweat gland ducts (sd) penetrate the base of the epidermal ridges (at the tips of the interpapillary pegs) and travel through all of the epidermal layers, including the stratum corneum (*arrowhead*) to release sweat from the body. Meissner corpuscles (*arrow*) and capillary loops are present in the dermal papillae of the papillary layer of dermis, whereas thick collagen fibers (cf) and larger blood vessels are found in its reticular layer (×16).

    b. The lipid-rich substance released from the membrane-coating granules in the strata spinosum and granulosum into the extracellular space coats the cells of the stratum corneum, forming a **lipid coat** around each cell.

    c. The cornified envelope in conjunction with the lipid coat constitutes the **compound cornified cell envelope**.

    The outermost layer of squames is continuously shed by **desquamation**. The rate of shedding matches the rate of cell renewal in the strata basale and the spinosum, thereby maintaining the thickness of the epidermis as well as the structural stability of the compound cornified cell envelope.

CLINICAL CONSIDERATIONS   **Psoriasis**

1. Psoriasis is a condition in which reddened, inflamed patches of skin, having a whitish, flaky layer on top, appear almost anywhere on the body.
2. It is caused by an **increase in mitotic activity** of cells in the malpighian layer of the epidermis (stratum basale and stratum spinosum) that have a **shorter than normal cell cycle**.
3. The fast-growing epidermis promotes increased blood flow to nourish the accelerated growth, and inflammation may occur (both causing redness).
4. In psoriasis, the epidermis is often renewed in only days rather than in about a month.

  C. Nonkeratinocytes in the epidermis

    1. Melanocytes (Figure 14.1) are present in the **stratum basale** and originate as melanoblasts from neural crest. Once melanoblasts reach the epidermis, they become **premelanocytes**, enter the stratum basale, and form hemidesmosomes with the basal lamina, but do not form adhesive junctions with the keratinocytes. Once premelanocytes bind **stem cell factor**, they may remain premelanocytes or may differentiate into melanocytes, which extend finger-like processes, known as **dendrites** that occupy some of the extracellular spaces among the cells of the stratum spinosum. The dendrites of a single melanocyte contact a number of stratum spinosum cells, and this group of cells is known as an **epidermal-melanin unit**.

      a. Melanocytes synthesize a **dark brown pigment, melanin** in oval-shaped organelles known as **melanosomes** under the influence of the pituitary hormone, **melanocyte-stimulating hormone** (MSH). MSH acts by binding to receptors on the melanocyte plasma membrane, which causes these cells to activate their **microphthalmia-associated transcription factor**, a signaling molecule that induces melanin synthesis in melanosomes. Melanosomes contain **tyrosinase**, a UV-sensitive enzyme directly involved in melanin synthesis.

      b. Mature melanosomes and their melanin are transported into the dendrites along microtubule pathways, powered by **myosin Va**, and at the proper location the melanosomes are transferred to **F-actin** pathways that deliver them to the dendrite's plasma membrane, where the melanosomes are released into the extracellular space.

      c. Cells of the stratum spinosum phagocytose the released melanosomes (Figure 14.3). Once inside the keratinocytes, the melanosomes migrate to the region of the nucleus and form a **physical barrier** between the keratinocyte's nucleus and the impinging UV rays of the sun, thus protecting the keratinocyte's chromosomes from possible damage from the UV radiation.

        (1) The number of melanocytes per unit area of skin appears to be the same in dark- and light-skinned people and accounts for approximately 3% of the entire epidermal cell population.

        (2) Pigmentation differences are due to the rate of melanin synthesis, melanosome size, content, rate of transfer, and degradation patterns.

    2. Langerhans cells are **dendritic cells** (so named because of their long processes) that originate in the bone marrow, travel in the bloodstream, exiting in the dermis and migrating into the epidermis. They are independent cell making no adhesive junctions to keratinocytes.

      a. Langerhans cells are located primarily in the **stratum spinosum** and contain characteristic paddle-shaped **Birbeck granules** that are associated with the integral protein **langerin**.

      b. The cell membranes of Langerhans cells also express various immune-related proteins, namely CD1a, MHC I and MHC II, C3b receptors, as well as receptors for IgG. The protein

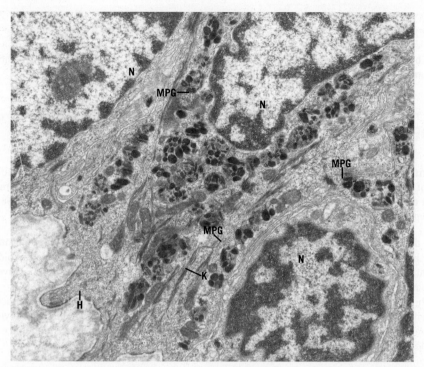

FIGURE 14.3. An electron micrograph of keratinocytes in the stratum basale of skin. Melanin pigment granules (MPG) are abundant in the cytoplasm, having been transferred to the cells via melanocyte processes. A few keratin filaments (K), mitochondria, and portions of nuclei (N) are observed. The base of keratinocytes in this layer attaches to the basal lamina by hemidesmosomes (H), and they attach to neighboring cells by way of desmosomes (×9,500).

CD1a, in association with langerin, defends the organism against the causative agent of leprosy, *Mycobacterium leprae*.

    c. These cells function as **antigen-presenting cells** in immune responses to contact antigens (contact allergies) and some skin grafts (see Chapter 12 Section II E and Section III).

    d. Once Langerhans cells phagocytize antigens, they leave the epidermis and travel to a lymph node, where they present the epitope to T cells and thereby initiate a **delayed-type hypersensitivity reaction**.

  3. **Merkel cells** are present in small numbers in the **stratum basale**, near areas of well-vascularized, richly innervated connective tissue.

    a. They possess desmosomes and keratin filaments, suggesting an epithelial origin.

    b. Their pale cytoplasm contains **small, dense-cored granules** that are similar in appearance to those in some cells of the diffuse neuroendocrine system (DNES) and are presumed to house neurosecretions.

    c. They receive afferent nerve terminals and are believed to function as **sensory mechanoreceptors**. They appear to be more abundant in areas of acute sensory perception, as at the tips of fingers.

D. Thick and thin skin are distinguished on the basis of the thickness of the epidermis.

  1. Thick skin has an epidermis that is 400 to 600 μm thick.

    a. It is characterized by a prominent stratum corneum, a well-developed stratum granulosum, and often a distinct stratum lucidum.

    b. It lines the palms of the hands and the soles of the feet.

    c. Thick skin **lacks** hair follicles, sebaceous glands, and arrector pili muscles.

  2. Thin skin has an epidermis that is 75 to 150 μm thick.

    a. It has a less prominent stratum corneum than thick skin and generally lacks a stratum granulosum and stratum lucidum, although it contains individual cells that are similar to the cells of these layers.

    b. Thin skin covers most of the body and contains hair follicles, sebaceous glands, and arrector pili muscles.

CLINICAL CONSIDERATIONS   **Epidermolysis bullosa** is a group of **hereditary** diseases of the skin characterized by **blister formation** following minor trauma. These diseases are caused by **defects in the keratinocyte intermediate filaments** that provide mechanical stability and in the **anchoring fibrils** that attach the epidermis to the dermis.

III. DERMIS

The dermis is the layer of the skin underlying the epidermis. It is of **mesodermal origin** and is composed of dense, irregular connective tissue that contains many **type I collagen fibers** and networks of thick **elastic fibers**. Although it is divided into a **superficial papillary layer** and a **deeper**, more extensive **reticular layer**, no distinct boundary exists between these layers (Table 14.1).

A. The **dermal papillary layer** is uneven (Figure 14.2) and forms **dermal ridges (dermal papillae)**, which interdigitate with the epidermal downgrowths (epidermal ridges) forming the epidermal/dermal junction. The papillary layer is composed of thin, loosely arranged connective tissue containing fibroblasts, type III collagen fibers, fine elastic fibers, and capillary loops. Also located in the papillary layer are **Meissner corpuscles**, fine-touch receptors that make it possible to specifically identify two different coins in your pocket simply by feeling them. Fine, unmyelinated nerve fibers course through the papillary layer to gain access to the extracellular spaces of the epidermis, where they function as pain receptors.

B. The deeper **dermal reticular layer** constitutes the major portion of the dermis. It is composed of **dense bundles** of **collagen fibers** and thick **elastic fibers**. In its deeper aspects, it may contain **Pacinian corpuscles** (Figure 14.4), which are pressure receptors, as well as **Krause end-bulbs**

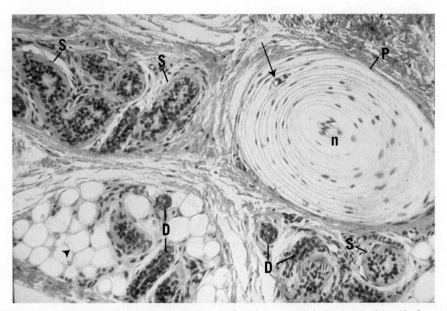

FIGURE 14.4. A light micrograph of eccrine sweat glands and a Pacinian corpuscle in the dermis of the skin. Sweat glands are also present in the hypodermis among adipose cells (*arrowhead*). The secretory units (S) of the sweat glands are wrapped by finger-like processes of myoepithelial cells (M) and stain more lightly than the ducts (D) that are lined by a stratified cuboidal epithelium. This Pacinian corpuscle (P) lies deep in the dermis and is composed of a centrally located nerve (n) surrounded by concentric layers of connective tissue. The nuclei of fibroblasts are seen, and so is a capillary (*arrow*), which helps to nourish the structure. Pacinian corpuscles are mechanoreceptors that respond to deep pressure (×150).

(formerly thought to be cold receptors, but their actual function is uncertain). Specialized diffuse receptors are discussed in Chapter 21 II.

C. Located at various levels in the dermis are the appendages of skin. These include the two types of sweat glands (eccrine and apocrine), sebaceous glands, hair follicles, and nails.

CLINICAL CONSIDERATIONS **Keloids** are swellings in the skin that result from increased collagen formation in hyperplastic scar tissue. They are most prevalent in African Americans.

IV. GLANDS IN THE SKIN (Figure 14.5)

A. The 3 to 4 million **eccrine sweat glands** (Figure 14.4) are **simple coiled tubular glands** consisting of a secretory unit and a single duct. These glands are present in skin throughout most of the body but not in the lips and certain regions of the external genitalia. Eccrine sweat glands function in controlling body temperature, conserving electrolytes, and excreting urea and lactic acid.

1. The **secretory unit of eccrine sweat glands** is approximately 0.4 mm in diameter, and is embedded in the dermis, and composed of three cell types.
   a. **Dark cells** line the lumen of the gland and contain many mucinogen-rich secretory granules.
   b. **Clear cells** underlie the dark cells, are rich in mitochondria and glycogen, and contain intercellular canaliculi that extend to the lumen of the gland. These cells secrete a watery, electrolyte-rich material.
   c. **Myoepithelial cells** lie scattered in an incomplete layer beneath the clear cells. They stain deeply with eosin and are easily identified in histological sections. Their contractions aid in expressing the gland's secretions into the duct.

2. The **duct** (Figure 14.4) **of eccrine sweat glands** is **narrow** and lined by **stratified cuboidal epithelial cells**, which contain many keratin filaments and have a prominent terminal web. The cells forming the external (basal) layer of the duct have many mitochondria and a prominent nucleus.
   a. The duct leads from the secretory unit through the superficial portions of the dermis to penetrate an **interpapillary peg** of the epidermis, where the duct cells end. Beginning from this point, the walls of the duct are formed by epidermal cells as the duct forms a tight spiral through the layers of the epidermis to open at the surface of the skin at a sweat pore to deliver sweat to the **sweat pore** on the skin surface (Figure 14.2).
   b. As the secreted material passes through the dermal region of the duct, its cells reabsorb some electrolytes and excrete other substances (such as urea, lactic acid, ions, and certain drugs).
   c. Eccrine glands are stimulated by parasympathetic innervation as a result of fluctuations in body temperature.

CLINICAL CONSIDERATIONS **Hyperhidrosis** is a disorder of excessive sweating caused by overperspiration from secretion by eccrine sweat glands in the skin. Treatment with drugs has been unsatisfactory in alleviating the symptoms of this condition, but injecting a highly diluted form of **Botox** directly into the skin on the palms of the hands, soles of the feet, or of the axillae offers relief. The toxin blocks sympathetic nerve impulses to the cells of the eccrine sweat glands and decreases their ability to secrete. A single injection of Botox may provide months of relief, and the injections can be repeated when excessive sweating resumes.

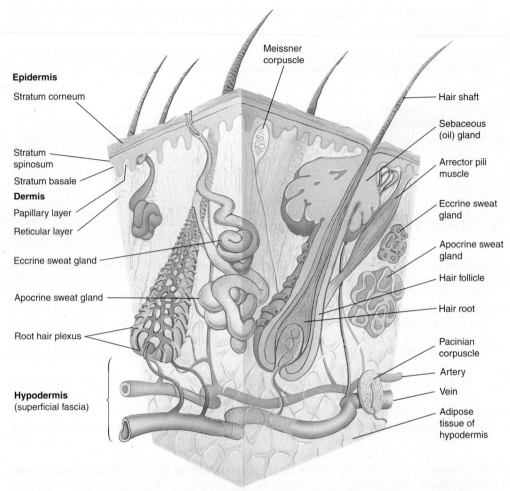

Skin and its appendages, **hair**, **sweat glands** (both **eccrine** and **apocrine**), **sebaceous glands**, and **nails**, are known as the **integument**. Skin may be **thick** or **thin**, depending on the thickness of its epidermis. Thick skin epidermis is composed of five distinct layers of **keratinocytes** (strata basale, spinosum, granulosum, lucidum, and corneum) interspersed with three additional cell types, **melanocytes**, **Merkel cells**, and **Langerhans cells**. Thin skin epidermis lacks strata granulosum and lucidum, although individual cells that constitute the absent layers are present.

FIGURE 14.5. A diagram illustrating skin and its derivatives. (From Gartner LP, Hiatt JL. *Color Atlas of Histology*. 5th ed. Baltimore, MD: Lippincott William & Wilkins; 2009:230.)

B. **Apocrine sweat glands** (Figure 14.5) include the **large, specialized sweat glands**, approximately 3 mm in diameter, located in various areas of the body (e.g., axilla, areola of the nipple, perianal region), and the ceruminous (wax) glands of the external auditory canal.
   1. These glands do not begin to function until puberty and are **responsive to hormonal influences**.
   2. Their large coiled secretory units are located in the dermis and hypodermis and are enveloped by scattered myoepithelial cells. Unlike in eccrine glands, the secretory units are composed of a single cell type.
   3. These glands empty their viscous, odorless secretions into hair follicles at a location superficial to the entry of sebaceous gland ducts. Bacteria act on these secretions to produce odors that are somewhat specific to each individual.
   4. Although the term **apocrine** implies that a portion of the cytoplasm becomes part of the secretion, electron micrographs have shown that the **cytoplasm does not become part of the secretions** of apocrine sweat glands.
   5. Apocrine glands are stimulated by sympathetic innervation usually in response to stressful conditions.

C. **Sebaceous glands** (Figure 14.5) are **branched acinar glands** that exhibit a lobular appearance. Clustered acini of one sebaceous gland empty into a single short duct.

1. The duct empties into the neck of a hair follicle.
2. Sebaceous glands are embedded in the dermis over most of the body's surface but are absent from the palms and soles. They are most abundant on the face, forehead, and scalp.
3. These **holocrine glands** release **sebum** (composed of an oily secretion and degenerating epithelial cells). As sebum continues to be produced, the cell undergoes apoptosis and/or necrosis; thus, the cellular debris becomes a component of the secretory product.
4. Sebum has a number of functions, such as maintaining the skin's barrier to aqueous fluids, guarding skin from oxidative stress, shielding skin from microorganisms, and maintaining the suppleness of skin and the luster of hair.

V. HAIR, HAIR FOLLICLE, AND ARRECTOR PILI MUSCLE (Figure 14.6)

A. **Hairs (hair shafts)** are one of the characteristics of mammals and are keratinized, thin, thread-like structures that extend for various lengths above the surface of the epidermis. Hair in mammals functions in thermal protection, and in some instances as camouflage, and as sensory organ, whereas in humans its function is more of a tactile sensory organ because when a hair shaft is disturbed, it transduces that sensory information to the nervous system. There are three types of human hairs, one of which are present prenatally and are gone shortly after birth, known as the lanugo, and two that are present postnatally, known as vellus hairs and terminal hairs.

1. **Lanugo** is an exceptionally fine, somewhat longish hair that covers almost the entire fetus and falls out shortly after birth.
2. **Vellus hairs** are present throughout the individual's life. They are almost invisible, but when viewed in sunlight at an angle, for instance, on a person's eyelids (on the skin of the eyelids, not

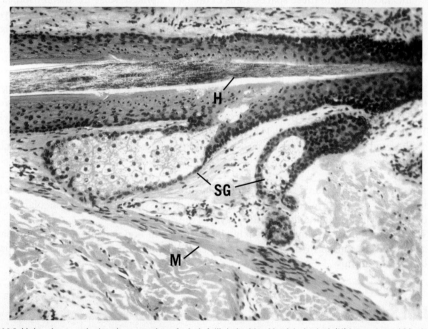

FIGURE 14.6. Light micrograph showing a portion of a hair follicle in thin skin. A hair shaft (H) is present within the follicle, and the surface of the skin is out of view at the right. Two sebaceous glands (SG) and an arrector pili muscle (M) are also observed. This muscle originates in the papillary layer of the dermis and passes obliquely to insert on the hair follicle. When it contracts, it causes the hair to stand more upright, makes the surface of the skin dimple (causing "goose flesh"), and compresses the sebaceous gland so that it expresses sebum into the shaft of the hair follicle (×50).

the eyelashes), they are evident as short, very fine, soft, and pale structures. Most of the human body is covered by vellus hairs.

3. **Terminal hairs** are the coarse, long, highly keratinized, dark hairs that one associates with the word "hair." These are present on the head, eyebrows, eyelashes, pubic hairs, etc. Most of the primate body is covered by terminal hair.

B. A **hair follicle** is an **invagination of the epidermis**, extending deep into the dermis.

1. The **hair shaft** is a long, slender filament in the center of the follicle that extends above the surface of the epidermis. It consists of an inner **medulla, cortex**, and **cuticle of the hair**. At its deep end, it is continuous with the **hair root**. The cuticle of the hair is surrounded by the **internal root sheath** (see below).

2. The **hair root** is the terminal expanded region of the hair follicle, located deep within the dermis where the hair is rooted. The hair root is deeply indented by a **dermal papilla**, which contains a capillary network necessary for sustaining the follicle. The hair root is separated from the dermal papilla by a basement membrane, and the two together constitute the **hair bulb**.

   a. The **hair root** contains keratinocytes that function as **stem cells** for hair shaft regeneration. Interestingly, these stem cells are present even in bald individuals, but the signaling molecules that induce them to form new hair are absent.

   b. The majority of the cells of the hair root comprise the **matrix**, whose cells form the **medulla** (the core of thick hairs) and the internal root sheath.

      (1) The **internal root sheath** lies deep to the entrance of the sebaceous gland. It is composed of the **Henle layer**, the **Huxley layer**, and the **cuticle of the internal root sheath** (not to be confused with the cuticle of the hair).

      (2) The **external root sheath** is a direct continuation of the stratum malpighii of the epidermis.

      (3) The **glassy membrane** is a **noncellular layer**, a thickening of the basement membrane. It separates the hair follicle from the surrounding dermal sheath.

   c. **Melanocytes** are located in the matrix, lying on the basement membrane. The long dendrites of these cells penetrate the extracellular space among cells of the cortex and deliver their melanosomes into these spaces. Cells of the cortex phagocytose the melanosomes, and it is in this fashion that hair acquires its color. As the individual ages, the tyrosinase synthesis by the melanocytes of the hair follicles diminishes and eventually ceases, resulting in the absence of melanin production, and hair loses its color and turns gray.

3. The average human head has approximately 150,000 hairs, which grow at a rate of 2 mm per day. Hair growth occurs in three phases; a growing phase, known as the **anagen phase**; a short respite from active growth, known as the **catagen phase**; and the terminal resting phase, known as the **telogen phase** when the hair falls out; that shed hair is known as a club hair because the removed hair possesses a club-shaped root. On a daily basis, approximately 50 to 100 hairs are lost from the head. Hairs in some regions of the body last longer than others. Hair on the head stays in place for as long as seven years, whereas hairs in the armpit fall out in less than half a year.

C. The **arrector pili muscle** attaches at an **oblique angle to the dermal sheath** surrounding a hair follicle.

1. It extends superficially to underlie sebaceous glands, passing through the reticular layer of the dermis and **inserting into the papillary layer** of the dermis.

2. The contraction of this **smooth muscle** elevates the hair and is responsible for formation of goose bumps, caused by depressions of the skin where the muscle attaches to the papillary layer of the dermis.

VI. NAILS (Figure 14.7)

Nails are located on the distal phalanx of each finger and toe.

A. Nails are hard keratinized plates that rest on the **nail bed** composed of the epidermis and underlying dermis of the skin.

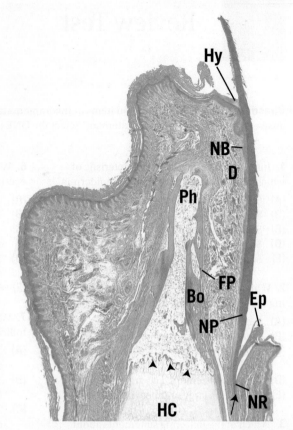

FIGURE 14.7. A fingernail on the dorsal surface of a distal phalanx (Ph) is illustrated. The highly keratinized nail plate (NP) extends deep into the dermis (D) to form the nail root (NR). The epidermis of the distal phalanx forms a continuous fold, resulting in the eponychium (Ep), or cuticle, the nail bed (NB) underlying the nail plate, and the hyponychium (Hy). The epithelium (*arrow*) surrounding the nail root is responsible for the continuous elongation of the nail. The dermis between the nail bed and the bone (Bo) of the distal phalanx is tightly secured to the fibrous periosteum (FP). The presence of hyaline cartilage (HC) and endochondral osteogenesis (*arrowheads*) indicates that this is a developing finger.

B. At the proximal end, each is covered by a fold of epidermis, called the **cuticle** or **eponychium**, which corresponds to the stratum corneum. The cuticle overlies the crescent-shaped whitish **lunula**.

C. At the distal (free) edge, each is underlain by the **hyponychium**, which is also composed of stratum corneum.

D. Nails grow as the result of mitoses of cells in the matrix of the **nail root**. Fingernails grow no more than 0.5 mm per week, and toenails grow a bit slower; interestingly, growth is faster in the summer than in any other time of the year.

CLINICAL CONSIDERATIONS

Warts (verrucae) are common **skin lesions** caused by a **virus**.

1. They may occur anywhere on the skin or on the oral mucosa, but are most common on the dorsal surfaces of the hands, often **close to the nails**.

2. Histological features of warts include marked epidermal hyperplasia, eosinophilic cytoplasmic inclusions, and deeply basophilic nuclei. By electron microscopy, many intranuclear viral particles can be observed in the keratinocytes.

Male pattern baldness (androgenic alopecia)

Male pattern baldness is a genetic condition that accounts for almost 95% of male baldness. It is recognizable by the loss of hair at both sides of the temple as well as at the crown of the head. Usually the two patterns occur simultaneously and result in a bald top with an open ring of hair on the side and back of the head. In men the hair loss can begin in the early thirties, but in most men it does not begin until the individual is in his fifties. A similar condition, **female pattern baldness**, is also evident in women, but not to the same extent as in men. The principal cause of male pattern baldness is the presence of dihydrotestosterone, the male sex hormone, which acts on the hair follicles, reducing their size and forcing it into dormancy.

Review Test

Directions: Each of the numbered items or incomplete statements in this section is followed by answers or completions of the statement. Select the ONE lettered answer that is BEST in each case.

1. Intercellular bridges are characteristic of which of the following layers of the epidermis?

(A) Stratum granulosum
(B) Stratum lucidum
(C) Stratum corneum
(D) Stratum spinosum
(E) Stratum basale

2. Which of the following statements concerning the stratum granulosum is true?

(A) It contains melanosomes.
(B) It lies superficial to the stratum lucidum.
(C) It is the thickest layer of the epidermis in thick skin.
(D) It contains keratohyalin granules.
(E) It contains large numbers of dividing cells.

3. Which of the following statements about Langerhans cells is true?

(A) They are commonly found in the dermis.
(B) They function as sensory mechanoreceptors.
(C) They function as receptors for cold.
(D) They play an immunological role in the skin.
(E) They are of epithelial origin.

4. Meissner corpuscles are present in which of the following regions of the skin?

(A) Dermal reticular layer
(B) Dermal papillary layer
(C) Hypodermis
(D) Stratum basale
(E) Epidermal ridges

5. Which of the following statements concerning thin skin is true?

(A) It does not contain sweat glands.
(B) It lacks a stratum corneum.
(C) It is less abundant than thick skin.
(D) It contains hair follicles.
(E) Its epidermis does not rest on a basement membrane.

6. Which of the following statements about eccrine sweat glands is true?

(A) They are absent in thick skin.
(B) They are holocrine glands.
(C) They have a narrow duct lined by a stratified cuboidal epithelium.
(D) They secrete an oily material called sebum.
(E) They empty into hair follicles.

7. Which of the following statements about hair follicles is true?

(A) They are always associated with an eccrine sweat gland.
(B) They are present in thin skin but not in thick skin.
(C) Their associated arrector pili muscle is composed of striated fibers.
(D) Their hair shaft inserts into the papillary layer of the epidermis.
(E) They do not extend into the dermis.

8. Which of the following statements concerning skin melanocytes is true?

(A) They synthesize a pigment that protects against damage caused by UV radiation.
(B) They are located only in the dermis.
(C) They produce keratohyalin granules.
(D) They may give rise to basal cell carcinoma.
(E) They originate from the mesoderm.

9. Which of the following statements concerning sebaceous glands is true?

(A) They do not begin to function until puberty.

(B) They employ the mechanism of holocrine secretion.

(C) They are present in thick skin.

(D) They secrete only in response to hormones.

(E) They produce a watery enzyme-rich secretion.

10. Which of the following is an appendage of skin?

(A) Meissner corpuscle

(B) Langerhans cell

(C) Krause end-bulb

(D) Pacinian corpuscle

(E) Nail

Answers and Explanations

1. **D.** Observations with an electron microscope show that intercellular bridges are associated with desmosomes (maculae adherentes), linking the processes of adjacent cells in the stratum spinosum. Desmosomes also link cells within the other epidermal layers, but these cells do not form processes characteristic of bridges. The keratinocytes of the stratum basale also contain hemidesmosomes, which attach the cells to the underlying basal lamina (see Chapter 14 II B).

2. **D.** The stratum granulosum contains a number of dense keratohyalin granules, but not melanosomes. It lies just deep to the stratum lucidum and is a relatively thin layer in the epidermis of thick skin. Only rarely would a cell undergo mitosis in this layer of the skin (see Chapter 14 II B).

3. **D.** Langerhans cells in the epidermis function as antigen-presenting cells by trapping antigens that penetrate the epidermis and transporting them to regional lymph nodes, where they are presented to T lymphocytes. In this way, these cells assist in the immune defense of the body. They originate in the bone marrow and do not arise from epithelium (see Chapter 14 II C).

4. **B.** Meissner corpuscles are encapsulated nerve endings present in dermal papillae, which are part of the papillary layer of the dermis. These corpuscles function as receptors for fine touch (see Chapter 14 III A).

5. **D.** In contrast to thick skin, which lacks hair follicles, thin skin contains many of them (see Chapter 14 II D).

6. **C.** Eccrine sweat glands are simple, coiled tubular glands that have a duct lined by a stratified cuboidal epithelium. They are found in both thick and thin skin and are classified as merocrine glands, meaning they release only their secretory product, which does not include cells or portions of cells (see Chapter 14 IV A).

7. **B.** Hair follicles are present only in thin skin. They are associated with sebaceous glands and arrector pili smooth muscle bundles (see Chapter 14 V).

8. **A.** Melanocytes are present in the stratum basale of the epidermis. They synthesize melanin pigment and transfer it to keratinocytes to protect against damage caused by UV radiation. Melanocytes sometimes give rise to a form of skin cancer called malignant melanoma. They derive from neural crest and migrate into the epidermis early during embryonic development (see Chapter 14 II C).

9. **B.** Sebaceous glands produce sebum, an oily material, and release it into the upper shaft of the hair follicle by a mechanism called holocrine secretion (which means the product and cellular debris are both released from the gland) (see Chapter 14 IV C).

10. **E.** The nail is one appendage of the skin. Other skin appendages are hair follicles, sweat glands, and sebaceous glands (see Chapter 14 VI).

15 Respiratory System

I. OVERVIEW—THE RESPIRATORY SYSTEM

A. The respiratory system includes the **lungs** and a series of **airways** that connect the lungs to the external environment.

B. The respiratory system can be functionally classified into two major subdivisions: a **conducting portion**, consisting of airways that deliver air to the lungs, and a **respiratory portion**, consisting of structures within the lungs in which oxygen in the inspired air is exchanged for carbon dioxide in the blood.

C. The components of the respiratory system possess characteristic lining epithelia, supporting structures, glands, and other features, which are summarized in Table 15.1.

II. CONDUCTING PORTION OF THE RESPIRATORY SYSTEM

This portion of the respiratory system includes the nose, nasopharynx, larynx, trachea, bronchi, and bronchioles of decreasing diameters, including and ending at the terminal bronchioles. These structures **warm, moisten**, and **filter the air** before it reaches the respiratory components, where gas exchange occurs.

A. Nasal cavity. The nasal cavity is subdivided by the median nasal septum into right and left nasal cavities, each leading to the paranasal sinuses, thus providing a large surface area for filtering, moistening, and warming the inspired air.

   1. The **nares** are the nostrils; their outer portions are lined by **thin skin**. They open into the vestibule.

   2. The **vestibule** is the first portion of the nasal cavity, where the epithelial lining becomes **nonkeratinized**. Posteriorly, the lining changes to **respiratory epithelium** (pseudostratified ciliated columnar epithelium with goblet cells).

      a. The vestibule contains **vibrissae** (thick, short hairs), which filter large particles from the inspired air.

      b. It has a richly **vascularized** lamina propria (many venous plexuses) and contains **seromucous glands**.

      c. Each nasal cavity contains bony shelves that originate from the lateral nasal wall and project into the nasal cavity. These are the **superior, middle**, and **inferior conchae**

| t a b l e **15.1** Comparison of Respiratory System Components |

Division	Support	Glands	Epithelium	Ciliated Cells	Goblet Cells	Special Features
Nasal cavity						
Vestibule	Hyaline cartilage	Sebaceous and sweat glands	Stratified squamous keratinized	No	No	Vibrissae
Respiratory	Bone and hyaline cartilage	Seromucous	Pseudostratified ciliated columnar	Yes	Yes	Large venous plexuses
Olfactory	Nasal conchae (bone)	Bowman glands	Pseudostratified ciliated columnar (tall)	Yes	No	Bipolar olfactory cells, sustentacular cells, basal cells, nerve fibers
Nasopharynx	Muscle	Seromucous	Pseudostratified ciliated columnar	Yes	Yes	Pharyngeal tonsil, entrance of eustachian tube
Larynx	Hyaline, elastic cartilage	Mucous, seromucous	Stratified squamous nonkeratinized, pseudostratified ciliated columnar	Yes	Yes	Vocal cords, striated muscle (vocalis), epiglottis
Trachea Primary bronchi	C-shaped hyaline cartilage rings	Mucous, seromucous	Pseudostratified ciliated columnar	Yes	Yes	Trachealis (smooth) muscle, elastic lamina, two mucous cell types, short cells, diffuse endocrine cells
Intrapulmonary bronchi	Plates of hyaline cartilage	Seromucous	Pseudostratified ciliated columnar	Yes	Yes	Two helically oriented ribbons of smooth muscle
Primary bronchioles	Smooth muscle	None	Simple ciliated columnar to simple cuboidal	Yes	Only in larger ones	Clara cells (club cells)
Terminal bronchioles	Smooth muscle	None	Simple cuboidal	Some	None	Clara cells (club cells)
Respiratory bronchioles	Some smooth muscle	None	Simple cuboidal except where interrupted by alveoli	Some	None	Occasional alveoli, Clara cells (club cells)
Alveolar ducts	Smooth muscle at alveolar openings, some reticular fibers	None	Simple squamous	None	None	Linear structure formed by adjacent alveoli, type I and II pneumocytes, alveolar macrophages
Alveoli	Reticular fibers, elastic fibers at alveolar openings	None	Simple squamous	None	None	Type I and II pneumocytes, alveolar macrophages

Modified with permission from Gartner LP, Hiatt JL. *Color Atlas of Histology*. 2nd ed. Baltimore, MD: Williams & Wilkins; 1994:240.

(turbinate bones). Their structure and placement within the nasal cavity divide it into separate regions, thereby introducing turbulence to the air flow. Since they are covered by respiratory epithelium, their presence increases the surface area for warming, filtering, and moistening the inspired air.

d. **Paranasal sinuses** are air-filled, hollowed out portions of the sphenoid, frontal, ethmoid, and maxillary bones. These air sinuses are lined by a thin respiratory epithelium, but the function of the paranasal sinuses is not known.

3. **Olfactory epithelium**
   a. **Overview**
      (1) The olfactory epithelium is located in the roof of the nasal cavity, on either side of the nasal septum and on the superior nasal conchae.
      (2) It is a tall, **pseudostratified columnar epithelium** consisting of olfactory cells, supporting (sustentacular) cells, and basal cells (stem cells).
      (3) It has a lamina propria that contains many **veins** and **unmyelinated nerves**, and houses **Bowman glands**.
   b. **Olfactory cells** are **bipolar nerve cells** characterized by a bulbous apical projection (**olfactory vesicle**) from which several modified cilia extend.
      (1) Olfactory cilia (olfactory hairs)
         (a) are very **long, nonmotile cilia** that extend over the surface of the olfactory epithelium. Their proximal third contains a typical **9 + 2 axoneme pattern**, but their distal two-thirds are composed of nine peripheral **singlet** microtubules surrounding a central pair of microtubules.
         (b) act as receptors for odor.
      (2) Supporting (sustentacular) cells
         (a) possess nuclei that are more apically located than those of the other two cell types.
         (b) have many **microvilli** and a prominent **terminal web** of filaments.
      (3) Basal cells
         (a) rest on the basal lamina but do not extend to the surface.
         (b) form an incomplete layer of cells.
         (c) are believed to be **regenerative** for all three cell types.
      (4) Bowman glands (serous glands) produce a **thin, watery secretion** that is released onto the olfactory epithelial surface via narrow ducts. Odorous substances dissolved in this watery material are detected by the olfactory cilia. The secretion also flushes the epithelial surface, preparing the receptors to receive new odorous stimuli.

B. **Nasopharynx**
   1. The nasopharynx, the posterior continuation of the nasal cavities, becomes continuous with the oropharynx at the level of the soft palate.
   2. It is lined by **respiratory epithelium**, whereas the oropharynx and laryngopharynx are lined by **stratified squamous nonkeratinized epithelium**.
   3. The lamina propria of the nasopharynx, located beneath the respiratory epithelium, contains **mucous** and **serous glands** as well as an abundance of lymphoid tissue known as **Waldeyer ring**, including the **pharyngeal tonsil**. When the pharyngeal tonsil is inflamed, it is called an **adenoid**.
   4. Opening into the right and left lateral walls of the nasopharynx are the auditory tubes (Eustachian tubes), each arising from its respective middle ear cavity.

C. **Larynx**
   1. **Overview**
      a. The larynx connects the pharynx with the trachea. It functions to produce sounds and close the air passage during swallowing.
      b. The wall of the larynx is supported by **hyaline cartilages** (thyroid, cricoid, and lower part of arytenoids) and **elastic cartilages** (epiglottis, corniculate, and tips of arytenoids).
      c. The laryngeal wall also possesses **skeletal muscle**, connective tissue, and **glands**.
   2. The **vocal cords** consist of skeletal muscle (the **vocalis muscle**), the **vocal ligament** (formed by a band of elastic fibers), and a covering of **stratified squamous nonkeratinized epithelium**.
      a. Contraction of the laryngeal muscles changes the size of the opening between the vocal cords, which affects the pitch of the sounds caused by air passing through the larynx.
      b. Inferior to the vocal cords, the lining epithelium changes to **respiratory epithelium**, which lines air passages down through the trachea and intrapulmonary bronchi.

3. **Vestibular folds (false vocal cords)** lie superior to the vocal cords.
   a. These folds of loose connective tissue contain glands, lymphoid aggregations, and fat cells.
   b. They are covered by **stratified squamous nonkeratinized epithelium**.

D. **Trachea and extrapulmonary (primary) bronchi**
   1. **Overview**: The trachea, the largest conducting section of the respiratory system, bifurcates into the right and left primary bronchi, each of which enters the hilum of the lung on its side.
      a. The walls of these structures are supported by **C-shaped hyaline cartilages** (C-rings), whose open ends face posteriorly. Smooth muscle (**trachealis muscle** in the trachea) extends between the open ends of these cartilages.
      b. Dense **fibroelastic** connective tissue is located between adjacent C-rings, permitting elongation of the trachea during inhalation.
   2. **Mucosa**
      a. The **respiratory epithelium** in the trachea possesses the following cell types.
         (1) Ciliated cells
            (a) have **long, actively motile cilia** that beat toward the mouth.
            (b) move inhaled particulate matter trapped in mucus toward the oropharynx, thus protecting the delicate lung tissue from damage.
            (c) also possess **microvilli**.
         (2) Mature goblet cells are goblet shaped and are filled with **large secretory granules, containing mucinogen droplets**, which are secreted onto the epithelial surface to trap inhaled particles.
         (3) Small granule-mucous cells (**brush cells**)
            (a) contain varying numbers of **small mucous granules**.
            (b) are sometimes called brush cells because of their many uniform **microvilli**.
            (c) actively **divide** and often replace recently desquamated cells.
            (d) may represent goblet cells after they have secreted their mucinogen.
         (4) Diffuse neuroendocrine cells
            (a) are also known as **small granule cells**, amine precursor uptake and decarboxylation (APUD cells), or **enteroendocrine cells**.
            (b) contain many small granules concentrated in their **basal** cytoplasm.
            (c) synthesize different **polypeptide hormones** and **serotonin**, which often exert a local effect on nearby cells and structures (**paracrine regulation**). The peptide hormones may also enter the bloodstream and have an **endocrine effect** on distant cells and structures.
         (5) Basal cells
            (a) are short cells that rest on the basal lamina, but do not extend to the lumen; thus, this epithelium is pseudostratified.
            (b) are stem cells that are able to **divide** and replace the other cell types.
      b. The **basement membrane** is a very thick layer underlying the epithelium.
      c. The **lamina propria** is a thin layer of connective tissue that lies beneath the basement membrane. It contains longitudinal **elastic fibers** separating the lamina propria from the submucosa.
   3. The **submucosa** is a connective tissue layer containing many **seromucous glands**.
   4. The **adventitia** contains **C-shaped hyaline cartilages** and forms the outermost layer of the trachea.

E. **Intrapulmonary bronchi (secondary bronchi)** (Figure 15.1)
   1. Intrapulmonary bronchi arise from subdivisions of the primary bronchi upon entering the hilum of the lung. It is at this level that the cartilaginous rings of the bronchi are replaced with plates of irregularly shaped hyaline cartilage.
   2. They divide many times and give rise to **lobar** and segmental bronchi.
   3. They are lined by **respiratory epithelium**.
   4. **Spiraling smooth muscle bundles** separate the lamina propria from the submucosa, which contains **seromucous glands**.

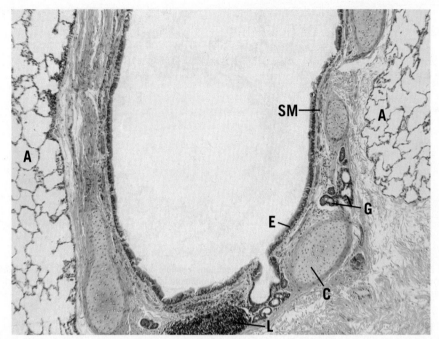

FIGURE 15.1. A light micrograph of an intrapulmonary bronchus cut in cross section. Lining its lumen is a pseudostrati-fied ciliated columnar epithelium with goblet cells (E). Beneath the epithelium in the lamina propria of loose, fibroelastic connective tissue are bundles of smooth muscle cells (SM) wrapped in a spiraling arrangement around the lumen. In the submucosal connective tissue outside of the smooth muscle are irregular plates of cartilage (C), seromucous glands (G), and lymphoid tissue (L). Alveoli (A) are evident in the nearby respiratory tissue (×75).

| CLINICAL CONSIDERATIONS | Lung cancer |

1. Lung cancer is the leading cause of death from cancer in men and women; most of it (90%) is a consequence of cigarette smoking.
2. Two types of lung cancer that are increased in smokers include squamous cell carcinoma and small cell (oat cell) carcinoma.
3. **Squamous cell carcinoma** typically arises in the bronchi, where cigarette smoking causes the respiratory epithelium to change to a stratified squamous epithelium (a metaplastic change). Then, a disorderly proliferation of cells showing great variability in nuclear size and shape occurs in the epithelium (dysplasia), followed by atypical changes that result in a carcinoma (a malignant neoplasm).
4. **Small cell (oat cell) carcinoma** is a highly aggressive carcinoma of bronchial origin whose incidence is greatly increased in smokers. It has a poor prognosis.

F. **Primary and terminal bronchioles lack glands** in their submucosa. Their walls contain **smooth muscle** rather than cartilage plates (Figure 15.2).
   1. **Primary bronchioles**
      a. Primary bronchioles have a diameter of 1 mm or less.
      b. They are lined by epithelium that varies from **ciliated columnar with goblet cells** in the larger airways to **ciliated cuboidal with Clara cells** in the smaller passages.
      c. They divide to form several terminal bronchioles after entering the **pulmonary lobules**.
   2. **Terminal bronchioles**
      a. Terminal bronchioles are the **most distal part of the conducting portion** of the respiratory system.

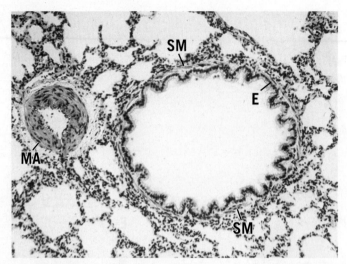

FIGURE 15.2. A light micrograph of a bronchiole in cross section. A simple columnar epithelium (E) lines its lumen, and smooth muscle cells (SM) support its wall. Surrounding the bronchiole is lung tissue with alveoli, and no cartilage or glands are present. Nearby, a muscular artery (MA) is evident (×75).

    b. They have a diameter of less than 0.5 mm.
    c. They are lined by a **simple cuboidal epithelium** that contains mostly **club cells** (formerly known as **Clara cells**), some ciliated cells, and no goblet cells.
    d. Function. Club cells have the following functions:
        (1) Club cells **divide**, and some of them differentiate to form ciliated and nonciliated cells.
        (2) They **secrete** a **surfactant-like** material that reduces **alveolar surface tension**, preventing the collapse of alveoli. They also produce **club cell secretory protein** whose function is assumed to be the protection of the respiratory epithelium.
        (3) They **metabolize airborne toxins**, a process that is carried out by cytochrome P450 enzymes in their abundant smooth endoplasmic reticulum (SER).

CLINICAL CONSIDERATIONS   **Asthma**

1. Asthma is marked by widespread **constriction of smooth muscle in the bronchioles**, causing a decrease in their diameter.
2. It is associated with **extremely difficult expiration** of air, **accumulation of mucus** in the passageways, and **infiltration of inflammatory cells**.
3. It is often treated with drugs, such as albuterol, that act to relax the bronchiolar smooth muscle cells and dilate the passageways and/or with corticosteroids, which are anti-inflammatory.
4. Recent studies have demonstrated that there are **taste receptors** on the smooth muscle cells of bronchioles of the lungs that respond to **bitter tastes**, and when stimulated by a bitter tastant, they cause bronchiolar smooth muscles to relax and the bronchioles to open to 90% of their normal volume. Current work is proceeding to develop aerosolized substances that can be used to stimulate these receptors.

III. OVERVIEW—RESPIRATORY PORTION OF THE RESPIRATORY SYSTEM (Figure 15.3)

This portion of the respiratory system includes the respiratory bronchioles, alveolar ducts, alveolar sacs, and alveoli, all in the lung. The **exchange of gases** takes place in this portion of the respiratory system.

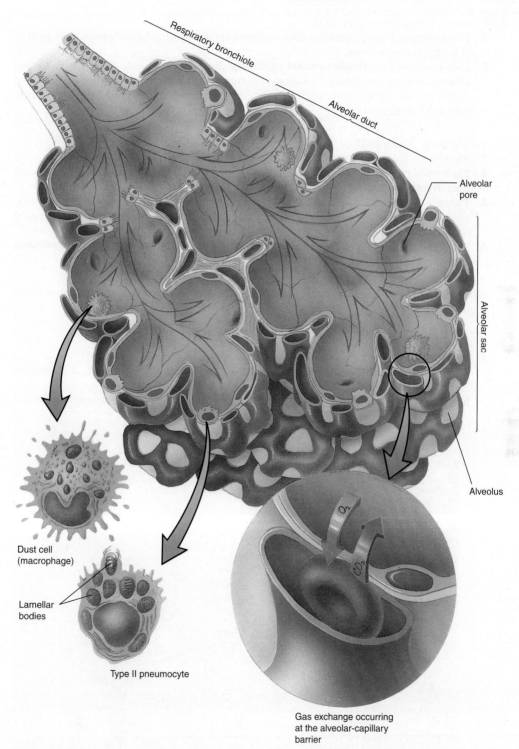

Respiratory bronchiole

Alveolar duct

Alveolar pore

Alveolar sac

Alveolus

Dust cell (macrophage)

Lamellar bodies

Type II pneumocyte

O_2

CO_2

Gas exchange occurring at the alveolar-capillary barrier

FIGURE 15.3. Components of the respiratory portion of the respiratory system, including a respiratory bronchiole, alveolar duct, and alveolar sac, are illustrated, as well as the exchange of oxygen (O_2) and carbon dioxide (CO_2) across the blood–gas barrier. (From Gartner LP, Hiatt JL. *Color Atlas of Histology.* 5th ed. Baltimore, MD: Lippincott William & Wilkins; 2009:251.)

A. **Respiratory bronchioles** (Figure 15.4)
  1. The respiratory bronchioles mark the transition from the conducting to the respiratory portion of the respiratory system.
  2. They are lined by a **simple cuboidal epithelium** that contains mostly **club cells** and some **ciliated cells**, except where their walls are interrupted by **alveoli**, the sites where gas exchange occurs and where the lining abruptly changes to a simple epithelium composed of highly attenuated squamous cells.

B. **Alveolar ducts** (Figure 15.5)
  1. Alveolar ducts are **linear passageways** continuous with the respiratory bronchioles.
  2. Their walls consist of **adjacent alveoli**, which are separated from one another only by an **interalveolar septum**.
  3. They are the most distal portion of the respiratory system to contain **smooth muscle cells**, which rim the openings of adjacent alveoli and which often appear as **knobs** in histological sections.
  4. Alveolar ducts are lined by **type II pneumocytes** and the highly **attenuated simple squamous epithelium** of **type I pneumocytes**.

C. **Alveolar sacs** are expanded outpouchings of numerous alveoli at the distal ends of alveolar ducts (Figure 15.5).

D. **Alveoli**
  1. **Overview**
     a. Alveoli are pouch-like evaginations about 200 μm in diameter in the walls of respiratory bronchioles, in alveolar ducts, and in alveolar sacs.
     b. They have thin walls, across which oxygen and carbon dioxide diffuse between the air and the blood.

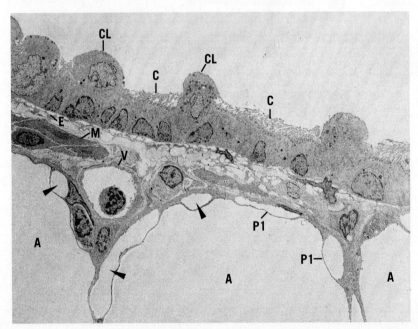

FIGURE 15.4. A low-magnification electron micrograph showing part of a terminal or respiratory bronchiole lined by a simple cuboidal epithelium composed of two cell types: Clara cells (CL) and ciliated cells (C). In the wall of the bronchiole, smooth muscle cells (M) and elastic tissue (E) are present. A venule (V) containing a white blood cell, several capillaries (*arrowheads*) cleared of blood cells, and alveoli (A) lined by the markedly thin cytoplasm of type I pneumocytes (P1) are also present (×1,500).

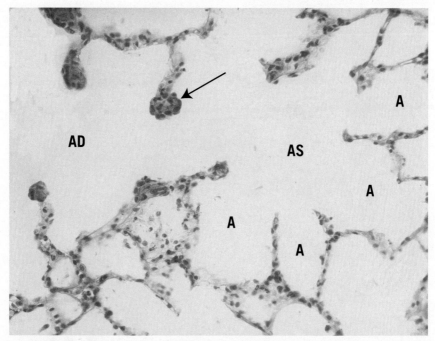

FIGURE 15.5. A light micrograph of an alveolar duct (AD) leading from a respiratory bronchiole into an alveolar sac (AS). The alveolar duct consists of adjacent alveoli, separated from one another only by an interalveolar septum. At the rims of the adjacent alveoli are a few smooth muscle cells (*arrow*) that appear as knobs in histological sections. Notice that the rims of alveoli (A) in the alveolar sac do not contain smooth muscle.

    c. They are separated from each other by **interalveolar septa** that may contain one or more **alveolar pores** (pores of Kohn). These pores permit equalization of pressure between alveoli.

    d. They are rimmed by **elastic fibers** at their openings (except in alveolar ducts, where they are rimmed by smooth muscle cells) and are supported by many **reticular fibers** in their walls.

    e. They are lined by a **highly attenuated simple squamous epithelium** composed of type I and type II **pneumocytes**.

  2. Alveolar cells

    a. Type I pneumocytes (type I alveolar cells)

      (1) cover about 95% of the alveolar surface and form part of the blood–gas barrier where exchange of oxygen and carbon dioxide occurs.

      (2) have an extremely **thin cytoplasm** that may be less than 80 nm thick (see Figure 15.4).

      (3) form **tight junctions** with adjacent cells.

      (4) may have **phagocytic** capabilities.

      (5) are **not** able to divide.

    b. Type II pneumocytes (type II alveolar cells; great alveolar cells; granular pneumocytes; septal cells) (Figure 15.6)

      (1) are **cuboidal** and are most often found **near septal intersections**.

      (2) bulge into the alveolus and have a free surface that contains short **microvilli** around their peripheral borders.

      (3) are able to **divide** and **regenerate** both types of alveolar pneumocytes.

      (4) form **tight junctions** with adjacent cells.

      (5) synthesize **pulmonary surfactant**, which is stored in cytoplasmic **lamellar bodies**.

        (a) Structure—Pulmonary surfactant. Pulmonary surfactant consists of **dipalmitoylphosphatidylcholine**, **phospholipids**, the four apolipoproteins, **surfactant-associated proteins** (known as **SP-A, SP-B, SP-C, and SP-D**), and **cholesterol**. It forms **tubular myelin** (a network configuration) when it is first released from lamellar bodies; it then spreads to produce a **monomolecular film** over the alveolar surface, forming a **lower aqueous phase** and a **superficial lipid phase**.

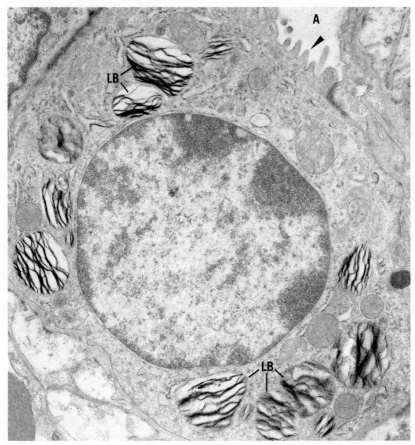

FIGURE 15.6. Electron micrograph of a type II pneumocyte that synthesizes surfactant and stores it in lamellar bodies (LB) in its cytoplasm. Type II pneumocytes are present mainly near the septal intersections and line only small portions of the alveoli (A). They possess microvilli (*arrowhead*) and are cuboidal in shape (×7,000).

(b) Function—Pulmonary surfactant. Pulmonary surfactant **reduces the surface tension** at the **air–liquid interface** of the alveolar surface, permitting the alveoli to expand easily during inspiration and preventing alveolar collapse during expiration. Additionally, surfactant reduces fluid accumulation in the alveoli. Moreover, SP-A and SP-D, apolipoproteins of the surfactant, participate in innate immunity by binding to bacterial and viral surfaces, and in that fashion **opsonizing** them. The opsonized microorganisms are recognized and phagocytosed by **macrophages (dust cells)** of the lung.

CLINICAL CONSIDERATIONS   **Hyaline membrane disease; infant respiratory distress syndrome**

1. Hyaline membrane disease is frequently observed in **premature infants (<28 weeks' gestational age)** who **lack adequate amounts of pulmonary surfactant**.
2. It is characterized by **labored breathing**, which results from difficulty expanding the alveoli because of a high alveolar surface tension.
3. If detected before birth, hyaline membrane disease can often be prevented by prolonging pregnancy and sometimes by administering **glucocorticoids** to the expectant mother a few days prior to delivery to help induce the synthesis of surfactant.

Spontaneous pneumothorax

A **spontaneous pneumothorax** is the collection of gas in the pleural cavity, the potential space between the visceral and parietal pleurae. It causes sudden sharp, severe chest pain on the same side as the affected lung and leads to shortness of breath. The condition occurs most often in young people who have no known underlying pulmonary disease. But computed tomography scans typically reveal **blebs near the lung surface that rupture**, allowing gas to invade the pleural space and causing the lung to collapse (either partially or completely). A minor lung collapse will often resolve on its own, but when the pneumothorax is larger, a needle or tube is usually inserted between the ribs to remove the gas over a period of a few days, which permits the lung to reinflate.

    c. **Alveolar macrophages (alveolar phagocytes; dust cells)** (see Figure 15.3)
       (1) are the principal mononuclear **phagocytes** of the alveolar surface.
       (2) remove inhaled dust, bacteria, and other particulate matter trapped in the pulmonary surfactant, thus providing a vital line of defense in the lungs.
       (3) migrate to the bronchioles after filling with debris. From there, they are carried via **ciliary action** to the upper airways, eventually reaching the oropharynx, where they are either swallowed or expectorated.
       (4) may also exit by migrating into the interstitium and leaving via lymphatic vessels.

CLINICAL CONSIDERATIONS **Asbestosis**

1. Asbestosis is a pulmonary disease caused by inhaling asbestos fibers (used in insulation materials, tiles, etc.).
2. The fibers deposit in the alveolar ducts and alveoli. The smaller fibers are phagocytosed by macrophages, but the larger ones penetrate the lung interstitium.
3. Activated macrophages release inflammatory mediators, which lead to **interstitial pulmonary fibrosis** in the walls of respiratory bronchioles, alveolar ducts, and alveoli.
4. **Asbestos bodies**, fibers 10 to 50 μm long encrusted with beads of protein, form in the interstitium and alveolar spaces. The asbestos bodies stain strongly for iron because of the hemoglobin protein released from small hemorrhages that accompany the fibrosis.

Emphysema

1. Emphysema results from **destruction of alveolar walls** and formation of large cyst-like sacs, reducing the surface area available for gas exchange.
2. It is marked by **decreased elasticity** of the lungs, which are unable to recoil adequately during expiration. In time, the lungs expand and enlarge the thoracic cavity (barrel chest).
3. Emphysema is associated with exposure to **cigarette smoke** and **other substances that inhibit** α_1-**antitrypsin**, a protein that normally protects the lungs from the action of **elastase** produced by alveolar macrophages.
4. It can be a hereditary condition resulting from a defective α_1-antitrypsin. In such cases, gene therapy with recombinant α_1-antitrypsin is being used in an effort to correct the problem, and it has recently been successful in boosting the availability of this protective protein.

  E. **Interalveolar septum**
    1. The interalveolar septum is the wall, or partition, between two adjacent alveoli.
    2. It is bounded on its outer surfaces by the extremely thin, simple, squamous epithelium lining the alveoli.
    3. It contains many **elastic and reticular fibers** in its thicker regions.
    4. It houses **continuous capillaries** in its central (interior) region.

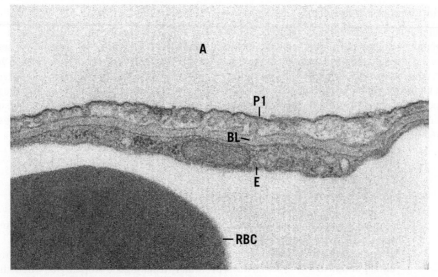

FIGURE 15.7. Electron micrograph showing the blood–gas barrier in the lung, which permits the exchange of gases between the alveolar airspace and the blood. Oxygen diffused from the alveolus (A) into the capillary containing erythrocytes (RBC) and carbon dioxide diffused from the capillary blood into the alveolus. The barrier shown here consists of the following three layers: the cytoplasm of a type I pneumocyte (P1), the fused basal laminae (BL) of a type I pneumocyte and a capillary endothelial cell, and the cytoplasm of the endothelial cell (E) ($\times$14,000).

   5. It accommodates the **blood–gas barrier**, which separates the alveolar airspace from the capillary lumen.
      a. **Structure—Blood–gas barrier** (Figure 15.7)
         (1) The thinnest regions of the barrier are 0.2 μm or less in thickness and consist of the following layers:
            (a) Type I pneumocytes and layer of surfactant lining the alveolar airspace
            (b) Fused basal laminae of type I pneumocytes and capillary endothelial cells
            (c) Endothelium of the continuous capillaries within the interalveolar septum
         (2) Thicker regions of the barrier measure as much as 0.5 μm across and have an **interstitial area** interposed between the two unfused basal laminae.
      b. **Function—Blood–gas barrier.** The blood–gas barrier permits the **diffusion of gases** between the alveolar airspace and the blood. **Oxygen** passes from the alveolus into the capillary, and **carbon dioxide** passes from the capillary blood into the alveolus.

CLINICAL CONSIDERATIONS   **Carbon monoxide poisoning**

   1. Carbon monoxide is an odorless, tasteless gas that **binds to hemoglobin** in red blood cells with **a greater affinity than does oxygen**. It is produced whenever fuel-burning appliances are used, which explains the importance of using carbon monoxide detectors.
   2. Individuals exposed to carbon monoxide are often unaware of the symptoms it may cause (such as nausea, headache, and sleepiness). Death may occur as the gas replaces oxygen in red blood cells of the lung and blocks the delivery of oxygen to tissues of the body.
   3. Treatment consists of exposing the patient to 100% oxygen (sometimes in a hyperbaric chamber) until oxygen displaces the carbon monoxide and recovery occurs.

IV. LUNG LOBULES

A. Lung lobules vary greatly in size and shape, but each has an apex directed toward the pulmonary hilum and a wider base directed outward.

B. Each lobule contains a **single primary bronchiole**, which enters at the apex and branches to form five to seven terminal bronchioles. The terminal bronchioles in turn divide, ultimately giving rise to alveoli at the base of the lobule.

V. PULMONARY VASCULAR SUPPLY

A. Pulmonary artery
   1. The pulmonary artery carries blood to the lungs to be **oxygenated**.
   2. It enters the root of each lung and extends branches along the divisions of the bronchial tree.
   3. It enters lung lobules, where **its branches follow the bronchioles** (see Figure 15.2).

B. Pulmonary veins
   1. In lung lobules, pulmonary veins run in the intersegmental connective tissue, **separated from the arteries**.
   2. After leaving the lobules, the pulmonary veins come close to divisions of the bronchial tree and **run parallel to branches of the pulmonary artery** as they accompany bronchi to the root of the lung.

C. Bronchial arteries and veins
   1. Bronchial arteries and veins provide nutrients to and remove wastes from the nonrespiratory portions of the lung (bronchi, bronchioles, interstitium, and pleura).
   2. They follow the branching pattern of the bronchial tree and form anastomoses with the pulmonary vessels near capillary beds.

VI. PULMONARY NERVE SUPPLY

The pulmonary nerve supply consists primarily of **autonomic fibers to the smooth muscle of bronchi and bronchioles**. Axons are also present in the thicker parts of the interalveolar septa.

A. **Parasympathetic stimulation** causes **contraction** of pulmonary smooth muscle.

B. **Sympathetic stimulation** causes **relaxation** of pulmonary smooth muscle and can be mimicked by certain drugs that cause dilation of bronchi and bronchioles.

Review Test

Directions: Each of the numbered items or incomplete statements in this section is followed by answers or completions of the statement. Select the ONE lettered answer that is BEST in each case.

1. Characteristics of olfactory epithelium include which one of the following?

(A) It is located in the inferior region of the nasal cavity.
(B) It is classified as simple columnar.
(C) It has an underlying lamina propria containing mucous glands.
(D) It has modified cilia, which act as receptors for odor.
(E) It is unable to regenerate.

2. Which of the following statements concerning terminal bronchioles is true?

(A) They are part of the conducting portion of the respiratory system.
(B) They function in gas exchange.
(C) They do not contain ciliated cells.
(D) They have cartilage plates present in their walls.
(E) They do not contain secretory cells.

3. The trachea possesses which one of the following components?

(A) Irregular cartilage plates in its wall
(B) Skeletal muscle in its wall
(C) An epithelium containing only two cell types
(D) A thick basement membrane underlying its epithelium
(E) Bowman glands in its lamina propria

4. Which of the following statements concerning respiratory bronchioles is true?

(A) No gas exchange occurs in them.
(B) They do not have alveoli forming part of their wall.
(C) They contain goblet cells in their lining epithelium.
(D) They are included in the conducting portion of the respiratory system.
(E) Ciliated cells comprise a portion of their lining epithelium.

5. True statements about asthma include which one of the following?

(A) It is due to a loss of lung elasticity.
(B) It eventually causes the lungs to expand and leads to a barrel chest.
(C) It is associated with difficulty expiring air from the lungs.
(D) It may be helped by gene therapy using recombinant α_1-antitrypsin.
(E) It is usually not associated with inflammation.

6. Which of the following statements concerning alveolar macrophages is true?

(A) They secrete α_1-antitrypsin.
(B) They secrete elastase.
(C) They originate from blood neutrophils.
(D) They may play a role in causing hyaline membrane disease.
(E) They secrete small amounts of surfactant.

7. Which one of the following disorders may in some cases be successfully treated with antielastase (α_1-antitrypsin)?

(A) Asbestosis
(B) Asthma
(C) Carbon monoxide poisoning
(D) Emphysema
(E) Hyaline membrane disease

8. Which one of the following is characterized by interstitial pulmonary fibrosis?

(A) Asbestosis
(B) Asthma
(C) Carbon monoxide poisoning
(D) Emphysema
(E) Hyaline membrane disease

9. Which one of the following is associated with a barrel chest?

(A) Asbestosis

(B) Asthma

(C) Carbon monoxide poisoning

(D) Emphysema

(E) Hyaline membrane disease

10. Which one of the following is frequently treated successfully with glucocorticoids?

(A) Asbestosis

(B) Asthma

(C) Carbon monoxide poisoning

(D) Emphysema

(E) Hyaline membrane disease

Answers and Explanations

1. **D.** The olfactory epithelium possesses nonmotile cilia, which act as receptors for odor. They are extensions of the bipolar nerve cells that form part of this tall, pseudostratified epithelium located in the roof of the nasal cavity. Bowman glands, which lie in the lamina propria beneath this epithelium, produce a watery secretion, which moistens the olfactory surface (see Chapter 15 II A).

2. **A.** Terminal bronchioles are the most distal components of the conducting portion of the respiratory system. They lack alveoli and thus do not function in gas exchange. They are lined by an epithelium composed of two cell types: secretory (Clara) cells and ciliated cells. Cartilage is not present in bronchioles (see Chapter 15 II F).

3. **D.** The pseudostratified ciliated columnar epithelium lining the trachea rests on a thick basement membrane and contains five cell types. The trachea possesses C-shaped cartilages with smooth muscle (the trachealis) extending between their ends. Bowman glands are found only in the nasal cavity and produce a thin watery secretion (see Chapter 15 II D).

4. **E.** Respiratory bronchioles have alveoli interrupting their walls, so some gas exchange takes place at this level. Their remaining walls are lined by a simple cuboidal epithelium consisting of Clara cells and ciliated cells. Respiratory bronchioles are categorized as part of the respiratory portion of the system (see Chapter 15 III A).

5. **C.** Asthma results from the constriction of smooth muscle in the bronchioles, which decreases their diameter and makes the expiration of air very difficult. Mucus accumulates in the airways, and inflammatory cells invade the bronchiolar walls (see Chapter 15 II F Clinical Considerations).

6. **B.** Alveolar macrophages secrete elastase. Normally, α_1-antitrypsin, a serum protein, interacts with elastase, thereby protecting the lung against damage that may lead to emphysema. Alveolar macrophages, like all macrophages, arise from blood monocytes; they do not secrete surfactant; and they are unrelated to the pathogenesis of hyaline membrane disease (see Chapter 15 III D Clinical Considerations).

7. **D.** Hereditary forms of emphysema are now being treated with recombinant α_1-antitrypsin, which has antielastase activity (see Chapter 15 III D Clinical Considerations).

8. **A.** Inhaling asbestos fibers causes interstitial pulmonary fibrosis in the walls of respiratory bronchioles, alveolar ducts, and alveoli. Asbestos bodies are a classic feature of asbestosis. After prolonged heavy exposure to asbestos, this disease may progress to mesothelioma (a malignant tumor) (see Chapter 15 III D Clinical Considerations).

9. **D.** A loss of lung elasticity in emphysema makes it difficult for the lungs to recoil normally during expiration. The lungs and thoracic cavity enlarge, producing a barrel chest (see Chapter 15 III D Clinical Considerations).

10. **E.** Glucocorticoids, which stimulate synthesis of pulmonary surfactant, are often administered to the expectant mother a few days prior to delivery to prevent or alleviate hyaline membrane disease in the premature infant (see Chapter 15 III D Clinical Considerations).

chapter 16

Digestive System: Oral Cavity and Alimentary Tract

I. OVERVIEW—THE DIGESTIVE SYSTEM

A. The digestive system comprises the **oral region** and **alimentary canal (esophagus, stomach,** and **small** and **large intestines)** and several **extrinsic glands**.

B. It consists of a hollow tube (highly modified in the oral cavity) of varying diameter, composed of a **mucosa, submucosa, muscularis externa,** and **serosa (**or **adventitia)**.

C. **Function.** The digestive system secretes **enzymes** and **hormones** that function in ingestion, digestion, and absorption of nutrients and in the elimination of indigestible materials.

II. ORAL REGION

The oral region includes the **lips**; **palate**; **teeth** and **associated structures**; **tongue**; major salivary glands; and lingual, palatine, tubal, and pharyngeal tonsils, where the tonsils (collections of lymphoid nodules) form Waldeyer tonsilar ring, to protect the entryways into the alimentary canal and the respiratory system. The oral region is lined in most places by a **stratified squamous epithelium** whose **epithelial ridges** interdigitate with tall **connective tissue papillae** (connective tissue ridges) of the subjacent connective tissue. The epithelial ridges and the connective tissue ridges are collectively known as the **rete apparatus**. The epithelium and connective tissue together form the mucosa. The oral cavity has three types of mucosae: **lining mucosa**, whose epithelium is nonkeratinized; **masticatory mucosa**, whose epithelium is keratinized; and **specialized mucosa**, whose nonkeratinized stratified squamous epithelium possesses taste buds. The dorsal surface of the tongue, hard palate, and gingivae are the only regions that possess masticatory mucosa; the dorsum of the tongue, soft palate, and regions of the pharynx possess specialized mucosa; the remainder of the oral cavity is lined by lining mucosa. The histology of the tongue is described at the end of Section II of this chapter.

A. **The lips** are divided into the **external (skin) region**, the **vermilion zone**, and the **internal (mucosal) region**. The first two regions are covered by stratified squamous keratinized epithelium, whereas the internal region is lined by a wet stratified squamous nonkeratinized epithelium.
   1. A dense irregular collagenous connective tissue core envelops skeletal muscle.
   2. **Sebaceous glands, sweat glands**, and **hair follicles** are present in the external region; **minor salivary glands** in the internal region; and occasional, nonfunctional sebaceous glands (known as **Fordyce granules**) in the internal region and vermilion zone.

B. **The palate** separates the nasal cavity from the oral cavity and is divided into an anterior **hard palate** (possessing a bony shelf in its core) and a posterior **soft palate** (possessing skeletal muscle in its core). At the posterior terminus of the soft palate is the **uvula**. Therefore, the palate has a nasal aspect and an oral aspect. The entire **nasal aspect** of the palate (with the exception of the uvula) is lined by **pseudostratified ciliated columnar epithelium** (respiratory epithelium).

1. The **hard palate** is lined on its oral aspect by stratified squamous **parakeratinized** to stratified squamous **keratinized** epithelium. It contains adipose tissue anteriorly and minor mucous salivary glands posteriorly in the oral aspect of its connective tissue, also known as the **mucoperiosteum**.

2. The **soft palate** is lined on its oral aspect by stratified squamous **nonkeratinized** epithelium. It contains minor mucous salivary glands in the oral aspect of its connective tissue.

CLINICAL CONSIDERATIONS

1. **Herpetic stomatitis** is caused by herpes simplex virus (HSV) type 1. In the dormant state, this virus resides in the trigeminal ganglia. HSV type 1 infection is very common and is transmitted by kissing. This infection is characterized by painful fever blisters on the lips or in the vicinity of the nostrils. These blisters exude a clear fluid or are covered by a scab.

2. **Angular cheilitis (perlèche)** is a painful condition, usually in patients older than 50 years of age, in which the corners of the mouth have short erythematous fissures and cracks that are inflamed and may become infected with *Candida albicans* or with occasional secondary bacterial colonization by *Staphylococcus aureus*. Licking the corner of the mouth exacerbates and prolongs the condition. Treatment is usually with an antifungal ointment, and in case of a secondary bacterial infection, an antibiotic regimen and behavioral modification, that is, having the patient resist the urge to lick the corners of the mouth.

3. **Cancers of the oral region** most commonly affect the lips, tongue, and floor of the mouth. These cancers initially resemble leukoplakia and are asymptomatic. Survival rate is high if these cancers are recognized and treated in the early stages.

C. **Teeth**

1. **Overview—Teeth**

   a. Teeth are composed of an internal soft tissue, the **pulp**, and three calcified tissues: **enamel** and **cementum**, which form the surface layer, and **dentin**, which lies between the surface layer and the pulp. As in bone, **calcium hydroxyapatite** is the mineral material in the calcified dental tissues.

   b. Teeth have an enamel-covered **crown**, a cementum-covered root, and a **cervix**, the region where the two surface materials meet.

2. **Components—Teeth**

   a. **Enamel**

   (1) has a highly calcified matrix with an organic component that is composed mostly of the fibrous keratin-like protein, **enamelin**, a substance that is elaborated by **ameloblasts** during formation of the crown and becomes calcified by the deposition of **calcium-hydroxyapatite crystals**. It consists of only 4% organic material and 96% inorganic material and, thus, is the most calcified tissue in the body.

   (2) is **acellular after tooth eruption** and therefore cannot repair itself.

CLINICAL CONSIDERATIONS

The bacterial flora of the oral cavity acts on food remnants lodged between teeth and in the gingival sulcus, the normally tiny crevice between the gum and the enamel of the tooth. As the bacteria metabolize the sugars in the food debris, they produce lactic acid that can dissolve enough of the calcium-hydroxyapatite crystals to form carious lesions (tooth decay), unless the individual practices good oral hygiene. The use of fluoride in the water supply (systemic application), as well as the addition of fluoride in toothpaste (topical application), makes enamel more resistant to bacterial acids by altering the hydroxyapatite crystals (fluoride replaces hydroxyl molecules). Moreover, the presence of fluoride on the enamel surface catalyzes its remineralization.

b. Dentin
(1) surrounds the central **pulp chamber** of the crown and **pulp (root) canal**.
(2) has a calcified matrix containing mostly **type I collagen fibers**.
(3) is manufactured by **odontoblasts**, which persist and continue to elaborate dentin for the life of the tooth.

c. Cementum
(1) has a mostly **type I collagen–containing** calcified matrix, which is produced by **cementoblasts**.
(2) is **continuously elaborated** even after tooth eruption, since it compensates for the decrease in tooth length resulting from abrasion of the enamel.

d. Dental pulp
(1) is a gelatinous, richly vascularized connective tissue containing **odontoblasts** in its peripheral layer (closest to the dentin), fibroblasts and mesenchymal cells, and thin types I and III collagen fibers.
(2) contains **afferent nerve fibers**. All sensations from the pulp are interpreted as pain in the central nervous system.

3. Crown formation
a. The crown begins to form 6 to 7 weeks after conception as a horseshoe-shaped band, the **dental lamina**, which is derived from the **oral epithelium**. A dental lamina develops in each jaw and projects into the underlying **ectomesenchyme**. The development of teeth, known as **tooth germs**, depends on the interaction, known as **epithelial–mesenchymal interaction**, between the epithelium and the ectomesenchyme (neural crest-derived mesenchymal tissue). This interaction is dependent on various signaling molecules produced by both the epithelium and the ectomesenchyme. A tooth germ has two components: the epithelially derived **enamel organ** and the ectomesenchymally derived **dental papilla** surrounded by the ectomesenchymally derived **dental sac**. The enamel organ is responsible for the formation of the **enamel** and **junctional epithelium**; the dental papilla will give rise to **dentin** and the **pulp**; and the dental sac will form the **attachment apparatus**, namely **cementum**, **periodontal ligament**, **bony alveolus**, and the connective tissue of the **gingiva**.
b. The crown forms **before** the root formation begins.
c. The sequential stages of crown formation of the tooth germ are **bud, cap, bell,** and **appositional stages**.
d. The ectomesenchyme releases **Activin βA** and **bone morphogenic protein 4 (BMP 4)**, stimulating the epithelium to form epithelial downgrowths, known as the **bud**, 10 buds along the maxillary and 10 buds along the mandibular dental laminae.
e. Each bud, in turn releases **fibroblast growth factor 4** as well as **BMP 2, BMP 4,** and **BMP 7**, which instruct the tooth germ to assume a specific shape (incisor, canine, premolar, or molar).

4. Root formation follows completion of the crown and is accompanied by tooth eruption.

D. Dental-supporting structures (Attachment apparatus)
1. The **periodontal ligament** is composed of a dense irregular collagenous connective tissue whose type I collagen fibers are arranged in five **principal fiber bundles**, which extend from cementum to bone (alveolar crest, horizontal, oblique, apical, and interradicular fiber groups), suspending the tooth in its **alveolus**.
2. **Gingivae (gums)** are covered by stratified squamous **keratinized** (or **parakeratinized**) epithelium; their collagen fibers are also arranged in five **principal fiber bundles** (alveologingival, dentogingival, circular, dentoperiosteal, and transseptal fiber groups).
3. **Alveolar bone** consists of an inner layer of compact bone (**cribriform plate**, or **alveolar bone proper**). There is also an outer layer (**cortical plate**) of compact bone with an intervening layer of cancellous bone (**spongiosa**).

E. Tongue
1. Overview—Tongue
a. The tongue is divided into an anterior two-thirds and a posterior one-third by the V-shaped **sulcus terminalis**, whose posteriorly pointing apex ends in the **foramen cecum**.
b. Its dorsal surface is covered by stratified squamous **parakeratinized** to **keratinized** epithelium, whereas its ventral surface is covered by stratified squamous **nonkeratinized**

| t a b l e | 16.1 | Summary of the Histological Features of the Oral Mucosa |

Mucosal Region	Type of Epithelium/Mucosa	Height of CT Papilla	Special Comments
Lip			
Skin aspect	Stratified squamous keratin	Medium	Hair, sebaceous and sweat glands
Vermilion zone	Stratified squamous keratin	High	Few sebaceous glands(?)
Mucosal aspect	Stratified squamous nonkeratinized	Medium	Mucous (mixed) minor salivary glands and Fordyce granules
Cheek			
Skin aspect	Stratified squamous keratinized	Medium	Hair, sebaceous and sweat glands
Mucosal aspect	Stratified squamous nonkeratinized	Medium	Mucous (mixed?) minor salivary glands and Fordyce granules
Gingiva			
Free and Attached	Masticatory mucosa	High	Tightly bound to the periosteum
Sulcular	Lining mucosa	Low	Lines the gingival sulcus
Junctional epithelium	Stratified squamous nonkeratinized	None	Attached to tooth surface and to gingival connective tissue by hemidesmosomes
Alveolar mucosa	Lining mucosa	Low	Some minor mucous salivary glands
Hard palate*			
Anterior lateral	Masticatory mucosa	High	Adipose tissue in the connective tissue
Posterior lateral	Masticatory mucosa	High	Minor mucous salivary glands in CT
Raphe	Masticatory mucosa	High	Tightly bound to periosteum
Soft palate*	Lining mucosa	Low	Elastic lamina; minor mucous salivary glands
Uvula	Lining mucosa	Low	Minor mucous salivary glands in CT
Floor of the mouth	Lining mucosa	Low	Minor mucous salivary glands in CT
Tongue			
Dorsal surface	Specialized mucosa embedded in masticatory mucosa	Low High	Taste buds; lingual papillae; serous, mucous, and mixed minor salivary glands
Ventral surface	Lining mucosa	Low	Sublingual folds

CT, connective tissue.

*The description in this table for the hard palate and soft palate is only for the oral aspect. The nasal aspect of both hard and soft palates is covered by a respiratory epithelium. However, the nasal aspect of the uvula is covered by a stratified squamous nonkeratinized epithelium.

epithelium (see Table 16.1). Both epithelial surfaces are underlain by a **lamina propria** and **submucosa** of dense irregular collagenous connective tissue.

c. The tongue possesses a **core of skeletal muscle**, which forms the bulk of the tongue.

2. **Lingual papillae** are located on the **dorsal surface of the anterior two-thirds** of the tongue.

a. **Filiform papillae** are short, narrow, **highly keratinized** structures, lacking taste buds.

b. **Fungiform papillae** are mushroom-shaped structures interspersed among the filiform papillae; they contain occasional **taste buds** on their superior aspect.

c. **Foliate papillae** are shallow longitudinal furrows on the lateral aspect of the posterior region of the anterior two-thirds of the tongue. Their taste buds degenerate shortly after the second year of life.

d. **Circumvallate papillae** are 10 to 15 large circular papillae, each of which is surrounded by a moat-like furrow. They lie just anterior to the **sulcus terminalis** and possess taste buds.

   (1) **Taste buds**

      (a) Each of the 2,000 to 8,000 taste buds located on the tongue is composed of 60 to 80 spindle-shaped cells that form a barrel-shaped **intraepithelial structure**. These structures are located on the superior surface of fungiform papillae, on the **lateral surfaces** of circumvallate papillae, and in the **walls** of the surrounding moat-like furrows. Each taste bud has a small opening, the **taste pore**, from which microvilli (**taste hairs**) project into the oral cavity (or into the moat surrounding the circumvallate papilla).

(b) Four different cells may be recognized, three of which are spindle shaped: dark cells (type I cells), light cells (type II cells), and intermediate cells (type III cells) have short life spans; the fourth type are the short, regenerative, basal cells. Types I, II, and III cells form **synapses** with **afferent nerve fibers** that deliver the taste information to the central nervous system.

(c) When basal cells divide, they give rise to a basal cell and a dark cell. As the dark cell matures, it becomes a light cell, and as it degenerates, it becomes an intermediate cell. These three cell types are **neuroepithelial** cells whose microvilli, the taste hairs, recognize one specific tastant. The process of going from a newly formed dark cell to a dead intermediate cell takes about 10 days. A particular taste bud contains a variety of neuroepithelial cells that recognize all tastants, but each taste bud appears to be specialized to respond to only one or two of the tastants.

(d) **Function.** Taste buds perceive salty, sour, bitter, sweet, and umami (glutamate receptor that senses delicious flavors) taste sensations, and some, in individuals who have the genetic capability, may specialize in tasting fats. The chemical moieties of the food substances that are recognized by taste buds are known as **tastants**.

(e) Salt and sour tastants stimulate sodium and hydrogen ion channels, respectively; sweet, bitter, and umami tastants stimulate G protein–linked receptors; and fatty tastants stimulate fatty acid transporters.

CLINICAL CONSIDERATIONS It appears that the more molecules of a particular tastant bind to a neuroepithelial cell, the stronger the taste sensation. Recently, it has been shown that the taste receptors also have binding sites for nontastant molecules that act as **enhancer molecules**. Therefore, when enhancer molecules bind along with tastants, the tastants are locked in the receptor for a longer period of time. Thus, the tastant–enhancer molecule combination augments the taste sensation so that the binding of only a few tastant molecules is interpreted as if many such tastant molecules were present.

The sense of taste is a complex interaction between the information that the brain receives from the taste buds; from sensory cells that determine the temperature, spiciness, and texture of the food; as well as from **retronasal olfaction**. The process of retronasal olfaction depends on olfactory cells located in the posterior aspect of the nasal cavity, and the odor that they perceive arises from the back of the mouth rather than the more commonly thought of **orthonasal olfaction**, where the odor is perceived via air entering the nasal cavity. An additional component of the perception of taste is the visual information that the brain gleans via the sense of sight. An unusually colored version of a particular food morsel may elicit a sense of disgust, a perceived altered taste, and the inability to consume the food substance.

---

(2) **Glands of von Ebner** are minor salivary glands that deliver their **serous secretion** into the furrow surrounding each papilla, assisting the taste buds in perceiving stimuli. These glands also deliver their saliva into the furrows of the foliate papillae.

3. The **muscular core of the tongue** is composed of bundles of **skeletal muscle fibers** arranged in three planes with **minor salivary glands** interspersed among them.

4. A **lingual tonsil** is located on the dorsal surface of the **posterior one-third** of the tongue.

III. DIVISIONS OF THE ALIMENTARY CANAL

Divisions of the alimentary canal are determined by the histophysiological variations of the layers (Table 16.2). The alimentary canal is said to have a general plan of histological organization, in that the lumen is lined by a **mucosa**, composed of **epithelium**, a loose, cellular connective tissue housing glands, known as the **lamina propria**, and the outer muscular layer of the mucosa known as the **muscularis mucosae**. The mucosa is surrounded by a denser connective tissue, the **submucosa** that houses glands, but only in the esophagus and the duodenum. The submucosa is surrounded by the

t a b l e   **16.2**   Selected Histological Features of the Alimentary Canal

Region	Epithelium	Lamina Propria	Layers of Muscularis Mucosae*	Submucosa	Layers of Muscularis Externa[†]
Esophagus	Stratified squamous	Esophageal cardiac glands	Longitudinal	Collagenous CT, esophageal glands proper	Inner circular, outer longitudinal
Stomach	Simple columnar, no goblet cells	Gastric glands	Inner circular, outer longitudinal, sometimes outermost circular	Collagenous CT, no glands	Inner oblique, middle circular, outer longitudinal
Small intestine	Simple columnar with goblet cells	Villi, crypts of Lieberkühn, Peyer patches in ileum (extend into submucosa), lymphoid nodules	Inner circular, outer longitudinal	Fibroelastic CT, Brunner glands in duodenum	Inner circular, outer longitudinal
Large intestine, cecum, colon	Simple columnar with goblet cells	Crypts of Lieberkühn (lack Paneth cells), lymphoid nodules	Inner circular, outer longitudinal	Fibroelastic CT, no glands	Inner circular, outer longitudinal (modified to form teniae coli)
Rectum	Simple columnar with goblet cells	Crypts of Lieberkühn (fewer but deeper than in colon), lymphoid nodules	Inner circular, outer longitudinal	Fibroelastic CT, no glands	Two layers: inner circular, outer longitudinal
Anal canal	Simple columnar cuboidal (proximal), stratified squamous nonkeratinized (distal to anal valves), stratified squamous keratinized (anus)	Sebaceous glands, circumanal glands, lymphoid nodules, rectal columns or Morgagni (involve entire mucosa), hair follicles (anus)	Inner circular, outer longitudinal	Fibroelastic CT with large veins, no glands	Inner circular (forms internal anal sphincter), outer longitudinal
Appendix	Simple columnar with goblet cells	Crypts of Lieberkühn (shallow), lymphoid nodules (large, numerous, and may extend into the submucosa)	Inner circular, outer longitudinal	Fibroelastic CT, confluent lymphoid nodules, no glands, fat tissue (sometimes)	Inner circular, outer longitudinal

CT, connective tissue.

*The muscularis mucosae is composed entirely of smooth muscle throughout the alimentary canal.

[†]The muscularis externa is composed entirely of smooth muscle in all regions except the esophagus. The upper third of the esophageal muscularis externa is all skeletal muscle; the middle third is a mixture of skeletal and smooth muscle; and the lower third is all smooth muscle.

muscularis externa, which, in turn, is covered by either a **serosa** or an **adventitia**. Variations of the components of these layers permit regional structural and functional specialization of the alimentary canal. Innervation of the alimentary canal is accomplished by the **enteric nervous system** (whose neurons are located in **Meissner [submucosal]** and **Auerbach [myenteric] plexuses**). The function of the enteric nervous system is modified by the **sympathetic** and **parasympathetic** components of the **autonomic nervous system** (See Chapter 9 IX).

A. **Esophagus**
   1. The esophagus is lined by a **stratified squamous nonkeratinized epithelium**.
   2. The lamina propria contains mucus-secreting **esophageal cardiac glands**.
   3. The **muscularis mucosae** varies in thickness and, in the esophagus, it is composed of a single longitudinal layer of smooth muscle.
   4. The submucosa houses mucus-secreting **esophageal glands proper**.
   5. The upper third of the **muscularis externa** is composed only of **skeletal muscle**; the middle third is composed of a combination of **smooth and skeletal muscle**; and the lower third is composed only of **smooth muscle**. The striated muscles are controlled by the **vagus nerve (CN X)**, whereas the smooth muscles are controlled by nerve fibers derived from the enteric nervous system.
   6. The **muscularis externa** of the esophagus conveys a **bolus** of food from the pharynx into the stomach by **peristaltic activity**. Two physiological **sphincters** (the pharyngoesophageal and the gastroesophageal) in the muscularis externa ensure that the **bolus** is transported in only one direction, toward the stomach.

B. **Stomach.** The **stomach acidifies** and converts the bolus into a thick, viscous fluid known as **chyme**. It also produces **digestive enzymes** and **hormones**.
   1. **General structure—Stomach**
      a. The stomach exhibits longitudinal folds of the mucosa and submucosa (called **rugae**), which disappear in the distended stomach. The gross anatomy of the stomach is divided into four regions (cardiac, fundic, body, and pyloric), but histologically, the stomach is said to have only three regions: the **cardiac region (cardia)**, where the esophagus joins the stomach; the bulk of the stomach, composed of the fundus and body, which are histologically identical and therefore referred to by histologists as the **fundic region** (**fundus**); and the **pyloric region (pylorus)**, where the stomach joins the small intestine.
      b. The lining of the stomach has many well-like openings, known as **gastric pits (foveolae)**, which are shallowest in the cardia and deepest in the pylorus (Figure 16.1). The gastric glands of the stomach mucosa deliver their secretions into the bases of the gastric pits.
         (1) Gastric mucosa
            (a) The **simple columnar** epithelium of the gastric mucosa is composed of mucinogen-producing **surface lining cells** (Figure 16.1), which are not goblet cells but produce a thick, viscous mucus, known as **visible mucus**, that lines the epithelial lining of the stomach and protects it from the highly acidic chyme and, therefore, from autodigestion. It also houses a very small number of taste cells that, similarly to the taste buds of the tongue, are capable of recognizing the taste sensations, especially bitter, umami, and sweet. These cells are described more fully in the section on the small intestine.
            (b) The **lamina propria** is a loose connective tissue housing smooth muscle cells, lymphocytes, plasma cells, mast cells, and fibroblasts. It contains **gastric glands**.
            (c) The **muscularis mucosae** is composed of a poorly defined inner circular layer, an outer longitudinal layer, and occasionally an outermost circular layer of smooth muscle.
         (2) Gastric submucosa
            (a) is composed of dense, irregular **collagenous** connective tissue.
            (b) contains fibroblasts, mast cells, and lymphoid elements embedded in the connective tissue.
            (c) houses **Meissner (submucosal) plexus**.
            (d) possesses arterial and venous plexuses that respectively supply and drain the vessels of the mucosa.

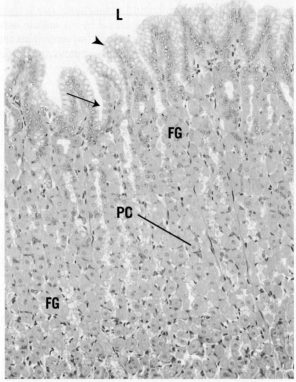

FIGURE 16.1. The gastric pits (*arrow*) of the fundic region of the stomach open into the lumen of the stomach (L), which is lined by mucus-producing surface lining cells (*arrowhead*). The lumina of the fundic glands (FG) open into the bottom of the gastric pits. Observe the large parietal cells (PC) that abound in the fundic glands (×132).

       (3) Gastric muscularis externa
          (a) is composed of **three layers** of smooth muscle: an incomplete inner oblique layer, a thick middle circular layer that forms the **pyloric sphincter**, and an outer longitudinal layer. **Auerbach (myenteric) plexus** is located between the middle circular and outer longitudinal smooth muscle layers.
          (b) is responsible for mixing of gastric contents and emptying of the stomach.
          (c) is affected by various characteristics of the chyme (e.g., lipid content, viscosity, osmolality, caloric density, and pH), which influence the **emptying rate** of the stomach and the rate of muscle contraction.
       (4) A serosa covers the external surface of the stomach.
   2. **Gastric glands** are simple branched tubular glands in the lamina propria of the **cardia**, **fundus**, and **pylorus**. Each gland consists of an **isthmus**, which connects the gland to the base of a gastric pit; a **neck**; and a **base**.
   a. **Cells of the fundic glands**
       (1) **Parietal (oxyntic) cells** (Figure 16.1)
          (a) These are pyramidal cells concentrated in the upper half of the gland.
          (b) They secrete **hydrochloric acid** (HCl) and **gastric intrinsic factor**. The latter is necessary for absorption of vitamin B_{12} in the ileum.
          (c) They possess a unique intracellular **tubulovesicular system**, many mitochondria, and secretory **intracellular canaliculi** (deep invaginations of the apical plasma membrane) lined by **microvilli**.
          (d) When the parietal cells are stimulated to secrete HCl, the number and length of microvilli increase and the complexity of the tubulovesicular system decreases (suggesting that tubulovesicular membranes are incorporated into the intracellular canaliculi, thus lengthening the microvilli).

(2) Chief (zymogenic) cells

(a) are pyramidal cells residing in the lower half of the **gland**.

(b) secrete **pepsinogen** (a precursor of the enzyme **pepsin**) and the precursors of two other enzymes, **rennin** and **lipase**.

(c) display an abundance of basal rough endoplasmic reticulum (RER), a supranuclear Golgi complex, and many apical zymogen (secretory) granules.

(3) Mucous neck cells

(a) are located in the neck of the gland (and may be able to divide).

(b) possess short microvilli, apical mucous granules, a prominent Golgi complex, numerous mitochondria, and some basal RER.

(c) produce **soluble mucus**, a slippery substance that lubricates the lining of the stomach.

(4) Diffuse neuroendocrine system (DNES) cells

(a) are also referred to as **enteroendocrine cells** or as **APUD cells** (**a**mine **p**recursor **u**ptake and **d**ecarboxylation cells).

(b) are of two major categories, **open** and **closed**. The DNES cells of the open category have short processes that reach the lumen; they are believed to be chemosensory, and they test the luminal content to release specific substances based on the circumstances. DNES cells of the closed category do not have processes that reach the lumen and, therefore, they are "closed off" from the luminal content.

(c) include more than a dozen types of cells that house many small hormone-containing granules, usually concentrated in the **basal** cytoplasm. Each particular enteroendocrine cell is believed to secrete only one hormone (Table 16.3).

(d) possess an abundance of mitochondria and RER and a moderately well-developed Golgi complex.

table **16.3**	Selected Hormones Secreted by Cells of the Alimentary Canal*		
Hormone	**Cell**	**Site of Secretion**	**Physiological Effect**
Cholecystokinin	I	Small intestine	Stimulates release of pancreatic enzymes, contraction of gallbladder (with release of bile)
Gastric inhibitory peptide	K	Small intestine	Inhibits gastric HCl secretion
Gastrin	G	Pylorus, duodenum	Stimulates gastric secretion of HCl, pepsinogen
Ghrelin	P/D1	Stomach, pancreas	Produces hunger sensations by adjusting the muscle tone of the muscularis externa as the stomach expands so that the gastric intraluminal pressure remains unchanged
Glicentin	GL	Stomach to colon	Stimulates hepatic glycogenolysis
Glucagon	A	Stomach, duodenum	Stimulates hepatic glycogenolysis
Motilin	Mo	Small intestine	Increases gut motility
Neurotensin	N	Small intestine	Inhibits gut motility, stimulates blood flow to ileum
Secretin	S	Small intestine	Stimulates bicarbonate secretion by pancreas and biliary tract
Serotonin, substance P	EC	Stomach to colon	Increases gut motility
Somatostatin	D	Pylorus, duodenum	Inhibits nearby enteroendocrine cells
Urogastrone[†]		Duodenum (Brunner glands)	Inhibits gastric HCl secretion, enhances epithelial cell division
VIP	VIP	Stomach to colon	Increases gut motility, stimulates intestinal ion, water secretion
Peptide YY	L	Ileum and colon	Produces the sensation of satiation

A, α-cell-like cell; D, δ-cell-like cell; EC, enterochromaffin-like cell; G, gastrin-producing cell; GL, glicentin-producing cell; HCl, hydrochloric acid; Mo, motilin-producing cell; N, neurotensin-producing cell; S, secretin-producing cell; VIP, vasoactive intestinal peptide.

*Some of these hormones are also secreted in other parts of the body and have additional physiological effects.

[†]Not produced by diffuse neuroendocrine system cell.

    (5) Regenerative cells are located primarily in the neck and isthmus; they replace all the epithelial cells of the gland, gastric pit, and luminal surface.

  b. Cardiac and pyloric glands are different from fundic glands in that they are coiled tubular mucus-secreting glands and lack chief cells.

 3. Gastric juice contains water, HCl, mucus, pepsin, lipase, rennin, and electrolytes. It is **very acidic** (pH 2.0) and facilitates the activation of pepsinogen to pepsin, which catalyzes the partial hydrolysis of proteins.

 4. Regulation of gastric secretion is effected by neural activity (vagus nerve) and by several hormones.

  a. Gastrin and **histamine**, released by enteroendocrine cells in the gastric and duodenal mucosa, together with acetylcholine released by parasympathetic nerve fibers of the vagus nerve, **stimulate HCl secretion**.

  b. Somatostatin, produced by enteroendocrine cells of the pylorus and duodenum, inhibits the release of gastrin and thus **indirectly inhibits HCl secretion**.

  c. Urogastrone (also known as **human epidermal growth factor**), produced by Brunner glands of the duodenum, and **gastric inhibitory peptide** along with **prostaglandins**, produced by enteroendocrine cells in the small intestine, **directly inhibit HCl secretion**.

C. Small intestine

 1. Overview—Small intestine

  a. The small intestine is approximately 7 m long and has three regions: the **duodenum** (proximal), **jejunum** (middle), and **ileum** (distal).

  b. Function. The small intestine secretes several **hormones**; it continues and largely completes the **digestion** of foodstuffs and **absorbs** the resulting metabolites.

 2. Luminal surface modifications—Small intestine. The luminal surface of the small intestine possesses plicae circulares, intestinal villi, and microvilli, which collectively increase the luminal surface area by a factor of 400 to 600.

  a. Plicae circulares (valves of Kerckring) are permanent spiral folds of the **mucosa** and **submucosa** that are present in the distal half of the duodenum, the entire jejunum, and the proximal half of the ileum. Plicae circulares *increase the surface area twofold to threefold.*

  b. Intestinal villi (Figures 16.2 and 16.3) are permanent evaginations that possess, in their connective tissue core (lamina propria), numerous plasma cells and lymphocytes,

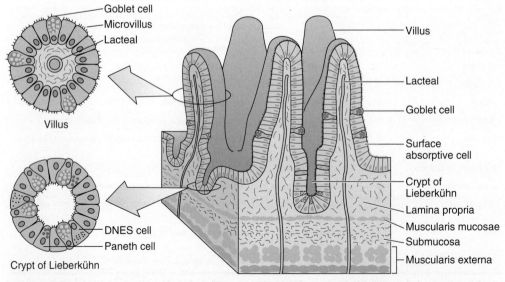

FIGURE 16.2. The spatial relationship of intestinal villi; crypts of Lieberkühn; and underlying muscularis mucosae, submucosa, and muscularis externa of the small intestine. Intestinal villi are evaginations of the epithelium and lamina propria. Each villus contains a single blind-ended lacteal and capillary loop. The submucosa, muscularis externa, and serosa are also depicted. DNES, diffuse neuroendocrine system.

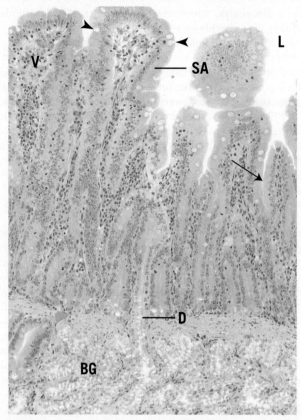

FIGURE 16.3. The villi (V) of the duodenum are covered mostly by surface absorptive cells (SA) as well as by goblet cells (*arrowheads*). The *arrow* is pointing to the approximate junction between the intervillar spaces that are continuous with the lumen (L) of the duodenum and the beginning of the crypts of Lieberkühn. The submucosa of the duodenum possesses Brunner glands (BG) whose ducts (D) open into the base of the crypts of Lieberkühn and, sometimes, into the intervillar spaces (×132).

fibroblasts, mast cells, smooth muscle cells, capillary loops, and a **single lacteal** (blind-ended lymphatic capillary). Villi *increase the surface area 10-fold.*

   c. **Microvilli** of the **apical** surface of the epithelial cells of each villus possess actin filaments that interact with myosin filaments in the terminal web. Microvilli *increase the surface area about 20-fold.*

3. **Mucosa of the small intestine**

   a. The **epithelium** of the mucosa of the small intestine is **simple columnar**. It is composed of goblet cells, surface absorptive cells, and some DNES cells that are of both types open and closed (Figure 16.3).

     (1) Goblet cells

       (a) are **unicellular glands** that produce **mucinogen**, which accumulates in membrane-bounded granules, distending the **apical** region (**theca**) of the cell. After being released, mucinogen becomes hydrated and is thus converted to **mucin**, a thick, viscous substance that acts as a **protective coating** of the epithelial lining of the lumen; mucin, when mixed with luminal contents is known as **mucus**).

       (b) have their nucleus and other organelles in the basal region (**stem**) of the cell.

       (c) increase in number from the duodenum to the ileum.

     (2) Surface absorptive cells

       (a) are tall columnar cells (Figure 16.3) with numerous mitochondria, smooth endoplasmic reticulum (SER) and RER, and a Golgi complex.

       (b) possess a layer of closely packed microvilli (**striated border**) on their free apical surface.

(c) have a **glycocalyx**, which overlies the microvilli and binds various enzymes, including disaccharidases and dipeptidases.

(d) have well-developed **tight junctions and zonula adherens**.

(3) DNES cells produce and secrete **gastrin, cholecystokinin, gastric inhibitory peptide**, and several other hormones (Table 16.3). Some of the open DNES cells possess the three genes for G protein–linked taste receptors similar to those of the taste buds located on the tongue. As in taste buds, sweet taste is coded for by T1R2 and T1R3, bitter by two copies of T2R subtypes, umami by T1R1 and T1R3. It is important to note that the taste cells of the gastrointestinal tract communicate with the islets of Langerhans, signaling the beta cells to release insulin once sweet taste is detected in the lumen.

b. **Lamina propria**

(1) occupies the cores of the villi and the interstices between the numerous **glands (crypts) of Lieberkühn** (Figure 16.3).

(2) consists of loose connective tissue with lymphoid cells, fibroblasts, mast cells, smooth muscle cells, nerve endings, and **lymphoid nodules**.

(3) also contains **lacteals** (blind-ended lymphatic vessels) and **capillary loops**.

(a) **Crypts of Lieberkühn** are simple tubular glands that extend from the intervillous spaces to the muscularis mucosae of the intestine. They are composed of goblet and oligomucous cells, columnar cells (similar to surface absorptive cells), DNES cells, regenerative cells, Paneth cells, intermediate cells, and M cells (M cells, the last of this group, are discussed under the category of lymphoid nodules).

1. **Paneth cells**, located at the base of the crypts of Lieberkühn, are pyramidal cells that secrete the antibacterial enzyme **lysozyme** stored in large, apical, membrane-bounded secretory granules. These cells also release other antibacterial agents, **defensins** and **tumor necrosis factor** α and display extensive RER (basally), a large supranuclear Golgi complex, and many mitochondria. These agents have the capability of killing bacteria as well as certain protozoa.

2. **Regenerative cells**, located in the basal half of the crypts of Lieberkühn, are thin, tall, columnar **stem cells** that divide to replace themselves and the other types of epithelial cells.

3. **Intermediate cells** make up the bulk of the epithelial lining of the crypts of Lieberkühn. These cells have regenerative properties; they are derived from regenerative cells, but have not as yet committed themselves to a certain cell line.

(b) **Lymphoid nodules** are usually small and solitary and are located in the lamina propria of the duodenum and jejunum. They increase in size and number in the ileum, where they form large contiguous aggregates, known as **Peyer patches**, which frequently extend through the muscularis mucosae into the submucosa.

1. **M (microfold) cells** are highly specialized, have an unusual shape, and lie in the epithelium over lymphoid nodules and Peyer patches. They are derived from undifferentiated cells of the crypts of Lieberkühn. They sample antigens as well as bacteria, viruses, and parasitic microorganisms. The endocytosed particles are conveyed via transcytosis to macrophages and lymphocytes that lie in the infoldings of the basal plasmalemma of M cells. These macrophages and the B and T lymphocytes are actually located in the lamina propria.

2. **Activated B lymphocytes** respond to antigenic challenge by forming more B cells, which enter the lymph and blood circulation, then home back to their original locations, where they populate the lamina propria and differentiate into immunoglobulin A (IgA) producing plasma cells.

3. **Plasma cells** manufacture monomeric immunoglobulin A (**IgA**). Two IgAs are bound to each other within the plasma cell by a protein, **protein J**, another product of the plasma cell, forming a dimeric variety of IgA. The IgA dimer then enters the lamina propria of the small intestine and binds to dimeric IgA receptors at the basal membrane of the surface absorptive cells. The **IgA–receptor complex** is endocytosed into the cell and is transported to an early endosome to be transported across the intestinal epithelium (**transcytosis**) to

the glycocalyx. Here a portion of the dimeric IgA receptor is cleaved from the complex, whereas the remainder of the receptor remains bound to the dimeric IgA as its secretory component, and the molecule is known as **secretory IgA (sIgA)**. Some of the sIgA remains as an immunological defense against bacteria and antigens in the lumen of the intestine. Much of the **sIgA** is reabsorbed by the surface absorptive cells and is transported into the lamina propria, where it enters blood vessels and goes to the liver, where it is internalized by hepatocytes to be secreted as part of bile. From the liver, sIgA enters the gallbladder to be released into the lumen of the duodenum to join the sIgA already present there to contribute to the immunological defense of the gastrointestinal tract. This process is referred to as the **enterohepatic circulation**.

   c. The **muscularis mucosae** is composed of an inner circular and an outer longitudinal layer of smooth muscle.

CLINICAL CONSIDERATIONS

   1. It is interesting to note that the immune system of the alimentary canal, under normal conditions, is tolerant of the normal bacterial flora and of epithelial cells lining the gut that are in close contact with bacteria. It has been shown that this tolerance is due to dendritic cells that inhibit T cells from initiating an immune response. However, if the conditions become inimical to health, as in an inflammatory reaction, the dendritic cells instruct the T cells to respond and elicit an immune reaction. In order to assist the dendritic cells in their function of dictating tolerance, stromal cells of lymph nodes present proteins produced by cells of the alimentary canal to naïve T cells, instructing them to be tolerant of those proteins unless instructed otherwise by dendritic cells.

   2. Tourists who have contracted the Shigatoxigenic group of *Escherichia coli* are at risk when they medicate themselves with antibiotics, such as Ciprofloxacin, that they take on their trips as a protective measure to cure their diarrhea. Unfortunately, when these *E. coli* die, they release enormous quantities of the Shiga toxin that can kill the patient. It is advisable for patients not to take Ciprofloxacin in case they have bloody diarrhea but seek competent medical advice.

---

    4. Submucosa of the small intestine
      a. consists of **fibroelastic** connective tissue containing blood and lymphatic vessels, nerve fibers, and **Meissner plexus**.
      b. also houses **Brunner glands** (Figure 16.3), which are present *only in the duodenum*. These glands produce an **alkaline fluid** and **urogastrone**. The former protects the duodenal epithelium from the acidic chyme; the latter is a polypeptide hormone (**human epidermal growth factor**) that enhances epithelial cell division and inhibits gastric HCl production.
    5. The **muscularis externa of the small intestine** is composed of **two** layers of smooth muscle: an inner circular and an outer longitudinal layer. The inner layer participates in the formation of the **ileocecal sphincter**. **Auerbach (myenteric) plexus** is housed between the two layers.
    6. External layer of the small intestine
      a. **Serosa** covers all of the jejunum and ileum and part of the duodenum.
      b. **Adventitia** covers the remainder of the duodenum.

  D. Large intestine
    1. Overview—Large intestine
      a. The large intestine consists of the **cecum, colon** (ascending, transverse, descending, and sigmoid colon), **rectum, anal canal**, and **appendix**.
      b. The large intestine contains some digestive enzymes received from the small intestine.
      c. It houses bacteria that produce **vitamin B$_{12}$** and **vitamin K**; the former is necessary for hemopoiesis and the latter for coagulation.
      d. The large intestine produces **abundant mucus**, which lubricates its lining and facilitates the passage and elimination of feces.

    e. Function. The large intestine functions primarily in the **absorption of electrolytes, fluids, and gases**. Dead bacteria and indigestible remnants of the ingested material are compacted into **feces**.

  2. Cecum and colon

    a. The **mucosa of the cecum and colon lacks villi** and possesses no specialized folds.

      (1) The **epithelium** of the mucosa of the cecum and colon is **simple columnar** with numerous goblet cells, surface absorptive cells, and occasional DNES cells.

      (2) The **lamina propria** is similar to that of the small intestine, possessing lymphoid nodules, blood and lymph vessels, and closely packed crypts of Lieberkühn, which lack Paneth cells.

        (a) Fibroblasts at the base of the crypts of Lieberkühn of the lamina propria undergo mitotic division and travel alongside of the epithelial components of the intestinal crypt, and as they reach the vicinity of the opening of the crypt, differentiate into cells with characteristics of macrophages. It is believed that these newly differentiated cells assist the monocyte-derived macrophages in their protective functions.

        (b) Lymphoid elements, members of the **gut-associated lymphoid tissues (GALT)**, composed of lymphoid nodules and cells, are richly represented in the lamina propria.

        (c) Interestingly, **lymphoid drainage** occurs rarely, if ever, from the lamina propria; thereby, the absence of lymphatic vessels greatly limits the capability of metastasis of malignant tumors from the mucosa of the colon.

      (3) The **muscularis mucosae** consists of an inner circular and outer longitudinal layer of smooth muscle cells.

    b. The **submucosa of the cecum and colon** is composed of **fibroelastic** connective tissue. It contains blood and lymphatic vessels, nerves, and **Meissner (submucosal) plexus**.

    c. The **muscularis externa of the cecum and colon** is composed of an inner circular and a modified outer longitudinal layer of smooth muscle. The outer layer is gathered into three flat, longitudinal ribbons of smooth muscle that form the **teniae coli**. When continuously contracted, the teniae coli form sacculations of the wall known as **haustra coli**. **Auerbach (myenteric) plexus** is housed between the two layers of smooth muscle.

    d. External layer of the cecum and colon

      (1) Adventitia covers the ascending and descending portions of the colon.

      (2) Serosa covers the cecum and the remainder of the colon. Fat-filled outpocketings of the serosa (**appendices epiploicae**) are characteristic of the transverse and sigmoid colon.

    e. The **lumen of the large intestine** houses trillions of microbes, approximately 10 times the number of cells in the entire human body. These microorganisms form a part of the body's **microbiome**, whose physiological balance has shown to reflect the health of the individual harboring them. It appears that there are three groups of intestinal flora, known as **enterotypes** that predominate in the human population, and each individual possesses a predominance of one of these enterotypes. How these enterotypes develop and what their significance is are not as yet understood.

CLINICAL CONSIDERATIONS

1. Malabsorption disorders may lead to malnutrition, resulting in wasting diseases, if major nutrients (carbohydrates, amino acids, ions) cannot be assimilated.

  a. Gluten enteropathy (nontropical sprue) results from the destructive effects of certain glutens (particularly of rye and wheat) on the intestinal villi, which reduce the surface area available for absorption. It is treated by eliminating wheat and rye products from the diet.

  b. Malabsorption of vitamin B$_{12}$ may cause pernicious anemia. It usually results from inadequate production of gastric intrinsic factor by the parietal cells of the gastric mucosa.

2. Cholera-induced diarrhea is caused by the action of cholera toxin, which blocks intestinal absorption of sodium ions and promotes excretion of water and electrolytes. It causes death shortly after onset unless the lost electrolytes and water are replaced.

3. Diverticulitis is a disease of the aging individual. As the person enters the fifth decade of life, the muscular layers of the large intestine begin to weaken, permitting the eventual formation of outpocketings (diverticula) of the mucosa and submucosa of the distal colon, mainly in the lower descending colon and the sigmoid colon. As materials become trapped in these diverticula, inflammation occurs in about 15% to 25% of individuals with diverticulosis, and it is this inflammation that is known as diverticulitis. Individuals suffering from diverticulitis exhibit abdominal pain (usually in the left lower quadrant of the abdomen), and if the inflammation is severe, fever, nausea, diarrhea, and cramps may also be experienced.

4. **Fecal transplant** is a relatively recent procedure used in patients whose normal bacterial flora has been decimated and usurped by pathogenic bacteria, such as *Clostridium difficile*. These individuals suffer from *C. difficile* colitis with a resultant bout of diarrhea that may last as long as several months. Although these patients are placed on a long-term antibiotic regimen, in many cases the colitis remains unresolved. It has been noted that if they receive a cleansing preparation such as the one used in preparation for a colonoscopy and then receive a fecal transplant from a healthy donor (usually a close member of the household), the colitis is resolved in a matter of days, the patient's intestinal flora returns to normal, and the diarrhea ceases.

5. **Certain intestinal microbes** have the ability to metabolize trimethylamine, a structure present in substances such as carnitine of red meat and lecithin present in egg yolk, liver, wheat germ, and pork, into **trimethylamine-N-oxide (TMAO)**, a substance that increases the risk of atherosclerosis and stroke. In fact, it has been shown that blood TMAO level is a relatively accurate indicator of impending heart attacks and strokes in individuals who otherwise display no risk factors for these conditions.

3. The **rectum** is similar to the colon but contains fewer and deeper crypts of Lieberkühn (Table 16.2).
4. The **anal canal** is the constricted continuation of the rectum.
   a. The **anal mucosa** displays longitudinal folds called **anal columns** (or **rectal columns of Morgagni**), which join each other to form **anal valves**. The regions between adjacent valves are known as **anal sinuses**.
      (1) Epithelium of the anal canal
         (a) is simple columnar changing to **simple cuboidal** proximal to the anal valves.
         (b) changes to **stratified squamous nonkeratinized** distal to the anal valves.
         (c) changes to **stratified squamous keratinized** (epidermis) at the anus.
      (2) The **lamina propria** is composed of **fibroelastic** connective tissue and contains sebaceous glands, circumanal glands, hair follicles, and large veins.
      (3) The **muscularis mucosae** consists of an inner circular and an outer longitudinal layer of smooth muscle, both of which terminate at the anal valves.
   b. The **anal submucosa** is composed of dense, irregular fibroelastic connective tissue that houses large veins.
   c. The **anal muscularis externa** is composed of an inner circular and an outer longitudinal layer of smooth muscle. The inner circular layer forms the **internal anal sphincter**.
   d. **Anal adventitia** attaches the anus to surrounding structures.
   e. The **external anal sphincter** is composed of **skeletal muscle**, whose superficial and deep layers invest the anal canal. It exhibits **continuous tonus**, thus maintaining a closed anal orifice. The degree of tonus is under **voluntary control**, so the retention or evacuation of feces normally can be controlled at will.

CLINICAL CONSIDERATIONS

1. **Colorectal carcinoma** is the second highest cause of cancer death in the United States. It most commonly affects individuals who are 55 years of age or older. It usually arises from adenomatous polyps and may be asymptomatic for many years. Rectal bleeding is frequently present. Colorectal carcinoma is probably related to diet. Diets high in fat and refined carbohydrates and low in fiber appear to be associated with colorectal carcinoma.

2. **Hemorrhoids** are very common in people older than 50 years. They present as rectal bleeding during defecation. Hemorrhoids are caused by the breakage of dilated, thin-walled vessels of venous plexuses either above (internal hemorrhoids) or below (external hemorrhoids) the anorectal line.

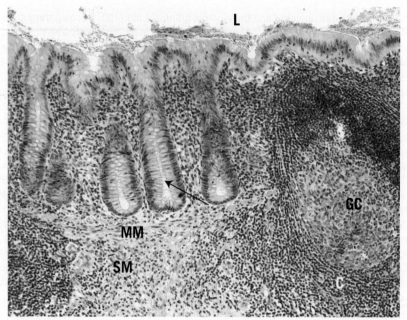

FIGURE 16.4. The histology of the appendix is similar to that of the colon, but it is smaller in diameter and has fewer crypts of Lieberkühn (*arrow*); its lumen (L) usually houses debris, and it is richly endowed with lymphoid elements with germinal centers (GC) and a corona (C). The muscularis mucosae (MM) is infiltrated by lymphocytes as is the submucosa (SM). Because this is an appendix from a human, the patient probably had appendicitis that would account for the great amount of lymphoid tissue (×270).

5. **Appendix**
   a. **Overview—Appendix**
      (1) The appendix is a short, tubular extension of the blind terminus of the cecum.
      (2) It has a narrow, stellate, or irregularly shaped lumen that often contains debris.
      (3) The wall is **thickened** by large aggregates of **lymphoid nodules** in the mucosa and even in the submucosa (in middle-aged and older individuals).
   b. **Mucosa of the appendix**
      (1) The **epithelium** is **simple columnar** and contains surface columnar cells and goblet cells (Figure 16.4).
      (2) The **lamina propria** displays **numerous lymphoid nodules** (capped by M cells) and lymphoid cells. It does not form villi but possesses **shallow crypts of Lieberkühn** with some goblet cells, surface columnar cells, regenerative cells, occasional Paneth cells, and numerous DNES cells, especially deep in the crypts.
      (3) The **muscularis mucosae** is composed of an inner circular and outer longitudinal layer of smooth muscle.
   c. The **submucosa of the appendix** is composed of **fibroelastic** connective tissue containing confluent lymphoid nodules and associated cell populations.
   d. The **muscularis externa of the appendix** is composed of an inner circular and an outer longitudinal layer of smooth muscle.
   e. The **serosa** completely surrounds the appendix.

CLINICAL CONSIDERATIONS

1. The **function** of the appendix is not known, although recent studies demonstrated a very high concentration of bacterial biofilm in this small portion of the gut. It has been suggested that the appendix acts as a reservoir for the normal bacterial gut flora, and in case of severe diarrhea, such as that caused by cholera toxins, when the normal bacterial population is decimated by the disease, reserve bacteria residing in the appendix are able to re-establish the normal intestinal flora.

2. **Appendicitis**, an inflammation of the appendix, is usually associated with pain and/or discomfort in the lower right abdominal region, fever, nausea, vomiting, and an elevated white blood count.

IV. DIGESTION AND ABSORPTION

A. **Carbohydrates**
   1. **Salivary and pancreatic amylases** hydrolyze carbohydrates to **disaccharides** and **polysaccharides**. This process begins in the oral cavity, continues in the stomach, and is completed in the small intestine.
   2. **Disaccharidases** present in the glycocalyx of the brush border of surface absorptive cells cleave disaccharides into monosaccharides, principally into glucose, fructose, and galactose.
   3. **Monosaccharides** are actively conveyed by transporters coupled to **Na$^+$** and located at the microvillar bases into surface absorptive cells and then discharged by the use of additional transporters at the base of the cells into the lamina propria, where they enter the circulation to be transported to the liver via the **hepatic portal vein system**.

B. **Proteins**
   1. **Pepsin** in the lumen of the stomach partially hydrolyzes proteins, forming a mixture of high-molecular-weight **polypeptides**. Pepsin activity is greatest at low pH.
   2. **Pancreatic proteases** within the lumen of the small intestine hydrolyze the polypeptides received from the stomach into very short polypeptides (composed of no more than three or four amino acids) and dipeptides.
   3. **Dipeptides** are cleaved into amino acids by dipeptidases present in the glycocalyx of the brush border of surface absorptive cells. Short polypeptides and amino acids are conveyed by transporters located at the base of the microvilli into surface absorptive cells. Amino acids and short polypeptides are discharged into the lamina propria by various transporters located at the base of the surface absorptive cells, where they enter the circulation to be transported to the liver via the **hepatic portal vein system**.

C. **Fats** are degraded by **pancreatic lipase** into **monoglycerides**, **free fatty acids**, and **glycerol** in the lumen of the small intestine (Figure 16.5).
   1. **Absorption of lipid digestion products** occurs primarily in the **duodenum** and **upper jejunum**.
      a. **Bile salts** act on the free fatty acids and monoglycerides, forming **water-soluble micelles**.
      b. **Micelles** and **glycerol** then enter the surface absorptive cells.
   2. **Formation of chyle**
      a. **Triglycerides** are resynthesized from monoglycerides and free fatty acids within the SER.
      b. **Chylomicrons** are formed in the Golgi complex by the complexing of the resynthesized triglycerides with proteins. Chylomicrons are transported to the lateral cell membrane and released by exocytosis; after crossing the basal lamina, they enter **lacteals** in the lamina propria to contribute to the formation of **chyle**.
      c. **Chyle** enters the submucosal lymphatic plexus by contraction of smooth muscle cells in the intestinal villi.
      d. The chyle travels via larger and larger lymph vessels into the largest lymph vessel, known as the **thoracic duct**, which empties into the junction of the left subclavian vein with the left internal jugular vein to enter into the **systemic circulation** at the left side of the heart.
   3. **Short-chain fatty acids** of less than 10 to 12 carbon atoms are not re-esterified but leave the surface absorptive cells directly and enter blood vessels of the lamina propria to be transported to the liver via the **hepatic portal vein system**.

D. **Water and electrolytes** are absorbed by surface absorptive cells of both the small and the large intestine, whereas **gases** are absorbed mostly in the large intestine.

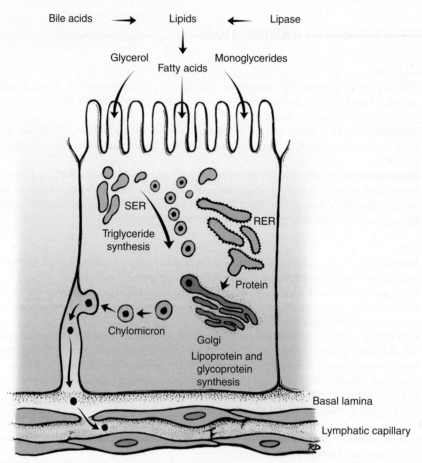

FIGURE 16.5. Absorption of lipids by surface absorptive cells of the small intestine and the formation of chylomicrons. SER, smooth endoplasmic reticulum; RER, rough endoplasmic reticulum.

Review Test

Directions: Each of the numbered items or incomplete statements in this section is followed by answers or completions of the statement. Select the ONE lettered answer that is BEST in each case.

1. The type of epithelium associated with the vermilion zone of the lips is

(A) stratified squamous nonkeratinized.
(B) pseudostratified ciliated columnar.
(C) stratified squamous keratinized.
(D) stratified cuboidal.
(E) stratified columnar.

2. Which of the following cell types is present in the gastric glands of the pyloric stomach?

(A) Goblet cells
(B) Mucous neck cells
(C) Paneth cells
(D) Basal cells
(E) Chief cells

3. Secretin and cholecystokinin are produced and secreted by cells in the lining of the alimentary tract. Which of the following statements about these two substances is true?

(A) They are produced by diffuse neuroendocrine cells (DNES cells) in the lining of the stomach and small intestine.
(B) They are digestive enzymes present within the lumen of the duodenum.
(C) They are produced by Paneth cells.
(D) They are hormones that have target cells in the pancreas and biliary tract.
(E) They are produced by Brunner glands and released into the lumina of the crypts of Lieberkühn.

4. If odontoblasts malfunction because of developmental anomalies, which of the following will be affected?

(A) Cementum
(B) Enamel
(C) Dentin
(D) Tooth crown only
(E) Tooth root only

5. Which of the following statements concerning the principal fiber bundles of the periodontal ligament is true?

(A) They are composed of elastin.
(B) They extend from the cementum to the enamel.
(C) They extend from the dentin to the cementum.
(D) They are composed of collagen.
(E) They extend from one tooth to the next.

6. A patient goes to the emergency department, and the physician notes one of the classic symptoms of appendicitis. Which of the following is that symptom?

(A) Apnea
(B) Vomiting of blood
(C) Depressed white cell count
(D) Rectal bleeding
(E) Abdominal pain

7. Passage of a bolus through the esophagus into the stomach is facilitated by which of the following?

(A) Peristaltic activity of the esophageal muscularis externa
(B) Peristaltic activity of the gastric muscularis mucosae
(C) Reflux through the pharyngoesophageal sphincter
(D) Smooth muscle in the esophageal muscularis mucosae
(E) Reflux through the gastroesophageal sphincter

8. The small intestine has three histologically distinct regions. Which of the following statements concerning the histological differences in the three regions is true?

(A) Peyer patches are present only in the ileum.

(B) Goblet cells are present only in the epithelium of the duodenum.

(C) Brunner glands are located in the duodenum and jejunum but not the ileum.

(D) Lacteals are present only in the lamina propria of the ileum.

(E) The muscularis mucosae contains three layers of smooth muscle in the ileum and two layers in the duodenum and jejunum.

9. Which of the following materials can be absorbed directly by the surface lining cells of the stomach?

(A) Vitamin B_{12}

(B) Polysaccharides

(C) Chylomicrons

(D) Triglycerides

(E) Alcohol

10. Which of the following is characteristic of angular cheilitis?

(A) Patients in the early 20s

(B) Presence of herpes virus

(C) Erythematous lesions at the corners of the mouth

(D) Apnea

(E) High blood levels of secretin

Answers and Explanations

1. **C.** The external aspect and vermilion zone of the lips are covered by thin skin, which contains a stratified squamous keratinized epithelium. The internal aspect of the lips is lined by a wet mucosa containing a stratified squamous nonkeratinized epithelium (see Chapter 16 II A).

2. **B.** Mucous neck cells are located in the neck of gastric glands in all parts of the stomach, whereas only fundic glands contain chief (zymogenic) cells (see Chapter 16 III B 2).

3. **D.** Secretin and cholecystokinin are hormones produced by enteroendocrine cells in the small intestine. Secretin stimulates bicarbonate secretion in the pancreas and biliary tract. Cholecystokinin stimulates the release of pancreatic enzymes and contraction of the gall bladder (see Chapter 16 III C 3).

4. **C.** Dentin is manufactured by odontoblasts (see Chapter 16 II C 2).

5. **D.** The principal fiber bundles of the periodontal ligament are composed of collagen fibers. They suspend a tooth in its alveolus, extending from the cribriform plate of the alveolar bone to the cementum on the root of the tooth. The fibers that extend from one tooth to the next are the transseptal fibers of the gingivae (see Chapter 16 II D 1).

6. **E.** Rectal bleeding or vomiting of blood often accompanies gastrointestinal pathologies but not appendicitis. Elevated, not depressed, white cell count and abdominal pain are classic signs of appendicitis (see Chapter 16 III D 5 Clinical Considerations).

7. **A.** The smooth muscle of the muscularis mucosae plays no role in the movement of a bolus through the esophagus. This movement is accomplished by peristalsis of the esophageal muscularis externa, which contains both skeletal and smooth muscle. The sphincters at the proximal and distal ends of the esophagus permit movement of food in only one direction, toward the stomach (see Chapter 16 III A 5).

8. **A.** The primary histological differences in the three regions of the small intestine are the presence of Peyer patches in the lamina propria of the ileum and the presence of Brunner glands in the submucosa of the duodenum. The duodenum and jejunum lack Peyer patches, and the jejunum and ileum lack Brunner glands. Goblet cells are present throughout the small intestine (see Chapter 16 III C 3).

9. **E.** Only a few simple substances, such as alcohol, can be absorbed by the epithelial lining of the stomach (see Chapter 16 III B 1).

10. **C.** The corners of the mouth have painful erythematous lesions (see Chapter 16 II B 2 Clinical Considerations).

chapter 17

Digestive System: Glands

I. OVERVIEW—EXTRINSIC GLANDS OF THE DIGESTIVE SYSTEM

A. The extrinsic glands of the digestive system include the **major salivary glands**, the **pancreas**, and the **liver** (with the associated **gallbladder**), all of which are outside the wall of the digestive tract.

B. These glands produce enzymes, buffers, emulsifiers, and lubricants that are delivered to the lumen of the digestive tract via a system of ducts.

C. They also produce hormones, blood proteins, and other products.

II. MAJOR SALIVARY GLANDS

A. Overview
1. The major salivary glands consist of three **paired exocrine** glands: the **parotid**, **submandibular**, and **sublingual**.
2. **Function.** They synthesize and secrete **salivary amylase**, **lysozyme**, **lactoferrin**, and **secretory component**.
   a. Secretory component is a *portion* of the **IgA dimer receptor molecule** located on the basal plasma membrane of the secretory cell and facilitates the transfer of the IgA dimer into the early endosome of the secretory cell. This portion of the receptor molecule remains bound to the IgA dimers, immunoglobulins that are produced by plasma cells in the connective tissue, forming a complex that resists enzymatic digestion in the saliva but can still perform its immune function.
   b. The serous secretory cells of major salivary glands also secrete histidine-rich, proline-rich, and cysteine-rich proteins. The cells of the striated ducts of these glands also release an enzyme **kallikrein** both into the lumen as well as into the connective tissue. In the lumen kallikrein begins the digestion of proline- and cysteine-rich proteins, whereas in the connective tissue kallikrein enters the bloodstream, where it converts **kininogens** into the vasodilator and bronchial smooth muscle contractant **bradykinin**.
   c. **Lysozyme** and **lactoferrin** are antimicrobial agents that control the bacterial flora of the oral cavity.
   d. **Amylase** begins the digestion of carbohydrates in the oral cavity.

B. **Structure.** The major salivary glands are **compound tubuloacinar** (tubuloalveolar) glands. They are further classified as **serous**, **mucous**, or **mixed** (both serous and mucous), depending on the type of secretory acini they contain. These glands are surrounded by a capsule of dense irregular collagenous connective tissue with septa that subdivide each gland into lobes and lobules. Neurovascular elements serving these glands are conveyed to the acinar cells within the connective tissue septa.

1. **Salivary gland acini**
   a. Salivary gland acini consist of pyramidal serous or mucous cells arranged around a central lumen that connects with an **intercalated duct**. Mucous acini may be overlaid with a crescent-shaped collection of serous cells called **serous demilunes**. Recently, it has been suggested that serous demilunes are fixation artifacts, in that a mixed acinus has both serous and mucous cells situated around a central lumen. During processing for microscopy, the mucous cells become swollen and squeeze the bulk of the serous cells to the periphery of the acinus, making them appear to form a serous cap covering the mucous cells. If the tissue is flash-frozen, so that swelling of the mucous cells is prevented, serous demilunes are not present. In spite of this finding, since in nonfrozen preparations serous demilunes are evident and since classical histology uses these artifactual structures as classifying characteristics, in this review book they will be treated as if they were actual structures.
   b. Acini of salivary glands possess **myoepithelial cells** that share the basal lamina of the acinar cells. The acinus and its associated intercalated and striated ducts form the **salivon**, the functional unit of a salivary gland.
   c. They release a **primary secretion** that resembles extracellular fluid. This secretion is modified in the ducts to produce the **final secretion**.
   d. Salivary glands are classified according to their types of acini.
      (1) **Parotid glands** consist of **serous acini** and are classified as serous.
      (2) **Sublingual glands** consist mostly of **mucous acini** capped with **serous demilunes**. They are classified as mixed.
      (3) **Submandibular glands** consist of both **serous** and **mucous acini** (some also have serous demilunes). They are classified as mixed.

2. **Salivary gland ducts**
   a. **Intercalated ducts** originate in the acini and join to form striated ducts. They may deliver **bicarbonate ions** into the primary secretion.
   b. **Striated (intralobular) ducts**
      (1) Striated ducts are lined by **ion-transporting cells** that remove sodium and chloride ions from the luminal fluid (via a sodium pump) and actively pump potassium and bicarbonate ions into it, thus transforming the initial saliva (**primary saliva**) produced by the acinar cells into **secondary saliva**, which leaves the striated duct and eventually enters the oral cavity.
      (2) Striated ducts converge in each lobule to form **intralobular ducts** that merge with each other to form **interlobular (excretory) ducts**, which run in the connective tissue septa. These ducts drain into the main duct of each gland, which empties into the oral cavity.

C. **Saliva**
   1. Saliva is a **hypotonic** solution produced at the rate of about 1 L per day.
   2. **Function**
      a. Saliva **lubricates** and **cleanses** the oral cavity by means of its water and glycoprotein content.
      b. It **controls bacterial flora** by the action of thiocyanate, lysozyme, lactoferrin, and IgA, as well as by its cleansing action.
      c. It initiates **digestion of carbohydrates** by the action of salivary amylase.
      d. It acts as a solvent for substances that stimulate the taste buds.
      e. It assists in the process of deglutition (swallowing).

CLINICAL CONSIDERATIONS

1. The flow of saliva is important not only for the easy swallowing of masticated food but also as a vehicle that facilitates the sensation of taste and the initiation of digestion as well as for the maintenance of proper oral health. Individuals who had radiation treatment for cancers of the head and/or neck and those who are being treated with chemotherapy frequently have xerostomia, dry mouth, because of reduced salivary gland function. Frequently, these patients have to use artificial saliva to maintain a moist oral environment. Usually, subsequent to the cessation of radiation therapy or chemotherapy, salivary gland function returns to normal.

2. **Sjögren syndrome** is believed to be an autoimmune disease whose symptoms are xerostomia, dry eyes, and generally dry mucous membranes. Although there is no cure for this painful and potentially debilitating disorder, eyedrops, the frequent intake of fluids, and/or the use of artificial saliva relieve some of the symptoms.

3. **Salivary calculus** is a calcification that is formed usually in the parotid gland. It may block the flow of saliva through the parotid duct. Occasionally, the blockage results in the backflow of saliva, with a concomitant painful swelling of the parotid gland. Frequently, a simple massage of the parotid duct can dislodge the stone; otherwise a surgical approach may be necessary.

4. **Mumps,** a viral infection, usually affects children 5 to 15 years of age but may affect adults as well. It is usually relatively benign in children, although it may cause considerable pain because of the swelling of the salivary glands. In adult males the virus may also cause swelling of the testes, and in addition to the considerable pain, it may result in sterility if both testes are involved. In others the pancreas may also become involved, causing pancreatitis with its attendant symptoms of abdominal pain and mild-to-severe nausea and vomiting. Fortunately, the symptoms subside within a week and there are no residual complications. In a few adults, less than 10% of the cases, the mumps virus may also cause meningoencephalitis that resolves itself in a week or so, but in a very small number of cases, serious, lifelong complications may result, including deafness and facial paralysis.

III. OVERVIEW—PANCREAS

The pancreas has a slender connective tissue capsule. This gland produces **digestive enzymes** in its exocrine portion and a number of **hormones** in its endocrine portion (**islets of Langerhans**). Blood flow into the pancreas is arranged in such a fashion that the acini receive arterial blood from vessels dedicated to these structures and the islets of Langerhans also receive blood dedicated to the islets. Additionally, acini also receive venous blood drained from the islets of Langerhans, so that hormones, such as somatostatin, released by those islet cells can reach the acinar cells immediately after release.

A. **The exocrine pancreas** is a **serous compound tubuloacinar** gland.
  1. **Pancreatic acinar cells**
     a. Pancreatic acinar cells are pyramidal serous cells arranged around a central lumen.
     b. They possess a round basal nucleus, abundant rough endoplasmic reticulum (RER), an extensive Golgi complex, numerous mitochondria, and many free ribosomes.
     c. **Zymogen (secretory) granules** are membrane bound and densely packed in the **apical** region of pancreatic acinar cells. They contain enzymes and proenzymes packaged in the Golgi complex.
     d. Their basal plasmalemma has receptors for cholecystokinin and acetylcholine.
  2. **Pancreatic ducts**
     a. The initial intra-acinar portion of the intercalated ducts is formed by **centroacinar cells**, which are low cuboidal with a pale cytoplasm.
     b. From the initial portion, the intercalated ducts converge into a small number of **intralobular ducts**, which in turn empty into large **interlobular ducts** that empty into the main (or accessory) pancreatic duct.
     c. The **main pancreatic duct** fuses with the common bile duct, forming the **ampulla of Vater**, which delivers secretions of the exocrine pancreas and the contents of the gallbladder into the duodenum at the **major duodenal papilla**.

3. **Exocrine pancreatic secretions**
   a. **Enzyme-poor alkaline fluid**
      (1) Enzyme-poor alkaline fluid is released in large quantities by **intercalated duct cells** stimulated by **secretin** in conjunction with **acetylcholine**.
      (2) Function. It probably **neutralizes** the acidic chyme as it enters the duodenum.
   b. **Digestive enzymes**
      (1) Digestive enzymes are synthesized and stored in the pancreatic **acinar cells**. Their release is stimulated by **cholecystokinin** (previously known as **pancreozymin**) and costimulated by acetylcholine released by postganglionic parasympathetic fibers.
      (2) Digestive enzymes are secreted as **enzymes** or **proenzymes** that must be activated in the intestinal lumen.
      (3) **Enzymes** include pancreatic amylase, pancreatic lipases, ribonuclease, and deoxyribonuclease; **proenzymes** include trypsinogen, chymotrypsinogen, procarboxypeptidase, and proelastase.
      (4) In order to protect themselves from the digestive enzyme trypsin, these cells manufacture **trypsin inhibitor** so that trypsinogen cannot be converted to trypsin within the cytosol.

B. **Islets of Langerhans (endocrine pancreas)** (Figure 17.1)
   1. Islets of Langerhans are richly vascularized spherical clusters (100–200 µm in diameter) of endocrine cells surrounded by a fine network of **reticular fibers**. They are scattered among the acini of the exocrine pancreas in an apparently random fashion.
   2. **Islet cells** (Table 17.1)
      a. Islet cells are of several types that can be differentiated from each other only by immunocytochemistry or by the use of special stains.
      b. They produce several polypeptide hormones, but *each cell type produces only one hormone.*

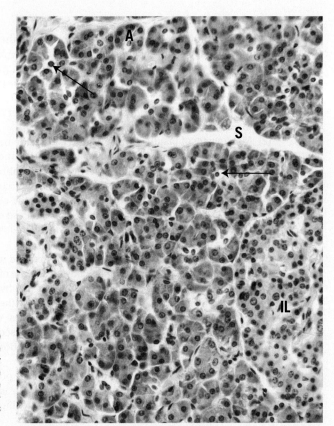

FIGURE 17.1. The islets of Langerhans (IL) represent the endocrine portion of the pancreas, whereas the acini (A), with their centroacinar cells (*arrows*), represent the exocrine portion of the pancreas. Observe the connective tissue septa (S) that subdivide the pancreas into lobes and lobules (×270).

t a b l e 17.1	Comparison of Secretory Cells in Islets of Langerhans				
Cell Type	Granule Characteristics	Relative Numbers	Location in Islets	Hormone	Function
Alpha (α)	Round; small halo between membrane and electron-dense core	~20%	Mostly at periphery	Glucagon	Elevate blood glucose levels
Beta (β)	Small; obvious halo between membrane, irregular dense core	~70%	Mainly central; present throughout	Insulin	Decrease blood glucose levels
Delta D cells (δ-cells)	Both D and D$_1$ cells are large and electron lucent	<5%	Scattered throughout	Somatostatin Vasoactive intestinal peptide	Inhibit hormone release by nearby cells; they also inhibit the release of pancreatic enzymes and HCl production by parietal cells in the stomach
D$_1$ cells (δ$_1$-cells)					Induce glycogenolysis; adjust gut motility and secretion of ions and water
Gastrin-producing	Small	Rare	Scattered throughout	Gastrin	Stimulate hydrochloric acid secretion
PP (F)	Small	Rare	Scattered throughout	Pancreatic polypeptide	Inhibit the release of exocrine pancreatic secretions as well as the release of bile from the gallbladder
Epsilon	Small	Rare	Scattered throughout	Ghrelin	Induce the feeling of hunger

PP, pancreatic polypeptide-producing cells.

3. **Islet hormones**
   a. **Glucagon** is produced by α-cells and acts to elevate the blood glucose level.
   b. **Insulin** is produced by β-cells and acts to *decrease the blood glucose level.*
      (1) **Mechanism of insulin release**. Increased blood glucose levels cause glucose to bind to transmembrane proteins (**glucose transporter protein 2 [GLUT-2]**) of β-cells, which induces these cells to release their stored insulin and, if necessary, synthesize more insulin. This uptake of glucose occurs in a manner that does not require the presence of insulin.
      (2) **Mechanism of insulin action**. Insulin causes the transport of glucose and amino acids into hepatocytes, fat cells, cardiac muscle cells, and skeletal muscle cells. It does so by binding to the extracellular moiety of transmembrane insulin receptors of these cells, which triggers a response from the intracellular component that includes the placing of **glucose transporter protein 4 (GLUT-4)** on the cell membranes of fat cells and skeletal muscle and cardiac muscle cells, and glucose enters these cells by way of GLUT-4. Unlike in the case of GLUT-2, this uptake of glucose occurs in a manner that requires the presence of insulin.
   c. **Somatostatin** and **vasoactive intestinal peptide** are produced by δ-cells and δ$_1$-cells (D cells and D$_1$ cells), respectively. Somatostatin **inhibits** the release of hormones by nearby secretory cells; it also inhibits the release of pancreatic enzymes and hydrochloric acid (HCl) production by parietal cells in the stomach and **reduces** the motility of the gastrointestinal tract and gallbladder by decreasing the contraction of their smooth muscles. Vasoactive intestinal peptide induces glycogenolysis in the liver and adjusts gut motility and secretion of ions and water.
   d. **Gastrin**, produced by G cells, **stimulates** (in conjunction with histamine and acetylcholine) gastric HCl secretion.
   e. **Pancreatic polypeptide**, produced by PP (pancreatic polypeptide-producing) cells, **inhibits** release of exocrine pancreatic secretions and the release of bile from the gallbladder.
   f. **Ghrelin**, produced by Epsilon cells, produces the feeling of hunger.

CLINICAL CONSIDERATIONS

1. Individuals who have low blood glucose and high blood insulin levels may be suffering from **insulinoma**, a tumor of the β-cells of the islets of Langerhans. Insulinomas are benign in 90% of the cases, and the condition is usually resolved by surgical excision of the tumor.

2. **Type 1 (insulin-dependent) diabetes mellitus (IDDM)**
   a. IDDM results from a **low level of plasma insulin**.
   b. It is characterized by **polyphagia** (insatiable hunger), **polydipsia** (unquenchable thirst), and **polyuria** (excessive urination).
   c. It usually has a **sudden onset** before 20 years of age and is distinguished by damage to and destruction of β-cells of the islets of Langerhans. Because of its early onset, IDDM is also known as **juvenile-onset diabetes mellitus**.
   d. It is treated with a combination of insulin therapy and diet.

3. **Type 2 (non–insulin-dependent) diabetes mellitus (NIDDM)**
   a. NIDDM does **not** result from low levels of plasma insulin and is **insulin resistant**, which is a major factor in its pathogenesis. The resistance to insulin is due to decreased binding of insulin to its plasmalemma receptors and to defects in postreceptor insulin action.
   b. It commonly occurs in overweight individuals older than 40 years.
   c. It is usually controlled by diet.
   d. Older individuals with type 2 diabetes often present with memory problems probably because **amyloid-β-derived diffusible ligands (ADDLs)** bind to the presynaptic membranes of the axons of certain neurons that are responsible for memory storage. This condition prevents the replenishment of **insulin receptors** of these axons, even though the receptors, synthesized in the soma, are available in the soma's cytoplasm. Apparently, the receptors are prevented from being transferred from the cytosol of the soma to the axoplasm of the axon. This makes these neurons insulin resistant and unable to regulate their glucose metabolism, and in turn, these neurons cannot function normally and the patient has memory loss and Alzheimer disease–associated dementia. Some researchers suggest this to be **type 3 diabetes**.

4. **Pancreatic cancer** is a malignant neoplasm, and most patients die within 6 months to 1 year after diagnosis. Most of the cases are **adenocarcinomas** in the head of the pancreas. Its incidence is three to four times greater in male patients than in female patients. Although its symptoms include anorexia, flatulence, fatty stool if the bile duct is obstructed, sudden loss of weight, weakness, back pain, and jaundice, exploratory biopsy is commonly required for a definitive diagnosis.

5. **Blood glucose level** in a fasting, nondiabetic individual should be between 80 and 110 mg per 100 mL (4.4 to 6.1 mmol per L) of blood. If the glucose levels rise above that level, the β-cells release insulin. If the blood glucose levels fall below that level, the α-cells release glucagon. Additional control mechanisms include the neurotransmitters released by the cells of the autonomic nervous system, namely: sympathetic fibers increase glucagon secretion and inhibit insulin secretion, whereas parasympathetic fibers increase both insulin and glucagon secretions in order to maintain a balanced homeostasis.

IV. LIVER

A. Overview
   1. The liver is composed of a single type of parenchymal cell, the **hepatocyte**.
   2. It is the largest gland in the body, weighing as much as 1.5 kg.
   3. It is surrounded by a dense, irregular collagenous connective tissue known as **Glisson capsule**, which gives rise to septa that subdivide the liver into its four lobes (right, left, caudate, and quadrate lobes) and its enormous number of lobules.
   4. **Function**. The liver produces **bile** and plasma proteins and has a myriad of other functions discussed in Sections E and F.

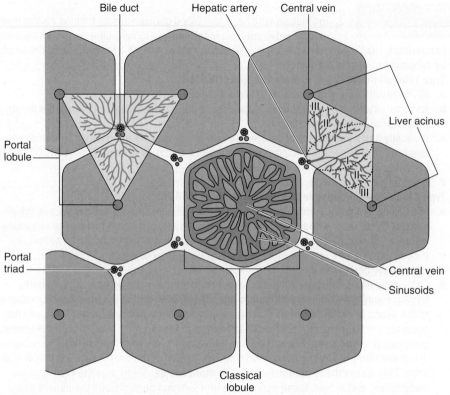

FIGURE 17.2. The defining characteristics of the classic liver lobule, portal lobule, and liver hepatic acinus of Rappaport. Observe the zonulation within the acinus of Rappaport. (Adapted with permission from Krause WJ, Cutts JH. *Concise Textbook of Histology.* 2nd ed. Baltimore, MD: Williams & Wilkins; 1986:331.)

B. Liver lobules (Figure 17.2)

1. The **classic liver lobule** is a hexagonal mass of tissue primarily composed of **plates of hepatocytes** (**liver cells**), which radiate from the region of the **central vein** toward the periphery (Figure 17.3).

a. Portal areas (portal canals or portal triads)

(1) The portal areas are regions of the connective tissue between lobules that contain branches of the portal vein, hepatic artery, lymph vessel, and bile duct.

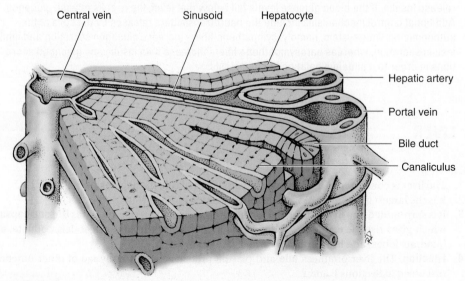

FIGURE 17.3. A portion of the classic liver lobule showing the area served by one portal triad.

(2) They are present at alternate corners of a classic liver lobule.

(3) Each portal area is surrounded by the **limiting plate**, a cylindrical plate of modified hepatocytes. A narrow space, known as the space of Moll, separates the limiting plate from the connective tissue elements of the portal area.

b. Liver sinusoids

(1) Liver sinusoids are sinusoidal capillaries that arise at the periphery of a lobule and run between adjacent plates of hepatocytes.

(2) They receive blood from the vessels in the portal areas and deliver it to the central vein.

(3) They are lined by **sinusoidal lining cells** (endothelial cells) that have large discontinuities between them, display **fenestrations**, and **lack basal laminae**.

(4) The lining of the sinusoid also contains **phagocytic cells** (**Kupffer cells**) derived from monocytes; these cells are interspersed among the sinusoidal lining cells but form no junctions with them. Kupffer cells remove debris, old erythrocytes, and cellular fragments from the bloodstream.

c. Space of Disse

(1) The space of Disse is the **subendothelial space** between hepatocytes and the cells lining the sinusoids.

(2) It contains the short microvilli of hepatocytes, reticular fibers (which maintain the architecture of the sinusoids), and occasional nonmyelinated nerve fibers.

(3) It also contains stellate-shaped **fat-storing cells** (**Ito cells**, also known as **perisinusoidal stellate cells**), which preferentially store vitamin A. However, when the liver is compromised, hepatocytes release **tumor growth factor β**, and in response, these fat-storing cells can divide, change their phenotype, and begin to synthesize collagen, leading to fibrosis and, if necessary, differentiate into **myofibroblasts** to control blood flow into the sinusoids.

(4) Function. The space of Disse functions in the exchange of material between the bloodstream and hepatocytes. Hepatocytes do not directly contact the bloodstream.

2. Portal lobule

a. The portal lobule, viewed in two dimensions, is a **triangular region** with three apices that are neighboring central veins and a center in a portal area (Figure 17.2).

b. It contains portions of **three** adjacent classic liver lobules.

c. The portal lobule is defined in terms of **bile flow**. In this concept of liver lobulation, the bile duct is in the center of the lobule.

3. Hepatic acinus of Rappaport

a. The hepatic acinus of Rappaport, viewed in two dimensions, is a **diamond-shaped region** encompassing triangular sections of **two** adjacent classic liver lobules (with apices that are the central veins) and is divided by the common distributing vessels (Figure 17.2).

b. This concept of liver lobulation is defined in terms of **blood flow** from the distributing vessels in a single portal area. This concept was established to explain the histologic appearance of pathologic changes that occur in liver disease.

c. The hepatic acinus of Rappaport can be divided into **three zones** on the basis of the proximity of the hepatocytes to the incoming blood.

C. Blood, bile, and lymph flow (Figure 17.3)

1. Blood flow into the liver is derived from two sources and is directed from the portal triads at the periphery of each classic liver lobule toward the central vein.

a. The **hepatic artery** brings oxygen-rich blood from the abdominal aorta and supplies 20% to 30% of the liver's blood.

b. The **portal vein** brings nutrient-rich blood from the alimentary canal and spleen; it supplies 70% to 80% of the liver's blood.

2. Blood flow out of the liver occurs via the **hepatic vein**, formed by the union of numerous sublobular veins, which collect blood from the **central veins** (Figure 17.4).

3. Bile flow is directed toward the periphery of the classic liver lobule (in the **opposite** direction of blood flow). Bile is carried in a system of ducts that culminate in the left and right **hepatic ducts**, which leave the liver and carry bile to the gallbladder.

a. Bile canaliculi

(1) The bile canaliculi are expanded intercellular spaces between adjacent hepatocytes that form tiny canals for the initial flow of bile.

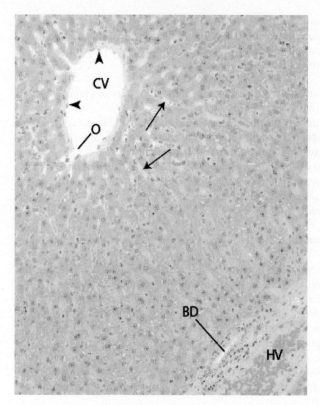

FIGURE 17.4. The central vein (CV) of the liver is lined by endothelial cells (*arrowheads*) that are continuous with those lining the liver sinusoid (*arrows*) where these sinusoids open (O) into the central vein. Observe the bile duct (BD) and a branch of the portal vein (HV) in a relatively large portal area (×132).

    (2) They receive the liver's **exocrine secretion** (bile) and carry it to the **canals of Hering** (bile ductules) at the very periphery of classic liver lobules. The canals of Hering are composed of both modified hepatocytes and low cuboidal **cholangiocytes (duct cells)**. Cholangiocytes of the canals of Hering or cells that resemble cholangiocytes and reside as cells of the canals of Hering can act as regenerative cells both of the liver as well as of bile ductules and bile ducts. It has been demonstrated that even if 50% of the liver is excised, it can regenerate to its previous size of 1.5 kg.

  b. Bile ducts

    (1) Bile ducts are located in the portal areas and are composed of a single layer of cuboidal-shaped cholangiocytes. The apical surface of each cholangiocyte faces the lumen of the bile duct and displays numerous short microvilli as well as a single, long primary cilium that monitors bile flow and bile composition within the bile duct.

    (2) They receive bile from the canals of Hering.

    (3) They enlarge and fuse to form the **hepatic ducts**, composed of a stratified epithelium of cholangiocytes, which leave the liver at the porta hepatis.

  4. Lymph in the liver collects in the space of Moll and is drained from there by branches of the lymph vessels located in the portal areas. As these lymph vessels coalesce, they increase in size and eventually form one or two larger lymph vessels that join the **thoracic duct** to return the lymph into the blood vascular system at the junction of the left subclavian and left internal jugular veins.

D. Hepatocytes

  1. Hepatocytes are large polyhedral cells (20–30 μm in diameter) that possess abundant RER and smooth endoplasmic reticulum (SER); numerous mitochondria, lysosomes, and peroxisomes; several Golgi complexes; and many lipid droplets and glycogen deposits.

  2. They usually contain one round central nucleus; about 25% of the cells are binucleated. Occasionally, nuclei are polyploid.

  3. Their average lifespan is approximately 5 months.

4. **Hepatocyte surfaces**
   a. **Hepatocyte surfaces facing the space of Disse** possess microvilli, which by increasing the surface area facilitate the transfer of materials (e.g., endocrine secretions into the blood and nutrients into the hepatocytes) between the hepatocytes and the blood.
   b. **Abutting surfaces of adjacent hepatocytes**
      (1) frequently delineate bile canaliculi, small, tunnel-like expansions of the intercellular space. The **bile canaliculi** are sealed off from the remaining intercellular space by **occluding junctions** located on each side of each canaliculus.
      (2) possess microvilli that extend into the bile canaliculus.
      (3) also have **gap junctions**.

E. **Hepatic functions carried out by hepatocytes**
   1. **Exocrine secretion** involves the production and release of 600 to 1,200 mL of **bile** per day. Bile is a fluid composed of bilirubin glucuronide (bile pigment), bile acids (bile salts), cholesterol, lecithin, phospholipids, ions, IgA, and water. Hydrophobic bilirubin, a breakdown product of hemoglobin, is converted into water-soluble bilirubin glucuronide (a nontoxic compound) in the SER of the hepatocytes.
   2. **Endocrine secretion** involves the production and release of several **plasma proteins** (e.g., prothrombin, fibrinogen, albumin, factor III, and lipoproteins) and urea. Hepatocytes can also manufacture and release nonessential amino acids.
   3. **Metabolites** are **stored** in the form of **glycogen** (stored glucose) and **triglycerides** (stored lipid).
   4. **Gluconeogenesis** is the conversion of amino acids and lipids into glucose, a complex process catalyzed by a series of enzymes.
   5. **Detoxification** entails the inactivation of various substances, such as drugs, noxious chemicals, and toxins, by enzymes, such as the **microsomal mixed-function oxidase** system, that catalyze the oxidation, methylation, or conjugation of such substances. These reactions usually occur in the SER or in peroxisomes, as in the case of alcohol.
   6. **IgA transfer** involves the uptake of IgA across the space of Disse and its release into bile canaliculi. IgA is transported through the hepatobiliary duct system to the intestine, where it serves an immunologic protective function. This process is referred to as the **enterohepatic circulation**.

F. **Hepatic functions carried out by cells other than hepatocytes**
   1. **Ito cells** store vitamin A.
   2. **Kupffer cells** phagocytose unwanted materials.

CLINICAL CONSIDERATIONS

1. **Hepatitis** is an inflammation of the liver, usually due to a viral infection but occasionally due to toxic materials.
   a. **Viral hepatitis A (infectious hepatitis)** is caused by hepatitis A virus, which is frequently **transmitted by the fecal–oral route**. It has a **short incubation period** (2–6 weeks), and is usually not fatal but may cause jaundice.
   b. **Viral hepatitis B (serum hepatitis)** is caused by hepatitis B virus, which is **transmitted by blood** and its derivatives.
      i. It has a **long incubation period** (6 weeks to 5 months).
      ii. Its clinical symptoms are similar to those associated with viral hepatitis A, but with more serious consequences, including cirrhosis, jaundice, and death.
   c. **Viral hepatitis C** is caused by hepatitis C virus and is responsible for most transfusion-related cases of hepatitis. It is also associated with **hepatocellular carcinoma**.
2. **Jaundice (icterus)**
   a. Jaundice is characterized by **excess bilirubin** in the blood and deposition of **bile pigment** in the skin and sclera of the eyes, resulting in a yellowish appearance.
   b. It may be hereditary or caused by pathologic conditions, such as excessive destruction of red blood cells (**hemolytic jaundice**), liver dysfunction, and obstruction of the biliary passages (**obstructive jaundice**).

V. GALLBLADDER

A. The gallbladder communicates with the common hepatic duct via the **cystic duct**, which originates at the neck of the gallbladder.

B. It has a muscular wall whose contraction, stimulated by **cholecystokinin** (possibly in conjunction with acetylcholine), forces bile from its lumen into the duodenum. The wall has four layers:
   1. The **mucosa** is composed of a **simple columnar epithelium** and a richly vascularized lamina propria. When the gallbladder is empty, the mucosa displays highly convoluted folds (Figure 17.5).
   2. The **muscle layer** is composed of a thin, oblique layer of **smooth muscle cells**.
   3. The **connective tissue layer** consists of dense irregular collagenous connective tissue and houses nerves and blood vessels.
   4. The **serosa** covers most of the gallbladder, but adventitia is present where the organ is attached to the liver.

C. **Function**. The gallbladder concentrates, stores, and releases bile. It removes approximately 90% of the bile's water content by the manipulation of the subepithelial connective tissue electrolyte levels. It does so by actively removing sodium, chloride, and bicarbonate ions from the epithelial cells using energy-requiring pumps in the epithelial cell's basal plasmalemma, which, in turn, causes water to leave the cell, passively, via aquaporin 1 and aquaporin 8 channels. In order to equilibrate the osmotic differences between the bile in the lumen of the gallbladder and the epithelial cells lining the lumen, water moves from the bile into the epithelial cells because of the processes just described.

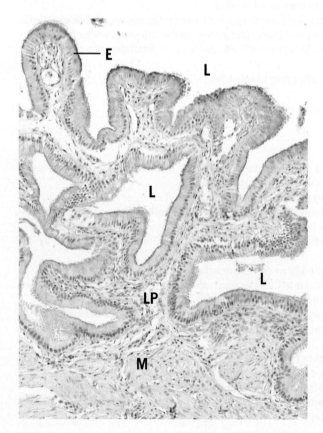

FIGURE 17.5. The mucosa of the empty gallbladder is highly folded, making the lumen (L) appear to be enclosed by the folds. The columnar epithelium (E) lining the lumen overlies a richly vascularized lamina propria (LP) that is surrounded by the smooth muscle (M) coat of the gallbladder (×132).

CLINICAL CONSIDERATIONS

1. Gallstones (biliary calculi)

    a. Gallstones are concretions, usually of fused crystals of **cholesterol**, which form in the gallbladder or bile duct.

    b. Accumulation of gallstones may lead to the blockage of the cystic duct, which prevents emptying of the gallbladder.

    c. Gallstones may have to be surgically removed if less-invasive methods fail to dissolve or pulverize them.

2. Inflammation of the gallbladder, whether **chronic** or **acute**, usually due to the presence of gallstones, obstructing the access to the cystic duct, is known as **cholecystitis**. Chronic cholecystitis is frequently the result of multiple bouts of acute cystitis. The acute form of the condition is quite painful, and the pain is experienced in the upper right quadrant of the abdomen and may be so severe as to induce nausea and vomiting. Frequently, the condition is treated by surgical removal of the gallbladder.

Review Test

Directions: Each of the numbered items or incomplete statements in this section is followed by answers or completions of the statement. Select the *one* lettered answer that is *best* in each case.

1. An 18-year-old man feels faint. Symptoms include constant hunger, thirst, and excessive urination. The probable diagnosis is

(A) viral hepatitis A.
(B) type 1 diabetes mellitus.
(C) type 2 diabetes mellitus.
(D) cirrhosis.
(E) mumps.

2. Which of the following statements concerning liver sinusoids is true?

(A) They are continuous with bile canaliculi.
(B) They are surrounded by a well-developed basal lamina.
(C) They are lined by nonfenestrated endothelial cells.
(D) They deliver blood to the central vein.
(E) They deliver blood to the portal vein.

3. A woman has yellow sclera and yellowish pallor. Blood test results indicate a low red blood cell count. The probable diagnosis is

(A) viral hepatitis A.
(B) viral hepatitis B.
(C) cirrhosis.
(D) hemolytic jaundice.
(E) type 2 diabetes mellitus.

4. Which of the following statements concerning the gallbladder is true?

(A) It synthesizes bile.
(B) It is lined by a simple columnar epithelium.
(C) Bile leaves the gallbladder via the common bile duct.
(D) It has no muscle cells in the walls.
(E) It is affected by the hormone secretin.

5. A patient complains to her physician about sudden weight loss, loss of appetite, weakness, and back pain. Because the patient's sclera and skin have a yellowish pallor, the doctor suspects

(A) type 2 diabetes.
(B) gallstones.
(C) pancreatic cancer.
(D) viral hepatitis A.
(E) viral hepatitis B.

6. Acinar cells of the exocrine pancreas secrete

(A) glucagon.
(B) lysozyme.
(C) insulin.
(D) plasma proteins.
(E) proteases.

7. Pancreatic α-cells secrete

(A) glucagon.
(B) lysozyme.
(C) insulin.
(D) plasma proteins.
(E) proteases.

8. Pancreatic β-cells secrete

(A) glucagon.
(B) lysozyme.
(C) insulin.
(D) plasma proteins.
(E) proteases.

9. Submandibular acinar cells secrete

(A) glucagon.
(B) lysozyme.
(C) insulin.
(D) plasma proteins.
(E) proteases.

10. Hepatocytes secrete

(A) glucagon.
(B) lysozyme.
(C) insulin.
(D) plasma proteins.
(E) proteases.

Answers and Explanations

1. **B.** The three classic signs of type 2 diabetes (juvenile onset) are polyphagia (excessive eating), polyuria (excessive urination), and polydipsia (excessive drinking). The condition occurs in young individuals, usually before 20 years of age (see Chapter 17 III B 3 Clinical Considerations).

2. **D.** Liver sinusoids are lined by fenestrated endothelial cells, lack a basal lamina, and deliver blood directly to the central vein (see Chapter 17 IV B 1 b).

3. **D.** Yellow skin and yellow sclera are indicative of jaundice. Because the patient had a low red blood cell count, the most probable diagnosis is hemolytic jaundice (see Chapter 17 IV E 6 Clinical Considerations).

4. **B.** The gallbladder is lined by a simple columnar epithelium (see Chapter 17 V).

5. **C.** Pancreatic cancer has all of the symptoms listed, namely, sudden weight loss, loss of appetite, weakness, back pain, and jaundice. Although jaundice is noted in hepatitis A and B and in the presence of obstructive jaundice caused by gallstones, sudden weight loss, loss of appetite, and weakness are not diagnostic of these diseases. Diabetes mellitus does not cause jaundice, loss of appetite, or weight loss (see Chapter 17 III B 3 Clinical Considerations).

6. **E.** Several proteases are synthesized by pancreatic acinar cells and are delivered via the pancreatic duct to the duodenum (see Chapter 17 III A 3).

7. **A.** Glucagon is produced by α-cells of the islets of Langerhans. They are the second most abundant secretory cells of the endocrine pancreas (see Chapter 17 III B 3).

8. **C.** Insulin is produced by pancreatic β-cells, which are the most abundant cell type of the islets of Langerhans (see Chapter 17 III B 3).

9. **B.** Lysozyme, an enzyme with antibacterial activity, is produced primarily by the submandibular salivary gland acinar cells (see Chapter 17 II B 1).

10. **D.** Hepatocytes synthesize several plasma proteins, including fibrinogen, prothrombin, and albumin (see Chapter 17 IV E 2).

chapter 18 The Urinary System

I. OVERVIEW—THE URINARY SYSTEM

A. **Structure.** The urinary system is composed of the paired **kidneys** and **ureters** and the **bladder** and **urethra**.

B. **Function.** The urinary system produces and excretes **urine**, thereby clearing the blood of waste products. The kidneys also regulate the electrolyte levels in the extracellular fluid, synthesize renin and erythropoietin, and convert the less reactive form of vitamin D_3 (25-OH-vitamin D_3) to its more active form known as **calcitriol [1,25-(OH)$_2$ vitamin D$_3$]**.

II. KIDNEYS

A. **General structure**
   1. Kidneys are paired bean-shaped organs enveloped by a thin **capsule** of connective tissue.
   2. Each kidney is divided into an outer **cortex** and an inner **medulla**.
   3. Each kidney contains about 2 million **nephrons.** A nephron and the collecting tubule into which it drains form a **uriniferous tubule.** Each collecting tubule drains a number of nephrons.

B. **The renal hilum** is a concavity on the medial border of the kidney. It houses arteries, veins, lymphatic vessels, nerves, and the renal pelvis.

C. **The renal pelvis** (Figure 18.1) is a funnel-shaped expansion of the upper end of the **ureter**. It is continuous with the **major renal calyces**, each of which in turn has several small tributaries, the **minor calyces**.

D. **The renal medulla** lies deep to the cortex, but sends extensions (**medullary rays**) into the cortex.
   1. **Renal (medullary) pyramids** are conical or pyramidal-shaped structures that compose the bulk of the renal medulla. The bases of the pyramids establish the corticomedullary junction. The apex of each pyramid forms the deepest portion of the medulla.
      a. Each kidney contains 10 to 18 renal pyramids.
      b. Each pyramid consists primarily of the thin limbs of **loops of Henle**, blood vessels, and **collecting tubules**.
   2. The **renal papilla** is located at the **apex** of each renal pyramid. It has a perforated tip (**area cribrosa**) that projects into the lumen of a minor calyx.

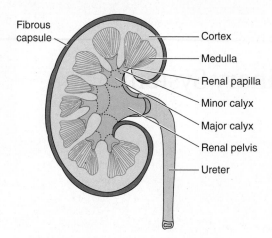

Fibrous capsule —
Cortex
Medulla
Renal papilla
Minor calyx
Major calyx
Renal pelvis
Ureter

FIGURE 18.1. The internal structure of a bisected kidney.

E. **The renal cortex** is the superficial layer of the kidney beneath the capsule. It consists primarily of **renal corpuscles** and **convoluted tubules**.
  1. **Renal columns of Bertin** are extensions of cortical tissue between adjacent renal pyramids.
  2. **Medullary rays** are groups of tubules that extend from the base of each renal (medullary) pyramid into the **cortex**. These tubules are the **straight portions** of the proximal and distal tubules as well as the **collecting ducts** that drain nephrons.

F. **The renal lobe** consists of a renal pyramid and its closely associated cortical tissue.

G. **The renal lobule** consists of a central medullary ray and the closely associated cortical tissue surrounding it, bounded on each side by an **interlobular artery**. Its many **nephrons** drain into the collecting tubules of the medullary ray.

H. **The renal interstitium** is the connective tissue compartment of the kidney. It is scanty in the cortex, occupying less than 10% of the cortical volume, and somewhat greater in the medulla, occupying about 20% of the medullary volume. The renal interstitium consists primarily of **fibroblasts** and **mononuclear cells** (probably macrophages). In the medulla, it consists of two additional cell types:
  1. **Pericytes** (see Chapter VI III B) are located along the blood vessels that supply the loops of Henle.
  2. **Interstitial cells** have long **processes** that extend toward (and perhaps encircle) capillaries and tubules in the medulla. These cells manufacture **medullipin I**, a vasodepressor hormone that is converted to **medullipin II** in the liver. Medullipin II is a vasodilator that acts to reduce blood pressure.

III. URINIFEROUS TUBULES (Table 18.1)

A. **Nephrons.** Nephrons consist of a **renal corpuscle, proximal tubule** (composed of the **proximal convoluted tubule** and the **pars recta of the proximal tubule), thin descending limb of Henle loop, Henle loop, thin ascending limb of Henle loop**, and **distal tubule** (composed of the **pars recta of the distal tubule,** the very short **macula densa**, and the **distal convoluted tubule**). Unfortunately for the student, the pars recta of the proximal tubule is also known as the **descending thick limb of Henle loop**, and the pars recta of the distal tubule is also known as the **ascending thick limb of Henle loop**.
  1. **Classification**. Nephrons can be classified as **cortical, midcortical**, and **juxtamedullary**, depending upon the location of the renal corpuscle. The renal corpuscles of cortical nephrons

table **18.1** Important Structural and Functional Characteristics of the Uriniferous Tubule

Region	Epithelium	Major Functions	Summary
Renal corpuscle	Simple squamous epithelium lining Bowman capsule: podocytes (visceral layer), outer (parietal layer)	Filters blood	Filtration barrier of fenestrated endothelial cells, fused basal laminae, filtration slits between podocyte secondary processes (pedicels)
Proximal convoluted tubule	Simple cuboidal epithelium with brush border; many compartmentalized mitochondria	Resorbs all glucose, amino acids, filtered proteins; at least 80% Na, Cl, H_2O	The activity of Na pumps in basolateral membranes, transporting Na^+ out of tubule, reduces volume of ultrafiltrate, maintains its isotonicity with blood
Loop of Henle, descending thick limb	Lined by simple cuboidal epithelium with brush border	Same as for proximal convoluted tubule	Same as for proximal convoluted tubule
Loop of Henle, descending thin limb	Simple squamous epithelium	Permeable to H_2O which exits ultrafiltrate and enters interstitium; Na, Cl enter ultrafiltrate	Ultrafiltrate becomes hypertonic with respect to blood; urea, from interstitium, also enters lumen of tubule
Loop of Henle, ascending thin limb	Simple squamous epithelium	Somewhat permeable to H_2O which enters ultrafiltrate from interstitium; Na, Cl exit ultrafiltrate	Ultrafiltrate remains hypertonic with respect to blood; urea, from interstitium, also enters lumen of tubule
Loop of Henle, ascending thick limb	Simple cuboidal epithelium; compartmentalized mitochondria	Impermeable to H_2O; Cl actively transported out of tubule into interstitium; Na follows	Ultrafiltrate becomes hypotonic with respect to blood; Cl pump in basolateral membranes is primarily responsible for establishing osmotic gradient in interstitium of outer medulla
JG apparatus macula densa	Simple cuboidal epithelium	Monitors level of Na (or decrease of fluid volume) in ultrafiltrate of distal tubule	Macula densa cells communicate with JG cells in afferent arteriole via gap junctions
JG cells in afferent arteriole	Modified smooth muscle cells containing renin granules	Cells synthesize renin, release it into bloodstream	Renin acts on plasma protein, to trigger events leading to formation of angiotensin II, release of aldosterone from adrenal gland
Distal convoluted tubule	Simple cuboidal cells; compartmentalized mitochondria	Cells respond to aldosterone by removing Na from ultrafiltrate	Ultrafiltrate more hypotonic in presence of aldosterone; K^+, NH_4^+, H^+ enter ultrafiltrate
Collecting tubules	Simple cuboidal epithelium; simple columnar epithelium	In absence of ADH, tubule impermeable to H_2O; hypotonic urine excreted	In presence of ADH, tubule permeable to H_2O, which is removed from filtrate, producing hypertonic urine

ADH, antidiuretic hormone; JG, juxtaglomerular.

are near the capsule, those of juxtamedullary nephrons are near the corticomedullary junction, and those of the midcortical nephrons are in between the other two. Juxtamedullary nephrons possess longer loops of Henle than do cortical or midcortical nephrons and are responsible for establishing the interstitial concentration gradient in the medulla. Even though only about 15% of all nephrons are juxtamedullary nephrons, the ensuing description is of a juxtamedullary nephron because once its structure and function are understood, the structure and function of the other two nephron types become self-evident.

2. A **renal corpuscle** (Figure 18.2) consists of the **glomerulus** and **Bowman capsule** and is the structure in which the **filtration of blood** occurs.

    a. Bowman capsule

        (1) The **parietal layer** is the simple squamous epithelium that lines the outer wall of the Bowman capsule.

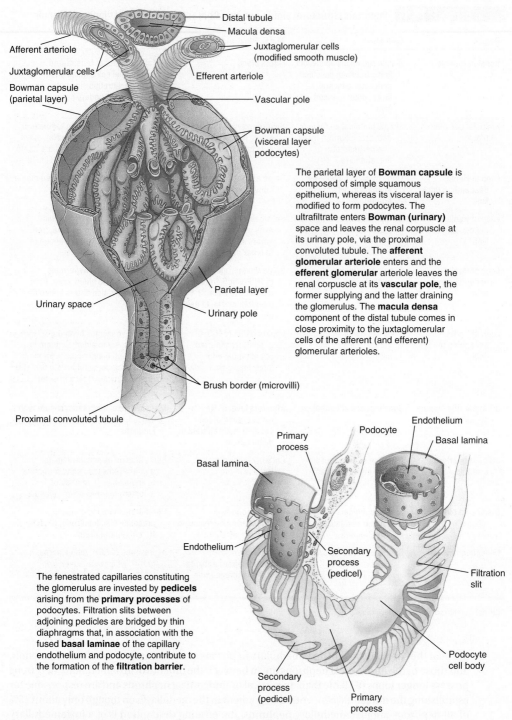

The parietal layer of **Bowman capsule** is composed of simple squamous epithelium, whereas its visceral layer is modified to form podocytes. The ultrafiltrate enters **Bowman (urinary)** space and leaves the renal corpuscle at its urinary pole, via the proximal convoluted tubule. The **afferent glomerular arteriole** enters and the **efferent glomerular** arteriole leaves the renal corpuscle at its **vascular pole**, the former supplying and the latter draining the glomerulus. The **macula densa** component of the distal tubule comes in close proximity to the juxtaglomerular cells of the afferent (and efferent) glomerular arterioles.

The fenestrated capillaries constituting the glomerulus are invested by **pedicels** arising from the **primary processes** of podocytes. Filtration slits between adjoining pedicels are bridged by thin diaphragms that, in association with the fused **basal laminae** of the capillary endothelium and podocyte, contribute to the formation of the **filtration barrier**.

FIGURE 18.2. A diagram illustrating components of the renal corpuscle. (From Gartner LP, Hiatt JL. *Color Atlas of Histology.* 5th ed. Baltimore, MD: Lippincott William & Wilkins; 2009:337.)

(2) The **visceral layer** (glomerular epithelium) is the modified simple squamous epithelium composed of **podocytes** that lines the inner wall of the Bowman capsule and envelops the glomerular capillaries.

(3) Bowman space (also known as **capsular space** or **urinary space**) is the narrow chalice-shaped cavity between the visceral and parietal layers into which the ultrafiltrate passes.

(4) The **vascular pole** is the site on Bowman capsule where the afferent glomerular arteriole enters and the efferent glomerular arteriole leaves the glomerulus.

(5) The **urinary pole** is the site on Bowman capsule where the capsular space becomes continuous with the lumen of the proximal convoluted tubule.

b. Podocytes are highly modified epithelial cells that form the **visceral layer** of Bowman capsule and synthesize **glomerular endothelial growth factor**, a signaling molecule that facilitates the formation and maintenance of the glomerular endothelial cells. Podocytes have complex shapes and possess several **primary processes** that give rise to many secondary processes called **pedicels**.

(1) Pedicels

  (a) Pedicels embrace the glomerular capillaries and interdigitate with pedicels arising from other primary processes.

  (b) Their surfaces facing Bowman space are coated with **podocalyxin**, a protein that is thought to assist in maintaining their organization and shape.

  (c) Pedicels possess $\alpha_3\beta_1$ **integrin** molecules that cause them to adhere to the basal lamina.

(2) Filtration slits are elongated spaces about 40 nm in width between adjacent pedicels. **A filtration slit diaphragm** bridges each filtration slit and is the principal structure that is the barrier responsible for the filtration of proteins.

  (a) Each slit diaphragm is composed of the extracellular portion of the transmembrane protein **nephrin** of one pedicel that contacts the extracellular portion of nephrin from the adjacent pedicel.

  (b) Within the cytoplasm of the pedicel, the intracellular moiety of nephrin binds to **podocin** as well as to **CD2-associated proteins** that in turn bind to **actin filaments** and in that manner stabilize the nephrin molecule.

c. The **renal glomerulus** is the **tuft of capillaries** that extends into the Bowman capsule.

(1) Glomerular endothelial cells

  (a) form the inner layer of the capillary walls.

  (b) have a thin cytoplasm that is thicker around the nucleus, where most organelles are located.

  (c) possess large **fenestrae** (60–90 nm in diameter) but **lack the thin diaphragms** that typically span the openings in other fenestrated capillaries.

(2) The **basal lamina** is **between** the podocytes and the glomerular endothelial cells and is manufactured by **both** cell populations. It is unusually **thick** (0.15–0.5 μm) and contains three distinct **zones**:

  (a) The **lamina rara externa**, an electron-lucent zone adjacent to the podocyte epithelium.

  (b) The **lamina densa**, a thicker, electron-dense intermediate zone of amorphous material.

  (c) The **lamina rara interna**, an electron-lucent zone adjacent to the capillary endothelium.

(3) The **mesangium** is the interstitial tissue between glomerular capillaries. It is composed of mesangial cells and an amorphous extracellular matrix elaborated by these cells.

  (a) Mesangial cells

   1. phagocytose large protein molecules and debris, which may accumulate during filtration or in certain disease states.

   2. can also **contract**, thereby decreasing the surface area available for filtration.

   3. possess **receptors for angiotensin II** and **atrial natriuretic peptide**.

   4. manufacture platelet-derived growth factor, endothelins, inteleukin-1, and prostaglandin E_2.

  (b) The **mesangial matrix**, manufactured by mesangial cells, is composed of type IV collagen, laminin, and proteoglycans and helps support glomerular capillaries.

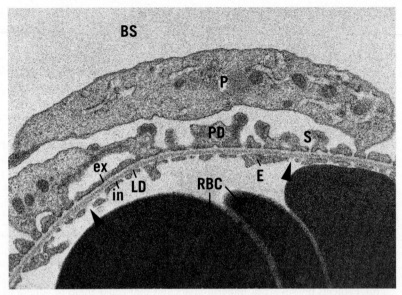

FIGURE 18.3. An electron micrograph of the renal filtration barrier. The primary process of a podocyte (P) in Bowman space (BS) gives off secondary processes, called pedicels (PD), which form a layer along the basal lamina enveloping the glomerular capillary. Between adjacent pedicels are the filtration slits (S) bridged by barely visible dense thin lines representing filtration slit membranes. The basal lamina consists of the lamina densa (LD), which is the major filtration barrier, and the laminae rara interna (in) and lamina rara externa (ex). Note the fenestrations (*arrowheads*) within the endothelial cells (E) lining the capillary, where red blood cells (RBC) are present (×14,000).

d. Renal filtration barrier (Figure 18.3)

  (1) Structure. The renal filtration barrier is composed of the **fenestrated endothelium** of the glomerular capillaries, the **basal lamina** (laminae rarae and lamina densa), and the **filtration slit diaphragm** bridging the filtration slits between adjacent pedicels .

  (2) Function. The renal filtration barrier **permits passage** of water, ions, and small molecules from the bloodstream into the capsular space but **prevents passage** of large and/or most negatively charged proteins, thus forming an **ultrafiltrate of blood plasma** in the Bowman space.

  (a) The **laminae rarae** contain **heparan sulfate**, a polyanionic glycosaminoglycan that assists in **restricting the passage of negatively charged proteins** into the Bowman space.

  (b) The **lamina densa** contains **type IV collagen** (composed of α_3, α_4, and α_5 chains rather than the α_1 and α_2 chains present in most other lamina densa), **perlacan, laminin, entactin,** and **agrin**. The negative charges of some of these macromolecules and the filtration slit diaphragm act as a **selective macromolecular filter**, preventing the passage of large protein molecules (molecular weight greater than 69,000 Da) into the Bowman space.

CLINICAL CONSIDERATIONS   **Glomerulonephritis**

  1. Glomerulonephritis is a type of nephritis characterized by **inflammation of the glomeruli**.
  2. It is sometimes marked by proliferation of podocytes, endothelial cells, and mesangial cells in the glomerular tuft; infiltration of leukocytes is also common.
  3. This disease often occurs **secondary to a streptococcal infection** elsewhere in the body, which is thought to result in deposition of immune complexes in the glomerular basal lamina. The immune complexes damage the glomerular basal lamina and markedly reduce its filtering ability.
  4. It may also result from immune or autoimmune disorders.

5. It is associated with production of urine-containing blood (**hematuria**), protein (**proteinuria**), or both; in severe cases, decreased urine output (**oliguria**) is common.
6. It occurs in acute, subacute, and chronic forms. The chronic form, in which the destruction of glomeruli continues, leads eventually to renal failure and death.

Chronic Renal Failure

1. Chronic renal failure can result from a variety of diseases (e.g., diabetes mellitus, hypertension, atherosclerosis) in which blood flow to the kidneys is reduced, causing a decrease in glomerular filtration and tubular ischemia.
2. It is associated with pathological changes (hyalinization) in the glomeruli and atrophy of the tubules, which impair virtually all aspects of renal function.
3. It is marked by **acidosis** and **hyperkalemia** because the acid–base balance cannot be maintained, and by **uremia** because of the inability to eliminate metabolic wastes.
4. If untreated, chronic renal failure leads to neurological problems, coma, and death.

Alport Syndrome

Mutation in the α_5 chain of the type IV collagen causes defective basal lamina formation in the kidney glomerulus (as well as in other regions of the body, such as the eye and inner ear). Since the mutation is X-linked, men are more seriously affected than women whose second X chromosome may not bear the same mutation. The effects on the kidney result in thickening of the basal lamina and the inability of the glomerular filtration to occur normally, and protein and blood begin to be present in the urine. Eventually, in many patients, the result is kidney failure, and dialysis is required to sustain life. In certain patients, kidney transplant is not viable because the transplanted kidney's normal type IV collagen may be perceived as antigenic by the host and the new kidney may be rejected by the immune system.

---

3. **Proximal convoluted tubule** (Figures 18.4 and 18.5)
   a. The proximal convoluted tubule is lined by a single layer of **irregularly shaped** (cuboidal to columnar) epithelial cells that have microvilli forming a prominent **brush border**. These cells exhibit the following structures:
      (1) Apical canaliculi, vesicles, and vacuoles (endocytic complex), which function in **protein absorption**.

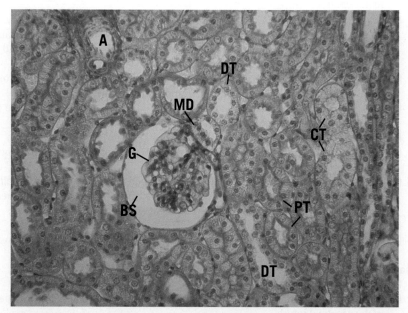

FIGURE 18.4. A light micrograph of components in the cortex of the kidney. A renal corpuscle showing Bowman space (BS) and a glomerulus (G); the macula densa (MD) of a juxtaglomerular apparatus; many proximal tubules (PT) with prominent brush borders, and a few distal tubules (DT) and collecting tubules (CT), as well as an artery (A) are illustrated (×150).

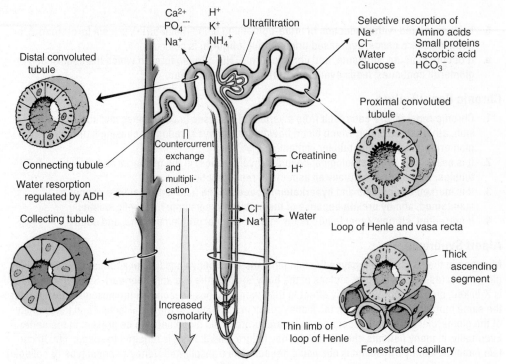

FIGURE 18.5. A uriniferous tubule showing its major structural and functional features and its vascular associations. ADH, antidiuretic hormone. (Adapted with permission from Williams PL, Warwick R, eds. *Gray's Anatomy*. 36th British ed. London: Churchill Livingstone; 1980:1393.)

(2) Prominent interdigitations along their lateral borders, which interlock adjacent cells with one another.

(3) Numerous **mitochondria** compartmentalized in the basal region by extensive infoldings of the basal plasma membrane, which supply energy for the **active transport of** Na^+ out of the tubule.

(4) Apically situated occluding junctions that block the paracellular pathway. And the apical cell membrane has **glucose transporters**, **Na^+K^+–ATPase pump**, and an apically positioned tubulovesicular system designed to endocytose small proteins and peptides that escaped into the ultrafiltrate.

(5) The basolateral cell membrane possesses **Na^+K^+–ATPase pump**, and, additionally, the basal cell membrane has glucose and amino acid transporters.

(6) Each cell also possesses a primary cilium that functions in monitoring the flow and composition of the ultrafiltrate.

b. **Function**

(1) The proximal convoluted tubule drains the Bowman space at the urinary pole of the renal corpuscle.

(2) It **resorbs** from the glomerular filtrate all of the glucose, amino acids, and small proteins and 60% to 80% of the sodium chloride and water and returns it into the peritubular capillary system to be distributed from there into the remainder of the body.

(3) It **exchanges** H^+ in the interstitium for HCO_3^- in the filtrate.

(4) It **secretes** organic acids (e.g., creatinine) and bases and certain foreign substances into the filtrate.

4. **Loop of Henle** (Figure 18.5)

a. **Descending thick limb of the Henle loop**

(1) The descending limb of the Henle loop is also known as the straight portion (**pars recta**) of the proximal tubule.

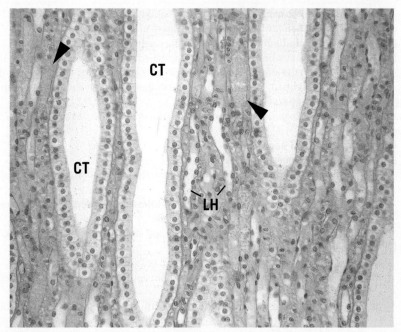

FIGURE 18.6. A light micrograph of components in the medulla of the kidney. Collecting tubules (CT) are lined by a simple columnar epithelium composed of cells displaying distinct lateral surfaces. The thin limbs of the loops of Henle (LH) are lined by a simple squamous epithelium whose cell nuclei bulge into the lumen, and capillaries (*arrowheads*) may be identified by the numerous red blood cells filling their lumens (×150).

    (2) It is lined by a simple **cuboidal** epithelium that has a prominent **brush border** and is similar to that lining the proximal convoluted tubule.

    (3) Its function is to resorb, exchange, and secrete in a manner similar to that of the proximal convoluted tubule.

  b. Thin limb of the Henle loop (Figure 18.6)

    (1) The thin limb of the Henle loop is composed of a descending segment, a loop, and an ascending segment, all of which are lined by simple **squamous** epithelial cells possessing a few short microvilli. The nuclei of these cells bulge into the lumen.

    (2) In juxtamedullary nephrons, the thin limb can be divided into **three** distinct portions on the basis of the four different types of simple squamous epithelial cells that form it, their organelle content, the depth of their tight junctions, and their permeability to water.

      (a) Cells of the **descending thin limb** possess many aquaporin 1 channels and, therefore, this segment is very permeable to water as well as being somewhat permeable to ions such as sodium and chloride.

      (b) **Henle loop** itself is similar to the ascending thin limb and is mostly impermeable to water.

      (c) **The ascending thin limb** is almost completely impermeable to water but possesses many sodium and chloride channels, which permit these ions to enter the cell from the lumen of the tubule and exit the cell into the renal interstitium. Additionally, urea enters the lumen of the ascending thin limb.

  c. Ascending thick limb of the Henle loop

    (1) The ascending thick limb of the Henle loop is also known as the straight portion (**pars recta**) of the distal tubule.

    (2) It is lined by **cuboidal** epithelial cells that possess only a few microvilli, an apical nucleus, and mitochondria compartmentalized within basal plasma membrane infoldings. These cells manufacture and release a glycoprotein known as **uromodulin** (Tamm–Horsfall glycoprotein) that reduces the ability of the kidney to form kidney stones and in some fashion reduces the possibility of urinary tract infections. Moreover, uromodulin also modulates the mechanism of urine concentration.

(3) It establishes a gradient of osmolarity in the medulla (see Section V).

(4) The ascending thick limb returns to the renal corpuscle of origin, where it is in close association with the afferent and efferent glomerular arterioles. In this region, the wall of the tubule is modified, forming the **macula densa**, which is part of the **juxtaglomerular apparatus (JG apparatus)**.

5. The **JG apparatus** (juxtaglomerular apparatus) is located at the **vascular pole** of the renal corpuscle.

   a. **Components of the JG apparatus**

   (1) **JG cells (juxtaglomerular cells)**

      (a) are **modified smooth muscle cells** that exhibit some characteristics of protein-secreting cells.

      (b) are located primarily in the wall of the **afferent arteriole**, but a few may also be present in the wall of the efferent arteriole.

      (c) synthesize **renin** (a proteolytic enzyme) and store it in secretory granules.

   (2) **Macula densa cells** (Figure 18.4)

      (a) are tall, narrow, closely packed epithelial cells of the **distal tubule**.

      (b) have elongated, closely packed nuclei that appear as a dense spot (macula densa) by light microscopy.

      (c) may **monitor the osmolarity and volume** of the fluid in the distal tubule and transmit this information to JG cells via the gap junctions between the two cell types. When the sodium concentration or the volume of the ultrafiltrate is reduced, the macula densa cells direct the JG cells to release their renin.

   (3) **Extraglomerular mesangial cells**

      (a) are also known as **polkissen** (pole cushion) or **lacis cells**.

      (b) lie between the afferent and efferent glomerular arterioles, but their functions are not understood.

   b. **Function.** The JG apparatus **maintains blood pressure** by the following mechanism:

   (1) A **decrease in extracellular fluid volume** (perhaps detected by the macula densa as decreased ultrafiltrate volume), a **decrease in blood pressure** at the afferent glomerular arteriole, or a **decrease in sodium concentration** of the ultrafiltrate stimulates JG cells to release renin into the bloodstream.

   (2) Renin acts on angiotensinogen (a large protein manufactured by hepatocytes of the liver) in the plasma. Renin cleaves the first 10 amino acids from angiotensinogen, converting it to the decapeptide **angiotensin I**. In capillaries of the lung and elsewhere, angiotensin-converting enzyme cleaves two amino acids from angiotensin I, converting it to **angiotensin II**, a potent vasoconstrictor that stimulates release of **aldosterone** in the adrenal cortex and the **release of antidiuretic hormone (ADH)** by the neurohypophysis.

   (3) Aldosterone stimulates the epithelial cells of the distal convoluted tubule to remove Na^+ and Cl^-. **Water follows the ions**, thereby **increasing the fluid volume** in the extracellular compartment, which leads to an increase in blood pressure.

   (4) ADH causes the epithelial cells (mainly the **principal cells**) of the collecting tubule to add **aquaporin 2 (AQP-2) channels** (as well as AQP-3 and AQP-4 channels) to their cell **membrane** and thus become permeable to water, releasing H_2O into the renal interstitium. As with the aldosterone mechanism discussed above, the increased extracellular fluid volume leads to elevation of the blood pressure.

6. **Distal convoluted tubule** (Figure 18.7)

   a. The distal convoluted tubule is continuous with the macula densa and is similar histologically to the ascending thick limb of the Henle loop.

   b. It is much shorter and has a wider lumen than the proximal convoluted tubule and **lacks a brush border**.

   c. **Function.** The distal convoluted tubule **resorbs Na^+** from the filtrate and actively transports it into the renal interstitium; this process is stimulated by **aldosterone**. It also transfers K^+, NH_4^+, and H^+ into the filtrate from the interstitium.

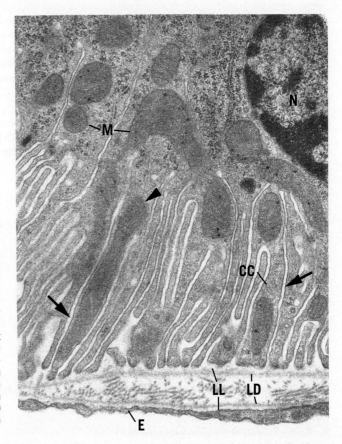

FIGURE 18.7. An electron micrograph of a cell in the distal convoluted tubule of the kidney. Elongated mitochondria (M) are located (*arrowhead*) within cytoplasmic compartments (CC) formed by deep infoldings of the basal plasma membrane where enzymes associated with ion transport are located. In between these extensive infoldings is extracellular space (*arrows*). These cells resorb Na^+ from the filtrate and actively transport it into the renal interstitium (aldosterone stimulates this process) and also transfer K^+, NH_4^+, and H^+ into the filtrate from the interstitium. Note the lamina densa (LD) and lamina lucida (LL), which form the basal lamina, the endothelial cell (E) lining a fenestrated capillary, and the apical nucleus (N) ($\times$6,000).

7. The **connecting tubule** is a short segment between the distal convoluted tubule and the collecting tubule into which it drains. It is lined by the following two types of epithelial cells:
   a. **Principal cells** have many infoldings of the basal plasma membrane. These cells **remove Na^+** from the filtrate and **secrete K^+** into it.
   b. **Intercalated cells** have many apical vesicles and mitochondria. These cells **remove K^+** from the filtrate and **secrete H^+** into it.

CLINICAL CONSIDERATIONS   **Nephrotoxic acute tubular necrosis** is the death of kidney tubule cells caused by their exposure to a toxic drug or molecule, rather than a lack of oxygen (**ischemic** acute tubular necrosis). When a person suffers a crush injury causing significant muscle trauma, myoglobin is released from the muscle and enters the bloodstream. The myoglobin is filtered through the glomeruli, but it is toxic to cells of the kidney tubules, causing nephrotoxic acute tubular necrosis. If the damage is not too severe, the kidney tubule cells may be able to replace themselves, but in severe cases, they cannot and the kidney may not completely recover.

B. **Collecting tubules** (Figure 18.5) have an embryological origin different from that of nephrons. They have segments in both the cortex and the medulla and converge to form larger and larger tubules.
   1. **Cortical collecting tubules** are located primarily within medullary rays, although a few are interspersed among the convoluted tubules in the cortex (**cortical labyrinth**). They are lined by a simple epithelium containing two types of **cuboidal** cells.
      a. **Principal (light) cells** possess a round central nucleus and a single **primary cilium**. It is these cells that are responsible for the ability of the collecting tubules to concentrate urine.

     b. Intercalated (dark) cells are less numerous than principal cells and possess microplicae (folds) on their apical surface and numerous apical cytoplasmic vesicles. There are two types of intercalated cells: α-**intercalated cells** that have the ability to release H^+ **ions** into the tubular lumen, thus acidifying urine, and β-**intercalated cells** that have the ability to release HCO_3^- **ions** into the tubular lumen, thus causing the urine to be more alkaline. α-Intercalated cells possess **hydrogen pumps**, and β-intercalated cells possess HCO_3^- **pumps** to fulfill their function.

  2. Medullary collecting tubules. In the **outer** medulla, medullary collecting tubules are similar in structure to cortical collecting tubules and contain both **principal** and **intercalated cells** in their lining epithelium. In the inner medulla, the collecting tubules are lined only by **principal cells** (Figure 18.6).

  3. Papillary collecting tubules (ducts of Bellini)

     a. Papillary collecting tubules are large collecting tubules (200–300 μm in diameter) formed from converging smaller tubules.

     b. They are lined by a simple epithelium composed of **columnar** cells that have a single **primary cilium**.

     c. They empty at the **area cribrosa**, a region at the apex of each renal pyramid that has 10 to 25 openings through which the urine exits into a minor calyx.

IV. RENAL BLOOD CIRCULATION

The renal blood circulation is extensive, with total blood flow through both kidneys of about 1200 mL/min. At this rate, all of the circulating blood in the body passes through the kidneys every 4 to 5 minutes.

A. Arterial supply to the kidney (Figure 18.8)

  1. Branches of the renal artery enter each kidney at the hilum and give rise to interlobar arteries.

  2. Interlobar arteries travel between the renal pyramids and divide into several **arcuate arteries**, which run along the corticomedullary junction parallel to the kidney's surface.

  3. Interlobular arteries

     a. Interlobular arteries are smaller vessels that arise from the arcuate arteries.

     b. They enter the cortical tissue and travel outward **between adjacent medullary rays**. Adjacent interlobular arteries delimit a renal lobule.

     c. They give rise to **afferent (glomerular) arterioles** and send branches to the interstitium just deep to the renal capsule.

  4. Afferent arterioles are branches of the interlobular arteries that **supply the glomerular capillaries**.

  5. Efferent arterioles arise from the glomerular capillaries and are associated with cortical, midcortical, and juxtaglomerular nephrons. They leave the glomerulus of cortical and midcortical nephrons and give rise to an extensive **peritubular capillary network** that supplies the cortical labyrinth, whereas those that leave the juxtaglomerular nephrons give rise to the **vasa recta**.

  6. Vasa recta

     a. The vasa recta arise from the efferent arterioles supplying **juxtamedullary nephrons**.

     b. These long, thin vessels (**arteriolae rectae**) follow a straight path into the medulla and renal papilla, where they form capillaries and then loop back and increase in diameter toward the corticomedullary boundary (**venulae rectae**).

     c. They are closely **associated with the descending and ascending limbs of Henle loops** and **collecting ducts**, to which they supply nutrients and oxygen.

     d. These vessels play a critical role in countercurrent exchanges with the interstitium.

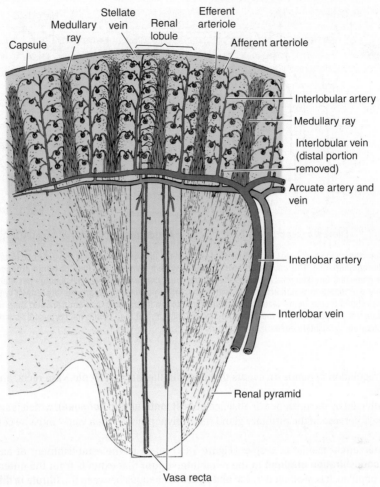

FIGURE 18.8. Blood circulation in the kidney. Arteries are shown in red and veins in blue. Adjacent interlobular arteries, which extend outward from the arcuate artery, define the boundaries of a renal lobule. (Reprinted with permission from Junqueira LC, Carneiro J, Kelley RO. *Basic Histology*. 9th ed. Stamford, CT: Appleton & Lange; 1998:375.)

B. Venous drainage of the kidney (Figure 18.8)

1. **Stellate veins** are formed by convergence of **superficial cortical veins**, which drain the outermost layers of the cortex.
2. **Deep cortical veins** drain the deeper regions of the cortex.
3. **Interlobular veins**
   a. Interlobular veins receive both stellate and deep cortical veins.
   b. They join **arcuate veins**, which empty into **interlobar veins**. These then converge to form a branch of the **renal vein**, which exits the kidney at the hilum.

V. REGULATION OF URINE CONCENTRATION

A. Overview

1. The regulation of urine concentration results in the excretion of large amounts of dilute (**hypotonic**) urine when water intake is high (**diuresis**) and of concentrated (**hypertonic**) urine when body water needs to be conserved (**antidiuresis**).

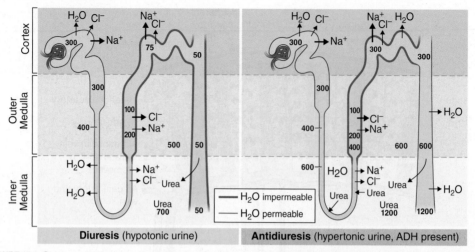

FIGURE 18.9. Summary of ion and water exchanges that occur in the uriniferous tubule in the absence (*left*) and presence (*right*) of antidiuretic hormone. The countercurrent multiplier system involving the loop of Henle produces an osmotic gradient in the medullary interstitium. Numbers refer to the local concentration in milliosmoles per liter. Segments of the tubule freely permeable to water are drawn with a thin line; impermeable segments are drawn with a thick line. In the distal convoluted tubule, some water follows sodium into the interstitium; sodium transport here is regulated by aldosterone. Note that the pars recta of the distal tubules actually contact their own renal corpuscles but they have been rotated in this diagram to facilitate easier identification.

2. This regulation depends on events that occur in the loops of Henle, vasa recta, and collecting tubules.
3. It is affected by the presence or absence of **ADH (antidiuretic hormone)**, which is secreted from the pars nervosa of the pituitary gland (neurohypophysis) when water must be conserved.

B. **The countercurrent multiplier system** (Figure 18.9) refers to the establishment of an **increasing osmotic concentration gradient** in the renal interstitium that extends from the outer medulla to the renal papillae. It is produced by **ion and water exchanges** between the **filtrate in different parts of the loop of Henle** and the **renal interstitium**:
  1. **In the descending limb of the loop of Henle,**
     a. the **isotonic** filtrate coming from the proximal convoluted tubules loses water to the interstitium and gains Na^+ and Cl^-.
     b. the filtrate becomes **hypertonic**.
  2. **In the ascending thin and thick limbs of the loop of Henle,**
     a. no water is lost from the filtrate because this part of the nephron is **impermeable to water** whether or not ADH is present.
     b. Cl^- is **actively transported** from the filtrate (in the ascending thick limb but passively in the ascending thin limb) into the interstitium, and Na^+ follows.
     c. an **osmotic gradient** is thus established in the **interstitium** of the outer medulla.
     d. the filtrate becomes **hypotonic**.
  3. **In the distal convoluted tubule,** active resorption of Na^+ from the filtrate may occur in response to aldosterone, resulting in some water loss as well.

C. Role of collecting tubules
  1. In the **absence of ADH**, the collecting tubules are **impermeable to water**. Thus, the hypotonic filtrate coming from the ascending limb of the loop of Henle is not changed, and **hypotonic** urine is excreted.
  2. In the **presence of ADH**, the collecting tubules add AQP-2 channels (as well as AQP-3 and AQP-4 channels) into their cell membranes of their **principal cells** and thus become **permeable to water**. Thus, the isotonic filtrate entering them from the distal convoluted tubules lose water, and **hypertonic** (concentrated) urine is produced.

CLINICAL CONSIDERATIONS

1. **Diabetes insipidus**
    a. Diabetes insipidus results from destruction of the supraoptic and paraventricular nuclei in the hypothalamus, which synthesize ADH (vasopressin) (see Figure 13.1).
    b. It is associated with a **decreased ability of the kidney to concentrate urine** in the collecting tubules because levels of ADH are reduced.
    c. Signs and symptoms include dehydration, excessive thirst (**polydipsia**), and excretion of **high volumes of dilute urine**.
2. **Diabetes mellitus**
    a. **Diabetes mellitus** is different from diabetes insipidus in that mellitus is a disease involving insulin formation and/or usage, whereas insipidus involves the release or the usage of ADH.
    b. In **type II diabetes mellitus**, podocytes lack **insulin receptors** and are, therefore, unable to regulate their glucose uptake. The lack of ability to normally endocytose glucose causes podocyte damage, resulting in the leakage of albumin and larger proteins into the ultrafiltrate and eventually in renal failure.

D. **Countercurrent exchange system** (Figure 18.10)
    1. The countercurrent exchange system involves passive ion and water exchanges between the renal interstitium and the blood in the vasa recta, the small straight vessels associated with the loops of Henle.
    2. This exchange acts to maintain the interstitial osmotic gradient created by changes taking place in the Henle loop.

E. **Effect of urea** (Figure 18.9) is to aid in the production and maintenance of the interstitial osmotic gradient, mostly in the inner medulla.
    1. **Urea** from the renal interstitium enters the uriniferous tubules at the loop of Henle, the ascending thin and thick limbs of Henle loop, and the collecting tubules of the outer medulla.
    2. **Urea concentrations** in the filtrate progressively increase as water is lost from the medullary collecting tubules, causing the urea to diffuse (passively) out into the interstitium and contributing to the interstitial osmolarity.

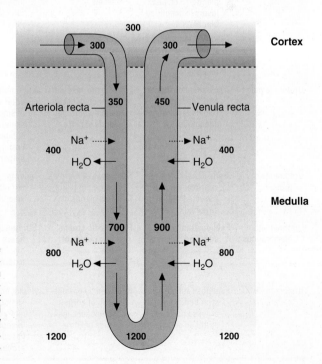

FIGURE 18.10. Countercurrent exchange mechanism. Summary of water and ion exchanges between the medullary interstitium and blood in the vasa recta. These countercurrent exchanges are *passive* and do not disturb the osmotic gradient in the interstitial tissue. Numbers refer to the local osmolarity per liter. (Adapted with permission from Junqueira LC, Carneiro J, Kelley RO. *Basic Histology.* 7th ed. Norwalk, CT: Appleton & Lange; 1992:390.)

3. A high-protein diet increases urea levels in the filtrate and its entrapment in the interstitium, thus enhancing the kidney's ability to concentrate the urine.
4. The ability of the kidney to concentrate urine depends mostly on the concentration of **sodium and chloride** in the renal interstitium of the **outer medulla**, but in the **inner medulla**, it is based mainly on the **urea** concentration in the renal interstitium.

VI. EXCRETORY PASSAGES

A. Overview (Table 18.2)
   1. The excretory passages include the minor and major **calyces** and the **renal pelvis**, located within each kidney, and the **ureters, urinary bladder**, and **urethra**, located outside the kidneys.

table **18.2** Features of Excretory Passages

Region	Epithelium	Lamina Propria	Muscularis	Comments
Calyces, minor, major	Transitional epithelium	Reticular, elastic fibers	A few inner longitudinal and outer circular smooth muscle fibers	Urine from collecting tubules (ducts of Bellini) empty into minor calyces.
Renal pelvis	Transitional epithelium	Reticular, elastic fibers	Inner longitudinal, outer circular layer of smooth muscle	Expanded upper portion of ureter receives urine from the major calyces.
Ureters	Transitional epithelium lines stellate lumen	Collagen, elastic fibers	Inner longitudinal, outer circular layer of smooth muscle; lower third has additional outermost longitudinal layer	Peristaltic waves propel urine, so it enters bladder in spurts.
Urinary bladder	Transitional epithelium: 5 or 6 cell layers in empty bladder; 3 or 4 cell layers in distended bladder Trigone: triangular region; apices are openings of ureters and urethra	Fibroelastic connective tissue rich in blood vessels	Three poorly defined layers of smooth muscle; inner longitudinal, middle circular, outer longitudinal	Plasmalemma of dome-shaped cells in epithelium has unique plaques, elliptical vesicles underlying remarkable (empty vs. full) transition. Trigone, unlike most of bladder mucosa, always presents smooth surface.
Urethra female	Transitional epithelium near bladder; remainder stratified squamous	Fibroelastic vascular connective tissue; mucus-secreting glands of Littre	Inner longitudinal, outer circular layer of smooth muscle; skeletal muscle sphincter surrounds urethra at urogenital diaphragm	Female urethra is conduit for urine. External sphincter of skeletal muscle permits voluntary control of micturition.
Urethra male prostatic	Transitional epithelium near bladder; pseudostratified or stratified columnar	Fibromuscular stroma of prostate gland; a few glands of Littre	Inner longitudinal, outer circular layer of smooth muscle	Conduit for urine and semen. Receives secretions from prostate glands, paired ejaculatory ducts.
Urethra male membranous	Pseudostratified or stratified columnar	Fibroelastic stroma; a few glands of Littre	Striated muscle fibers of urogenital diaphragm form external sphincter	Conduit for urine and semen. External sphincter of skeletal muscle permits voluntary control of micturition.
Urethra male cavernous	Pseudostratified or stratified columnar; at fossa navicularis stratified squamous	Replaced by erectile tissue of corpus spongiosum; many glands of Littre	Replaced by sparse smooth muscle, many elastic fibers in septa lining vascular spaces in erectile tissue	Conduit for urine and semen. Receives secretions of bulbourethral glands present in urogenital diaphragm.

2. These structures generally possess a three-layer wall composed of a **mucosa of transitional epithelium** (except in the urethra) lying on a lamina propria of connective tissue, a **muscularis (smooth muscle)**, and an **adventitia**.

B. Ureter

1. The ureter conveys urine from the renal pelvis of each kidney to the urinary bladder.
2. It has a **transitional epithelium** that is thicker and contains more cell layers than that of the renal calyces.
3. It possesses a **two-layer muscularis** (an inner longitudinal and outer circular layer of smooth muscle) in its upper two-thirds. The lowest third possesses an additional outer longitudinal layer of smooth muscle.
4. It contracts its muscle layers, producing **peristaltic waves** that propel the urine, so that it enters the bladder in spurts.

C. Urinary bladder. (Figure 18.11) The **urinary bladder** possesses a **transitional epithelium** with a morphology that differs in the relaxed (empty) and distended states, a thin lamina propria of **fibroelastic** connective tissue, and a **three-layer muscularis**.

1. **Epithelium of the relaxed bladder** is five to six cell layers thick and has **rounded** superficial **dome-shaped cells** that bulge into the lumen. These cells contain unique **plaques** (having a highly ordered substructure) in their thick luminal plasma membrane and flattened **elliptical vesicles** in their cytoplasm.
2. **Epithelium of the distended bladder**
   a. The epithelium of the distended bladder is only three to four cell layers thick.
   b. It has **squamous** superficial cells.
   c. It is much thinner and has a larger luminal surface than the relaxed bladder; this results from insertion of the elliptical vesicles into the luminal plasma membrane of the surface cells.

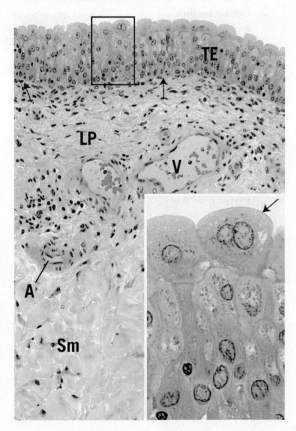

FIGURE 18.11. A light micrograph of the urinary bladder in a relaxed (empty) state. It is lined by transitional epithelium (TE) with dome-shaped surface cells and is separated from the underlying connective tissue by a basal lamina (*arrows*). A lamina propria (LP) of cellular, loose connective tissue may be distinguished from the submucosa (Sm) of dense connective tissue possessing many large collagen fibers. Note the venules (V) and an arteriole (A) present in the lamina propria (×132). *Inset.* The *boxed region* of transitional epithelium is here shown at higher magnification to demonstrate the large, dome-shaped surface cells (*arrow*), one of which is binucleated (×540). The transitional epithelium undergoes marked changes. In contrast to the relaxed state of the bladder shown here, when the bladder is distended and full of urine, the dome-shaped surface cells become squamous due to the insertion of unusual "elliptical-shaped vesicles" into their plasma membrane, and the entire epithelium is often reduced to only three cell layers in thickness.

Bladder cancer is two to three times more common in men than in women.
More than 90% of bladder cancers originate in the transitional epithelium
lining the organ. The most common sign of bladder cancer is blood in the urine **(hematuria)**, which
may not be visible to the naked eye. Frequent urination and/or pain during urination are sometimes
present, but often the disease is symptomless. **Cystoscopy** is used to examine the lining of the bladder, to take tissue samples in order to characterize the tumor, and to determine the extent to which it
has penetrated into the bladder wall. Superficial bladder cancer (limited to the epithelial layer) has a
5-year survival rate of about 85%, but invasive bladder cancer has a less favorable prognosis.

D. **Urethra**
1. **Overview**
   a. The urethra conveys urine from the bladder to outside the body. In men, the urethra also
      carries semen during ejaculation.
   b. It has a **two-layer muscularis** consisting of an inner longitudinal and an outer circular layer
      of smooth muscle.
   c. It is surrounded at some point by an **external sphincter of skeletal muscle**, which permits
      its voluntary closure.
2. **Male urethra**
   a. The male urethra is about 20 cm long and is divided into **prostatic, membranous**, and
      cavernous portions.
   b. It is lined by **transitional epithelium** in the prostatic portion and by **pseudostratified** or
      stratified columnar epithelium in the other two portions. The **fossa navicularis**, located at
      the distal end of the cavernous urethra, is lined by **stratified squamous epithelium**.
   c. It contains mucus-secreting **glands of Littre** in the lamina propria.
3. **Female urethra**
   a. The female urethra is much shorter (4–5 cm long) than the male urethra.
   b. It is lined primarily by **stratified squamous epithelium**, although patches of pseudostratified
      columnar epithelium are present.
   c. It may contain **glands of Littre** in the lamina propria.

Review Test

Directions: Each of the numbered items or incomplete statements in this section is followed by answers or completions of the statement. Select the ONE lettered answer that is BEST in each case.

1. Which of the following statements concerning the structure of medullary rays is true?

(A) They contain arched collecting tubules.
(B) They contain proximal convoluted tubules.
(C) They do not extend into the renal cortex.
(D) They lie at the center of a renal lobule.
(E) They contain thin limbs of the loops of Henle.

2. Which one of the following structures is located in the renal cortex?

(A) Vasa recta
(B) Thin limbs of the loops of Henle
(C) Afferent arterioles
(D) Interlobar veins
(E) Area cribrosa

3. Which of the following structures is present in the male urethra but is not present in the female urethra?

(A) Stratified squamous epithelium
(B) Transitional epithelium
(C) Glands of Littre
(D) External sphincter of skeletal muscle
(E) Connective tissue layer underlying the epithelium

4. Which of the following statements concerning cortical collecting tubules is always true?

(A) They are lined by a simple epithelium containing two types of cells.
(B) They are also known as the ducts of Bellini.
(C) They empty on the area cribrosa.
(D) They are permeable to water.
(E) They are continuous with the ascending thick limb of the Henle loop.

5. A 35-year-old woman had surgery to remove a cerebral tumor. A month after the procedure, she reports being excessively thirsty and drinking several liters of water per day. She must also urinate so frequently that she avoids leaving the house. Laboratory tests indicate that her urine has very low specific gravity. What is the most likely diagnosis of this woman's condition?

(A) Acute renal failure
(B) Glomerulonephritis
(C) Chronic renal failure
(D) Diabetes insipidus
(E) Urinary incontinence

6. The countercurrent multiplier system in the kidney involves the exchange of water and ions between the renal interstitium and

(A) the blood in the vasa recta.
(B) the blood in the peritubular capillary network.
(C) the filtrate in the proximal convoluted tubule.
(D) the filtrate in the loop of Henle.
(E) the filtrate in the medullary collecting tubule.

7. As the glomerular filtrate passes through the uriniferous tubule, ions and water are exchanged (actively or passively) with the renal interstitium, resulting in the filtrate being isotonic, hypotonic, or hypertonic relative to blood plasma. During a condition of antidiuresis, which part of the uriniferous tubule would contain a hypertonic filtrate?

(A) Ascending thick limb of the loop of Henle
(B) Bowman (capsular) space
(C) Cortical collecting tubule
(D) Medullary collecting tubule
(E) Proximal convoluted tubule

8. As the glomerular filtrate passes through the uriniferous tubule, ions and water are exchanged (actively or passively) with the renal interstitium, resulting in the filtrate being isotonic, hypotonic, or hypertonic relative to blood plasma. During a condition of antidiuresis, which part of the uriniferous tubule would contain an isotonic filtrate?

(A) Ascending thick limb of the loop of Henle
(B) Bottom of descending thin limb of loop of Henle
(C) Bowman (capsular) space
(D) Medullary collecting tubule
(E) Papillary collecting tubule

9. As the glomerular filtrate passes through the uriniferous tubule, ions and water are exchanged (actively or passively) with the renal interstitium, resulting in the filtrate being isotonic, hypotonic, or hypertonic relative to blood plasma. During a condition of antidiuresis, which one of the following parts of the uriniferous tubule would contain a hypotonic filtrate?

(A) Bowman (capsular) space
(B) Cortical collecting tubule
(C) Distal portion of the ascending thick limb of the loop of Henle
(D) Medullary collecting tubule
(E) Proximal convoluted tubule

10. As the glomerular filtrate passes through the uriniferous tubule, ions and water are exchanged (actively or passively) with the renal interstitium, resulting in the filtrate being isotonic, hypotonic, or hypertonic relative to blood plasma. During a condition of antidiuresis, which part of the uriniferous tubule would contain a hypertonic filtrate?

(A) Bottom of descending thin limb of loop of Henle
(B) Bowman (capsular) space
(C) Distal portion of the ascending thick limb of the loop of Henle
(D) Pars recta of the proximal tubule
(E) Proximal convoluted tubule

Answers and Explanations

1. **D.** A medullary ray contains the straight portions of tubules projecting from the medulla into the cortex, giving the appearance of striations or rays. A renal lobule consists of a central medullary ray and its closely associated cortical tissue (see Chapter 18 II E).

2. **C.** Afferent arterioles, which arise from interlobular arteries and supply the glomerular capillaries, are located in the renal cortex (see Chapter 18 III A 5).

3. **B.** Only the male urethra contains transitional epithelium (in the prostatic portion). Stratified squamous epithelium lines most of the female urethra and the distal end of the cavernous urethra in men. Mucus-secreting glands of Littre are always present in the male urethra and may be present in the female urethra (see Chapter 18 VI D).

4. **A.** Cortical collecting tubules are lined by a simple epithelium containing principal (light) cells and intercalated (dark) cells. They are permeable to water only in the presence of ADH; in the absence of this hormone, they are impermeable to water. The large papillary collecting tubules, called ducts of Bellini, empty on the area cribrosa at the apex of each renal papilla (see Chapter 18 III B).

5. **D.** This woman has diabetes insipidus. Surgical removal of the cerebral tumor likely damaged her hypothalamus, which in turn greatly reduced or eliminated the production of ADH. Therefore, her kidney collecting tubules and distal tubules fail to resorb water, resulting in the production of vast quantities of dilute urine and causing excessive thirst (see Chapter 18 V C Clinical Considerations).

6. **D.** The countercurrent multiplier system in the loop of Henle involves ion and water exchanges between the filtrate and the interstitium. It establishes an osmotic gradient in the interstitium of the medulla, which is greatest at the papilla (see Chapter 18 V B).

7. **D.** The filtrate that enters the cortical collecting tubules is nearly isotonic. When antidiuretic hormone is present (antidiuresis), water is removed from the filtrate in the collecting tubules, making the filtrate hypertonic by the time it reaches the medullary collecting tubules (see Chapter 18 V C).

8. **C.** Filtration of blood in the renal corpuscle yields an isotonic ultrafiltrate that enters the Bowman (capsular) space (see Chapter 18 V B).

9. **C.** The ascending thick limb of the loop of Henle is impermeable to water even in the presence of ADH, but it actively transports Cl^- from the filtrate into the interstitium (Na^+ follows passively). As a result, the filtrate becomes hypotonic as it approaches the distal convoluted tubule (see Chapter 18 V B).

10. **A.** The filtrate remains isotonic from the Bowman space throughout the proximal tubule, including the pars recta (also called the thick descending limb of the loop of Henle). As it passes through the descending thin limb of the loop of Henle, the filtrate loses water to the interstitium and gains Na^+ and Cl^-, becoming hypertonic (see Chapter 18 V B).

Female Reproductive System

I. OVERVIEW—FEMALE REPRODUCTIVE SYSTEM

A. The female reproductive system consists of the paired **ovaries** and **oviducts**; the **uterus, vagina,** and **external genitalia**; and the paired **mammary glands**, although technically, the mammary glands are part of the integument since they are highly modified sweat glands.

B. The female reproductive system undergoes marked changes at the onset of puberty, which is initiated by **menarche**.

C. It exhibits monthly menstrual cycles and menses from puberty until the end of the reproductive years, which terminate at **menopause**.

II. OVARIES (Figures 19.1 and 19.2)

A. Overview and embryonic development
   1. Overview
      a. Ovaries are covered by a simple cuboidal epithelium called the **germinal epithelium**.
      b. Deep to the germinal epithelium, the ovaries possess a capsule, the **tunica albuginea** that is composed of a dense, irregular collagenous connective tissue.
      c. Each ovary is subdivided into a **cortex** and a **medulla**, which are not sharply delineated.
   2. Development
      a. Embryonic development of the gonads is a function of the **SRY gene** (**sex-determining region on the Y** chromosome). If the Y chromosome is present, the SRY gene is expressed producing the **SRY protein**, which is the **testis-determining factor**, resulting in the formation of testes. In the absence of the Y chromosome, **ovaries** will be developed.
      b. During the sixth week of embryogenesis, **primitive germ cells** leave the **yolk sac** to enter the gonadal ridges. Once there, they undergo cell division and increase their number. The gonadal ridges still do not have distinguishing male or female characteristics and, therefore, they are referred to as **indifferent gonads**.
      c. Approximately 6 weeks later (fourth month of development), cells, perhaps supplemented by cells of the germinal epithelium, migrate to the primitive germ cells, surrounding each germ cell, now referred to as an **oogonium**, to form a single layer of cells known as **follicular cells** around each oogonium. Only about 500,000 oogonia will be surrounded by follicular cells; oogonia that have no follicular cell sheath undergo **apoptosis**.

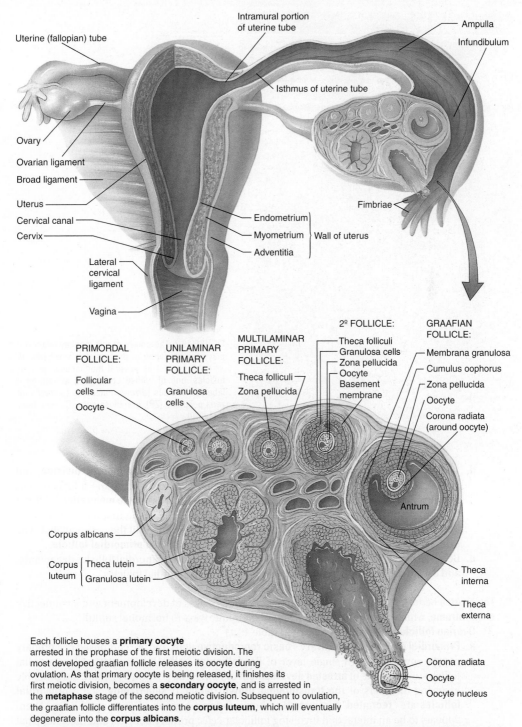

Each follicle houses a **primary oocyte** arrested in the prophase of the first meiotic division. The most developed graafian follicle releases its oocyte during ovulation. As that primary oocyte is being released, it finishes its first meiotic division, becomes a **secondary oocyte**, and is arrested in the **metaphase** stage of the second meiotic division. Subsequent to ovulation, the graafian follicle differentiates into the **corpus luteum**, which will eventually degenerate into the **corpus albicans**.

FIGURE 19.1. Structural features of the ovary. Follicles and corpus luteum are in different stages of development. Each follicle houses a *primary oocyte* arrested in the prophase of the first meiotic division. The most developed graafian follicle releases its oocyte during ovulation. As that primary oocyte is being released, it finishes its first meiotic division, becomes a *secondary oocyte*, and is arrested in the *metaphase* stage of the second meiotic division. Subsequent to ovulation, the graafian follicle differentiates into the *corpus luteum*, which will eventually degenerate into the *corpus albicans*. (Reprinted with permission from Gartner LP, Hiatt JL. *Color Atlas of Histology*. 3rd ed. Baltimore, MD: Lippincott Williams & Wilkins; 2000:342.)

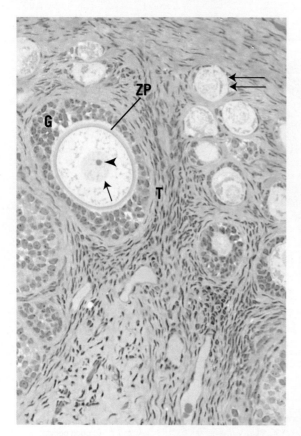

FIGURE 19.2. The cortex of this monkey ovary displays the presence of primordial follicles (*double arrows*) as well as several multilaminar primary follicles, one of whose constituent structures is labeled. Nucleus (*arrow*), nucleolus (*arrowhead*), zona pellucida (ZP), granulosa cells (G), and theca (T) (×270).

    d. The oogonia that are surrounded by follicular cells begin their **first meiotic division**, and are known as **primary oocytes**. In response to the meiotic division, the follicular cells manufacture and release a meiosis-preventing factor known as **oocyte maturation inhibitor (OMI)** that arrests the primary oocyte in the diplotene stage of the first meiotic division, and the primary oocytes remain in that arrested development until they are ovulated. The primary oocyte and its sheath of follicular cells are known as the **primordial follicle**.

    e. Between birth and the 11th year of life, more than 60% of the primordial follicles degenerate, and each ovary will be left with approximately 80,000 primordial follicles.

B. The ovarian cortex consists of **ovarian follicles** in various stages of development and a connective tissue **stroma**, which contains cells that respond in unique ways to hormonal stimuli.

  1. **Ovarian follicles** (Figures 19.1 and 19.2; Table 19.1)

    a. **Primordial follicles** are the ovary's **basic reproductive units** and are composed of a **primary oocyte** enveloped by a single layer of flat **follicular cells** (Figure 19.2). All primordial follicles are in a state of **arrested development** until in some unknown fashion, but probably involving members of the **transforming growth factor β superfamily**, some **primordial follicles** are "recruited" (**activated**) to begin to form a group of growing follicles. There appears to be an interaction involving follicular cells, primary oocytes, and mesenchymal cells of the ovarian cortex and, possibly, **insulin** and **follicle-stimulating hormone (FSH)** may also have a role in the recruitment of primordial follicles.

      (1) Primary oocytes

        (a) display a prominent, acentric, vesicular-appearing nucleus (**germinal vesicle**) possessing a single nucleolus.

        (b) have many Golgi complexes, mitochondria, profiles of rough endoplasmic reticulum (RER), well-developed annulate lamellae, as well as **cortical granules**

table **19.1**	Stages in the Development of Ovarian Follicles				
Stage	Zona Pellucida	Follicular Cell Layer (Granulosa)	Liquor Folliculi	Theca	Hormone Dependency
Primordial follicle	Not present	Single layer of flat cells	Not present	Not present	Dependent on local factors
Unilaminar primary follicle	Present	Single layer of cuboidal cells	Not present	Not present	Dependent on local factors
Multilaminar primary follicle	Present	Multiple layers of granulosa cells	Not present	Interna, externa present	Dependent on local factors
Secondary follicle	Present	Spaces among granulosa cells	Accumulates in spaces among granulosa cells	Interna, externa present	FSH dependent
Graafian follicle	Present	Forms membrana granulosa, cumulus oophorus	Fills the antrum	Interna, externa present	FSH dependent until becomes dominant follicle

FSH, follicle-stimulating hormone.

located just beneath the oocyte plasmalemma that contain enzymes that cleave proteins.

   (c) as stated above, become **arrested in prophase (dictyate stage) of meiosis I** by paracrine factors **OMI** produced by the follicular cells during fetal life and remain in this stage until ovulation (perhaps for as long as 40 years).

  (2) Follicular cells are

   (a) attached to one another by **desmosomes**.

   (b) separated from the surrounding stroma by a basal lamina.

b. Growing follicles

  (1) Primordial and primary follicles are **not dependent on FSH** for their development; instead, local factors such as **epidermal growth factor, insulin-like growth factor (IGF), activin**, and **Ca²⁺ ions**, stimulate the development of primordial and primary follicles. However, some authors are suggesting that even these early follicles may be FSH dependent.

  (2) Primary follicles are of two types, unilaminar and multilaminar. They possess an amorphous layer **(zona pellucida)** surrounding and produced by the primary oocyte (although some authors suggest that the follicular cells also make a contribution to its formation). The zona pellucida (ZP) separates the follicular cells from the primary oocyte. Follicular cells begin to express **FSH receptors** on their plasmalemma surface, and they also form gap junctions with each other as well as with the microvilli of the primary oocyte. A basal lamina is present at the interface of the follicular cells with the stroma.

   • **The zona pellucida** is a glycoprotein covering of the primary oocyte.

   • It is composed of four glycoproteins, known as ZP 1, ZP 2, ZP 3, and ZP 4.

   • **ZP 3** permits the binding of spermatozoon and facilitates the occurrence of the **acrosome reaction**.

   • **ZP 2** is also responsible for binding spermatozoon. After fertilization (discussed in Section VI below) has occurred, the ovum secretes the enzyme **ovastacin**, which degrades ZP 2, preventing the binding of additional spermatozoa to the zona pellucida.

   • **ZP 1** functions in cross-linking ZP 2 with ZP 3, thus preventing more spermatozoa from binding.

   • The function of **ZP 4** is not known.

   (a) Unilaminar primary follicles

    1. develop from primordial follicles.

    2. are composed of a single layer of **cuboidal** follicular cells surrounding the primary oocyte.

(b) Multilaminar primary follicles (Figure 19.2)
1. develop from unilaminar follicles by proliferation of follicular cells.
2. proliferate because of the protein **activin**, a product of the primary oocyte. Activin also promotes the release of FSH and its binding to FSH receptors. Additionally, the primary oocyte releases the growth factors **bone morphogenic protein 15 (BMP-15)** and **growth differentiation factor 9 (GDF-9),** both of which induce granulosa cell proliferation.
3. consist of several layers of follicular cells; these follicular cells are now also known as **granulosa cells**.
4. are circumscribed by two layers of stromal cells: an inner cellular layer (**theca interna**) and an outer fibro-muscular layer (**theca externa**). The theca interna is separated from the granulosa cells by a basal lamina.
5. Granulosa cells secrete **stem cell factor** (**kit-ligand**) that binds to kit ligand receptors on the surface of the **primary oocyte plasmalemma** as well as to kit ligand receptors on the surface of the **theca interna cell membranes**. The binding to **primary oocyte** kit ligand receptors is responsible for growth of the primary oocyte, and binding to kit ligand receptors on the **theca interna cells** facilitates their organization around the developing follicles.
6. Cells of the theca interna manufacture **androstenedione** (male sex hormone) and express **luteinizing hormone (LH) receptors** on their cell membranes.
7. Androstenedione penetrates the basal lamina and enters the granulosa cells, where the enzyme **aromatase** converts the male hormone into **estradiol**, the female hormone.

CLINICAL CONSIDERATIONS Mutations that affect the normal **connexin** synthesis result in the absence of graafian follicle formation as well as the inability of the oocyte to undergo meiotic division, with consequential female infertility. The most probable cause of the defects is the inability to exchange various necessary factors between follicular cells and the primary oocyte via the faulty gap junctions.

(3) **Secondary (antral) follicles**
(a) **Secondary follicles** are established when **liquor folliculi**, an exudate of plasma containing various hormones, such as activin, estradiol, follistatin, inhibin, and progesterone, and oocyte maturation iunhibitor (OMI), begins to accumulate in the spaces between granulosa cells. It is the OMI, synthesized by the granulosa cells, that prevents the oocyte from becoming larger than 125 μm in diameter and from completing its first meiotic division. The fluid-filled spaces will begin to coalesce, eventually to form a single large cavity called an antrum.
(b) Secondary follicles are **dependent on FSH**.
(c) As stated above, narrow **processes** extend from the granulosa cells into the zona pellucida.
(d) Granulosa cells contact each other via gap junctions and also form gap junctions with the cell membrane of the primary oocyte.
(e) Just as in the normal development of the primary follicle, the conversion from primary to secondary follicles is greatly dependent on **BMP-15** and **GDF-9**.
(f) Both granulosa cells and theca interna cells express LH receptors on their plasma membranes; additionally, granulosa cells also express FSH receptors on their cell membranes.
c. **Graafian (mature) follicle**
(1) The dominant graafian follicle is the one follicle among the secondary follicles that **will ovulate**. It is **FSH independent** and manufactures the hormone **inhibin** that shuts off FSH release by the basophils of the anterior pituitary gland, causing atresia of the other developing follicles (secondary and nondominant graafian follicles).

(2) It measures approximately 2.5 cm in diameter and is evident as a large bulge on the surface of the ovary.

(3) The primary oocyte is positioned off center on a small mound of granulosa cells (**cumulus oophorus**) that projects into the hyaluronic acid-rich **liquor folliculi-**containing **antrum** of the follicle. Granulosa cells surround the zona pellucida. Those contacting the zona pellucida are known as the **corona radiata**. Other granulosa cells line the antrum, forming the **membrana granulosa**.

(4) Theca interna cells, in response to luteinizing hormone (LH) binding to their LH receptors, manufacture **androstenedione (androgen)**, which is transferred to granulosa cells. The granulosa cells, under the influence of FSH binding to their FSH receptors, transform androstenedione into testosterone and, by the use of the enzyme **aromatase**, convert the testosterone into **estradiol (estrogen)**.

(5) The **theca externa** is composed of collagenous connective tissue enriched with a plethora of smooth muscle cells. It is also richly supplied with many blood vessels, which provide nourishment to the theca interna.

(6) Ovulation

    (a) An LH surge from the pituitary gland, along with the local factor manufactured by the primary oocyte, **maturation promoting factor** (a complex of **cyclin-dependent kinase** and **cyclin B**), triggers the **primary oocyte** to complete its first meiotic division just prior to **ovulation**, forming a **secondary oocyte** and the **first polar body**. The second meiotic division is triggered by the presence of local meiosis-inducing factors but is blocked at metaphase.

    (b) Ovulation also occurs in response to the LH surge. The secondary oocyte and its **corona radiata** cells leave the ruptured follicle at the ovarian surface to enter the fimbriated end of the oviduct.

    (c) The remnant of the graafian follicle becomes the **corpus hemorrhagicum** that is transformed into the **corpus luteum of menstruation**, a temporary structure that may remain functional for a couple of weeks and then degenerates into the **corpus albicans**. If the woman is pregnant, then the corpus hemorrhagicum becomes transformed into the **corpus luteum of pregnancy**, which remains functional for several months, and then it also degenerates into the **corpus albicans**.

(7) Time Period of Folliculogenesis. Although from the prior description of folliculogenesis it appears as if the entire process occurs within a single menstrual cycle, that is not the case. In fact, once a primordial follicle is recruited for development, almost a year is required before ovulation can occur, and it takes approximately 290 days to go from primordial to a completely developed secondary follicle and another 60 days or so for that follicle to become ovulated.

CLINICAL CONSIDERATIONS Some women experience a sudden abdominal (or pelvic) pain in the middle of their menstrual cycle that lasts 2 or 3 hours (although it may last as long as 48–72 hours or even longer), and they have attributed that to the process of ovulation. Although this attribution was not universally accepted, it is now known that the sudden **surge of LH** is followed by a similar surge in **prostaglandin F$_{2\alpha}$**, a pharmacologic agent that causes sudden, cramp-like contraction of the ovarian, fallopian tube, or uterine smooth muscle fibers. It is this violent contraction that is responsible for the pain experienced by some women. Other causes, such as painful distension of the ovarian follicles or the rupture of the tunica albuginea of the ovary, may also contribute to the ovulation pain.

---

2. The **corpus hemorrhagicum** is formed from the remnants of the graafian follicle. After the cumulus oophorus leaves the ovary, a little blood enters and forms a clot in the former antrum, and within a short period of time macrophages and connective tissue elements enter the region, and the macrophages dispose of the blood clot and other cellular debris. Once the macrophages have performed their function, the corpus hemorrhagicum, under the influence of various hormones, is converted into the corpus luteum. The hormones responsible for this transformation are: estrogens, prolactin, LH, human chorionic gonadotrophin (hCG), and insulin-like growth factors I and II (IGF-I and IGF-II).

3. **Corpus luteum**
   a. **Overview**
      (1) The corpus luteum is formed from the corpus hemorrhagicum. As the corpus hemorrhagicum collapses upon itself, its cellular components become greatly modified.
      (2) The corpus luteum is composed of **granulosa lutein cells** (modified granulosa cells) and **theca lutein cells** (modified theca interna cells).
      (3) The basement membrane between the theca interna and the former membrana granulosa disintegrates, and blood and lymph vessels arising from the theca interna invade the former membrana granulosa.
      (4) The formation of this richly vascularized **temporary endocrine gland** is dependent on LH.
   b. **Granulosa lutein cells**
      (1) Granulosa lutein cells are large (30 μm in diameter), pale cells that possess an abundance of smooth endoplasmic reticulum (SER), RER, many mitochondria, a well-developed Golgi complex, and lipid droplets.
      (2) They are derived from cells of the membrana granulosa.
      (3) Function. Granulosa lutein cells manufacture **progesterone** and convert androgens formed by the theca lutein cells into **estrogens**.
   c. **Theca lutein cells**
      (1) These small (15 μm in diameter) cells are concentrated mainly along the periphery of the corpus luteum.
      (2) They are derived from cells of the theca interna.
      (3) Function. Theca lutein cells manufacture **progesterone** and **androgens** and small amounts of estrogen.

4. The **corpus albicans** is the remnant of the degenerated corpus luteum. Its formation is due to the hypoxic conditions present in the corpus luteum as fibroblasts manufacture an overabundance of collagen. The fibrotic event elicits the arrival of **T cells** that release **interferon**-γ, a chemoattractant for macrophages, which release **tumor necrosis factor** α, a cytokine that drives both granulosa lutein and theca lutein cells into apoptosis. As the cell death and fibrosis progresses, the corpus albicans contracts and becomes a small scar on the surface of the ovary.

5. **Atretic follicles**
   a. **Atretic follicles** are follicles (in various stages of maturation) that are undergoing degeneration.
   b. They are commonly present in the ovary.
   c. After a dominant graafian follicle ovulates, the remaining graafian and secondary follicles degenerate because the **dominant follicle** releases **inhibin** that shuts off FSH production by the basophils of the anterior pituitary gland.
   d. They often show pyknotic changes in the nuclei of the granulosa cells and other degenerative changes.

C. The **ovarian medulla** contains large blood vessels, lymphatic vessels, and nerve fibers in a loose connective tissue stroma. They also possess a small number of **estrogen**-secreting **interstitial cells** and a few **androgen**-secreting **hilar cells**.

D. **Hormonal regulation** (Figure 19.3)
   1. **Control of follicle maturation and ovulation**
      a. The primary oocyte of unilaminar primary follicles secretes **activin**, which facilitates proliferation of granulosa cells. Granulosa cells secrete **stem cell factor** (**kit-ligand**) that binds to kit ligand receptors on the surface of the **primary oocyte plasmalemma** as well as to kit ligand receptors on the surface of the **theca interna cell membranes**. The binding to **primary oocyte** kit ligand receptors is responsible for growth of the primary oocyte, and binding to kit ligand receptors on the **theca interna cells** facilitates their organization around the developing follicles.
      b. Both the normal development of the primary follicle and the conversion from primary to secondary follicles is greatly dependent on **BMP-15** (bone morphogenic factor 15) and **GDF-9** (growth differentiation factor 9).

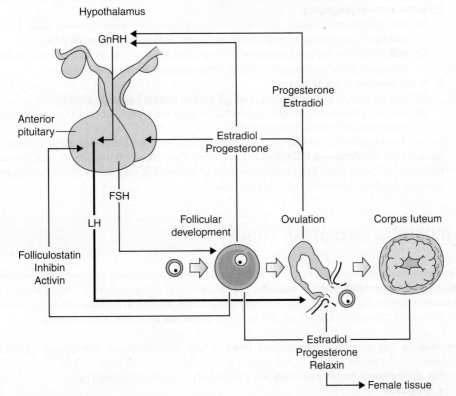

FIGURE 19.3. The hormonal relationship between the hypophysis and the reproductive system. The preferred term for gonadotropin-releasing hormone (GnRH) is LHRH, luteinizing hormone–releasing hormone. FSH, follicle-stimulating hormone; LH, luteinizing hormone. (Adapted with permission from Gartner LP, Hiatt JL. *Color Textbook of Histology*. Philadelphia, PA: Saunders; 1997:389.)

    c. Luteinizing hormone–releasing hormone (LHRH) (also known as gonadotropin-releasing hormone or GnRH) from the hypothalamus causes the release of FSH and LH from the pars distalis of the pituitary gland.

    d. FSH stimulates the growth and development of secondary (but, according to most authors, not earlier stage) ovarian follicles and the appearance of LH receptors on the granulosa cell plasmalemma. The regulation of FSH and LH is influenced by the following:

        (1) Theca interna cells manufacture androgens, which are converted to estrogens by granulosa cells.

        (2) Granulosa cells also secrete inhibin, follistatin, and activin, all of which (in addition to estrogen) regulate FSH secretion.

        (3) By approximately day 14 of the menstrual cycle, estrogen blood levels are sufficiently high to facilitate a sudden, brief surge of LH.

    e. Surge of LH

        (1) A surge of LH triggers the **primary oocyte** of the **dominant** graafian follicle to complete meiosis I and to enter meiosis II, where it is arrested at metaphase.

        (2) The dominant graafian follicle is no longer FSH dependent, and it releases the hormone **inhibin** that shuts off FSH release by the anterior pituitary, causing **atresia** of all developing FSH-dependent follicles.

        (3) The LH surge initiates ovulation of the secondary oocyte from the graafian follicle.

        (4) The LH surge promotes formation of the corpus luteum.

  2. Fate of the corpus luteum

    a. Luteal hormones

        (1) Progesterone, the major hormone secreted by the corpus luteum, inhibits the release of LH by suppressing the release of LHRH, but promotes the development of the uterine endometrium.

        (2) Estrogen inhibits the release of FSH by suppressing the release of LHRH.

        (3) Relaxin facilitates parturition.

b. **In the event of pregnancy,**

(1) the syncytiotrophoblast of the developing placenta manufactures **hCG** (human chorionic gonadotropin) and **human chorionic somatomammotropin (hCS)**.

(2) **hCG** maintains the corpus luteum of pregnancy for about 3 months, at which time the placenta takes over the production of progesterone, estrogen, and relaxin.

c. **In the absence of pregnancy,**

(1) neither LH nor hCG is present, and the **corpus luteum begins to atrophy**.

(2) lack of estrogen and progesterone also triggers the release of FSH from the pituitary, thus reinitiating the menstrual cycle.

3. In each menstrual cycle, only about five maturing follicles reach the graafian follicle stage; and usually only the **dominant follicle** undergoes ovulation. As mentioned above, the dominant follicle is FSH independent; it produces a surge of **inhibin** that suppresses FSH production and leads to atrophy of the other maturing follicles.

III. OVIDUCTS (FALLOPIAN TUBES)

Each of the two **oviducts** is about 12 cm in length and is subdivided into four regions: the **infundibulum**, which has a **fimbriated end**; the **ampulla**, which is its longest region (about 7 cm in length) and is the most common site of fertilization; the **isthmus**; and the **intramural portion**, which traverses the wall of the uterus. The wall of each oviduct consists of a **mucosa, muscularis**, and **serosa**.

A. The mucosa has extensive **longitudinal folds** in the infundibulum. The degree of folding progressively decreases in the remaining three regions of the oviduct (Figure 19.4).

1. The **epithelium** is **simple columnar** and consists of peg cells and ciliated cells.

a. **Peg cells**

(1) **Peg cells** (Figure 19.4) secrete a **nutrient-rich medium** that nourishes the spermatozoa (and preimplantation embryo), as well as cytokines that aid in the **capacitation** of spermatozoa.

(2) The presence of progesterone increases the number of peg cells.

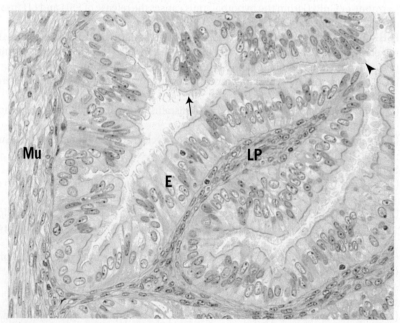

FIGURE 19.4. The mucosa of the ovary is highly convoluted, forming fingerlike processes, whose epithelial lining (E) is composed of two cell types, ciliated columnar cells (*arrow*) and peg cells (*arrowhead*). The richly vascularized lamina propria (LP) and the surrounding smooth muscle (Mu) coat are clearly evident (×270).

      (3) Their cytoplasm contains abundant RER, a well-developed Golgi complex, and many apical electron-dense secretory granules.

    b. Ciliated cells

      (1) Ciliated cells (Figure 19.4) possess many cilia, which beat mostly toward the lumen of the uterus.

      (2) The number of cilia and the intensity of their motion are increased by the presence of estrogen.

      (3) Function. Ciliated cells aid in the transport of the developing embryo to the uterus.

  2. The **lamina propria** (Figure 19.4) consists of loose connective tissue containing reticular fibers, fibroblasts, mast cells, and lymphoid cells.

B. Muscularis

  1. The muscularis is composed of an ill-defined inner circular and an outer longitudinal layer of smooth muscle.

  2. Function. By contracting rhythmically, the muscularis probably assists in moving the developing embryo toward the uterus.

C. The serosa, which is composed of a simple squamous epithelium overlying a thin connective tissue layer, covers the outer surface of the oviduct.

IV. UTERUS

The uterus has three regions, the **fundus, body (corpus)**, and **cervix**.

A. The uterine wall consists of the **endometrium, myometrium**, and **adventitia** (or serosa).

  1. Endometrium

    a. Overview

      (1) The endometrium (Figure 19.5), composed of an epithelial lining and a gland-rich connective tissue stroma, undergoes hormone-modulated cyclic alterations during the **menstrual cycle**, varying in thickness from less than 1 mm to 7 mm.

      (2) It is lined by a **simple columnar** epithelium containing **secretory** and **ciliated cells**.

      (3) Its stroma resembles mesenchymal connective tissue, with **stellate cells** and an abundance of **reticular fibers**. Macrophages and leukocytes are also present. The stroma houses the **simple tubular glands** of the endometrium.

    b. Layers of the endometrium

      (1) The **functional layer (functionalis)** is the thick superficial layer of the endometrium that is sloughed and reestablished monthly as a result of hormonal changes during the menstrual cycle.

      (2) The **basal layer (basalis)** is the deeper layer of the endometrium that is about 1 mm or less in thickness and is preserved during menstruation. It has **endometrial glands**, which have basal cells that provide a source for **reepithelialization** of the endometrium after the functional layer is shed.

    c. The **endometrial vascular supply** consists of two types of arteries derived from vessels in the **stratum vasculare** of the myometrium.

      (1) Coiled arteries extend into the functional layer and undergo pronounced changes during various stages of the menstrual cycle.

      (2) Straight arteries do not undergo cyclic changes and terminate in the basal layer.

CLINICAL CONSIDERATIONS **Endometriosis** is a condition in which the pelvic peritoneal cavity contains uterine endometrial tissue. It is associated with hormone-induced changes in the ectopic endometrium during the menstrual cycle. As the endometrium is shed, bleeding occurs in the peritoneal cavity, causing severe pain and the formation of cysts and adhesions. It may lead to **sterility** because the ovaries and oviducts become deformed and embedded in scar tissue. The factors that contribute to the occurrence of endometriosis are not known.

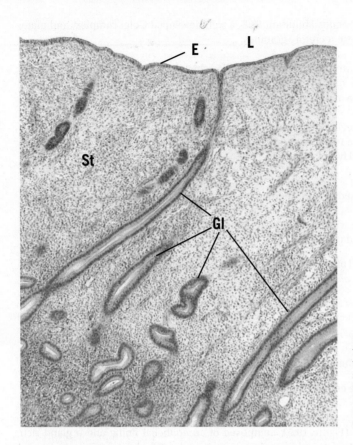

FIGURE 19.5. The uterine mucosa is in the process of being rebuilt during the follicular phase. The connective tissue stroma (St) is well developed, and uterine glands (Gl) are being formed and are beginning to become coiled. A simple columnar epithelium (E) lines the lumen (L) of the uterus (×53).

2. **Myometrium**
    a. The myometrium is the thick smooth muscle tunic of the uterus.
    b. It is composed of inner and outer longitudinal layers and a thick middle circular layer. The circular layer is richly **vascularized** and is often referred to as the **stratum vasculare**.
    c. The myometrium thickens during pregnancy because of the hypertrophy and hyperplasia of individual smooth muscle cells.
    d. Near the end of pregnancy, the myometrium develops many gap junctions between its smooth muscle cells. These junctions coordinate contraction of the muscle cells during parturition.
    e. At parturition, the myometrium undergoes powerful contractions triggered by the hormone **oxytocin** and by **prostaglandins** (both of which are increased at term).
    f. After parturition, the myometrium shrinks because many of the smooth muscle cells become deprived of estrogen and, therefore, undergo **apoptosis**.

3. **External covering**
    a. **Serosa** is present over surfaces of the uterus bulging into the peritoneal cavity.
    b. **Adventitia** is present along the retroperitoneal surfaces of the uterus.

B. **The menstrual cycle begins** on the day menstrual **bleeding appears**. At this time, the blood levels of **estrogen**, **progesterone**, **FSH**, and **LH** are very low.
    1. **Menstrual phase (days 1–4)** is characterized by a **hemorrhagic discharge (menses)** of the functional layer of the endometrium.
        a. It is triggered by **spasms of contraction** and **relaxation** of the coiled arteries (caused by low levels of progesterone and estrogen). Long-term (2–3 days) **vasoconstriction** of these arteries causes ischemia and eventual necrosis.
        b. Vasoconstriction is followed by sudden, intermittent **vasodilation** of the coiled arteries, which ruptures their walls, flooding the stroma with blood, detaching the functional layer, and dislodging the necrotic tissue.

    c. Because the basal layer is supplied by short straight vessels that do not undergo prolonged vasoconstriction, it is not sloughed and does not become necrotic.

    d. During the menstrual phase of the menstrual cycle, blood clotting is inhibited.

2. The **proliferative (follicular) phase** (Figure 19.5), **days 4 to 14**, follows the menstrual phase and involves **renewal of the entire functional layer**, including the repair of glands, connective tissue, and vascular elements (specifically, the coiled arteries). During the proliferative phase, the levels of **estrogen** in the blood continue to rise, and this is the principal hormone responsible for the stage of proliferation.

    a. The epithelium that lines the luminal surface of the uterus is renewed by mitotic activity of cells remaining in the uterine glands of the basal layer of the endometrium.

    b. Glands are straight and lined by a simple columnar epithelium.

    c. Stromal cells divide, accumulate glycogen, and enlarge.

    d. Coiled arteries extend approximately two-thirds of the way into the endometrium.

    e. At the end of the proliferative phase, the endometrium is approximately 3 mm in thickness.

3. The **secretory (luteal) phase (days 15–28)** begins shortly after ovulation and is characterized by a **thickening of the endometrium**, resulting from edema and secretion by the endometrial glands. **Progesterone**, and to a certain degree **estrogen**, are the principal hormones driving the secretory phase.

    a. Glands become **coiled**; their lumina become filled with a secretion of **glycoprotein material** and **glycogen**; and their cells accumulate large amounts of **glycogen**, in the basal aspect of their cytoplasm.

    b. Coiled arteries become not only more highly coiled but also longer, extending into the superficial aspects of the functional layer.

    c. At the end of the secretory phase, the endometrium is somewhat edematous and is approximately 6 to 7 mm in thickness.

CLINICAL CONSIDERATIONS   **Uterine prolapse** is a condition in which the uterine ligaments, namely the round ligament, broad ligament, uterosacral ligaments, and the ligament of the ovary, are no longer able to maintain the normal anatomical position of this organ, and the uterus slides down and frequently bulges into the vagina. The uterus may occupy only the upper one-third of the vagina or may slide all the way down to protrude through the vaginal orifice between the labia minora and majora. Uterine prolapse usually occurs in older women, but may also be present in younger women who had very large babies and a prolonged, difficult delivery. Extensive prolapse of the uterus may interfere with urination as well as with defecation. The usual treatment for uterine prolapse is surgical reattachment or, in more extreme cases, hysterectomy.

V. CERVIX

A. The cervix does not participate in menstruation, but its **secretions change** during various stages of the menstrual cycle.

B. The cervical wall is composed mainly of dense collagenous connective tissue interspersed with numerous elastic fibers and a few smooth muscle cells.

C. The cervix has a **simple columnar (mucus-secreting) epithelium** except for the inferior portion (continuous with the lining of the vagina), which is covered by a **stratified squamous nonkeratinized epithelium**.

D. Branched **cervical glands** secrete a serous fluid near the time of ovulation that facilitates the entry of spermatozoa into the uterine lumen. During pregnancy, cervical glands produce a thick, viscous secretion that hinders the entry of spermatozoa (and microorganisms) into the uterus.

E. Prior to parturition, the cervix dilates and softens as a result of the lysis of the collagen fiber bundles in response to the hormone **relaxin**.

> **CLINICAL CONSIDERATIONS**
>
> 1. In a **Papanicolaou (Pap) smear**, epithelial cells are scraped from the lining of the cervix (or vagina) and are examined to detect cervical cancer. A Pap smear shows **variation in cell populations** with stages of the menstrual cycle.
> 2. **Carcinoma of the cervix** originates from stratified squamous nonkeratinized epithelial cells. It may be contained within the epithelium and not invade the underlying stroma (**carcinoma in situ**), or it may penetrate the basal lamina and metastasize to other parts of the body (**invasive carcinoma**). It occurs at a relatively high frequency, but may be cured by surgery if discovered early (by Pap smear), before it becomes invasive.

VI. FERTILIZATION AND IMPLANTATION

A. Fertilization

1. Fertilization usually takes place within the ampulla **of the oviduct**, and occurs when a spermatozoon penetrates the corona radiata and the zona pellucida and pierces the plasma membrane of a **secondary oocyte**.

   a. Before a spermatozoon is capable of fertilizing, it must undergo **maturation**, and **capacitation**, and **hyperactivity**.

   (1) Maturation occurs in the male reproductive tract. Prior to maturation, the spermatozoon cannot travel in a forward direction; instead, it travels only in a circular fashion.

   (2) Capacitation occurs in the female reproductive tract. While the sperm is in the male reproductive tract, it is unable to undergo capacitation because the concentration of the prostate-manufactured **fertilization-promoting peptide (FPP)** is too high. Once the sperm arrives in the female reproductive tract, the concentration of FPP is reduced to a suitable level (because it becomes diluted by the vaginal secretions), and the sperm is prompted to begin the process of capacitation.

   (a) Cholesterol molecules are removed from the acrosomal plasmalemma, making the membrane less rigid.

   (b) Special Ca^{2+} **ion channels** open in the plasma membrane of the spermatozoon flagella, permitting the influx of calcium ions.

   (c) Elevated levels of intraflagellar calcium ions induce the formation of **cAMP**, which causes the spermatozoon to become hyperactive.

   (3) Hyperactivity is merely the ability of the spermatozoon to swim faster and more vigorously, making it easier for the sperm to penetrate the zona pellucida to contact the oocyte.

   b. Once the spermatozoon has undergone capacitation, it is capable of fertilizing the egg, but in order to do so it must undergo the **acrosome reaction, bind to ZP3**, and **fuse to the plasma membrane of the secondary oocyte**.

   (1) The acrosome reaction and **binding to ZP3** occur when the spermatozoon contacts the zona pellucida. Hydrolytic enzymes, especially **acrosin**, are released from the acrosome, reduce the viscosity of the zona pellucida just ahead of the spermatozoon, permitting it to reach the secondary oocyte.

   (2) Fusion of the spermatozoon membrane and the secondary oocyte plasmalemma occurs due to the presence of **fertilin**, an integral protein in the spermatozoon membrane with **CD9 molecules** and **integrins** of the secondary oocyte's plasmalemma.

   c. The **secondary oocyte** responds to the contact by the spermatozoon by undergoing the **cortical reaction, resuming the second meiotic division**, and forming the **female pronucleus**.

   (1) The **cortical granules** of the secondary oocyte, located just deep to the cell membrane, fuse with the cell membrane, releasing their enzymes into the zona pellucida. The ZP proteins form a complex with each other, which transforms the gelatinous nature of the zona pellucida into a highly viscous substance that stops other spermatozoa from reaching the secondary oocyte, thus preventing **polyspermy**.

(2) The contact of spermatozoon with the secondary oocyte permits the entry of the **spermatozoon's nucleus (male pronucleus)** and **centrosome** to enter the secondary oocyte's cytoplasm, triggering the oocyte to **complete its second meiotic division**, forming the **second polar body** and thus transforming the secondary oocyte into the **ovum**.

(3) The now haploid nucleus of the ovum is known as the **female pronucleus**. The two haploid pronuclei travel toward each other, shed their nuclear envelopes, their chromosomes intermingle as they form a **diploid cell**, known as the **zygote**. Immediately after the intermingling of the chromosomes, the centrosome, contributed by the spermatozoon, forms a mitotic spindle apparatus, and the zygote undergoes its **first mitotic** division. The two newly formed daughter cells are the first two cells of the new embryo. It should be noted that all centrosomes of the new individual are derived from the father, and all of the mitochondria are derived from the mother.

B. Implantation

1. The **zygote** undergoes mitotic cell division (known as **cleavage** during the early stages of embryogenesis) and is transformed into a multicellular structure called a **morula**, which requires about 3 days to travel through the oviduct and enter the uterus.

2. The **conceptus** (the preimplantation embryo and its surrounding membranes) acquires a fluid-filled cavity and becomes a blastocyst.

3. The **blastocyst** implants in the endometrium of the uterus and is surrounded by an inner cellular layer, the **cytotrophoblast**, and an outer multinucleated layer, the **syncytiotrophoblast**.

4. The **syncytiotrophoblast** further invades the endometrium in the wall of the uterus by the sixth day after fertilization. Formation of the placenta then begins.

CLINICAL CONSIDERATIONS

1. Ectopic (tubal) pregnancy is the **implantation** of the early **embryo** in an abnormal site (e.g., **wall of the oviduct**). It can be **fatal** without immediate medical intervention.

2. Teratomas are germ cell tumors that fall into three groups: mature, monodermal, and immature.

a. Mature teratomas are benign (although occasionally they may become malignant) and are usually present in young women. These are cysts with walls that frequently contain hair and other epidermal structures such as sebaceous glands, as well as bone, tooth, and cartilage fragments.

b. Monodermal teratomas are rare tumors that are also known as specialized teratomas. The two most frequent types of these tumors are struma ovarii and ovarian carcinoid. **Struma ovarii** is an ovarian tumor composed of well-developed thyroid follicles that produce thyroid hormone and may be responsible for hyperthyroidism. **Ovarian carcinoid** is a tumor that usually produces serotonin (5-OH-tryptamine).

c. Immature teratomas are fast-growing malignant tumors with a histology that resembles that of fetal rather than mature tissues. They are usually present in adolescents and very young women.

VII. PLACENTA

The placenta is a **transient** structure, consisting of a **maternal portion** and a **fetal portion**.

A. Structure

1. At birth it is approximately 18 cm in diameter, 2.5 cm thick, and weighs about 600 g.

2. As the placenta begins its development, the **cytotrophoblasts** and **syncytiotrophoblasts** form the **chorion**, and in response, the endometrium of the uterus forms the **decidua**.

3. The chorion develops into the **chorionic plate**, which gives rise to the **chorionic villi**.

4. The decidua has three regions—**decidua basalis**, **decidua capsularis**, and **decidua parietalis**— but only the decidua basalis forms the majority of the maternal portion of the placenta.
5. Maternal blood vessels invade the decidua basalis, forming large blood-filled spaces known as **lacunae**.
6. Chorionic villi of the developing fetus become vascularized, and capillary beds form within the villi. The chorionic villi grow into the lacunae, and receive nutrients and oxygen from and deliver waste products and carbon dioxide into the maternal blood of the lacunae.
7. This transfer of nutrients and waste products occurs across a barrier, the **placental barrier**, interposed between the maternal blood and fetal blood. The narrowest placental barrier is composed of the following (the presence of connective tissue elements between the two basal laminae enlarges the thickness of the placental barrier):
   a. Endothelial cells of the fetal capillaries
   b. Basal lamina of the fetal capillary endothelium
   c. Basal lamina of the cytotrophoblasts
   d. Cytotrophoblasts
   e. Syncytiotrophoblasts

B. **Function** (See Table 19.2)
   1. The placenta permits the exchange of various materials between the maternal and fetal circulatory systems. This exchange occurs **without** mixing of the two separate blood supplies.
   2. It secretes **progesterone, hCG** (human chorionic gonadotropin), **chorionic thyrotropin**, and **hCS (human chorionic somatomammotropin)**, a lactogenic and growth-promoting hormone as well as endothelial growth factor, IGF-I and II, fibroblast growth factor, colony-stimulating

t a b l e **19.2** Hormones Produced by the Placenta		
Hormone	Cells Producing Hormone	Function of Hormone
hCG	Cytotrophoblasts	Maintains corpus luteum
hCS (also known as human placental lactogen)	Syncytiotrophoblasts	Regulates glucose metabolism; stimulates proliferation of mammary gland duct
IGF I and IGF II	Cytotrophoblasts	Stimulates growth and proliferation of cytotrophoblasts
EGF	Early (4–5 weeks): cytotrophoblasts Late (6–12 weeks): syncytiotrophoblast	Stimulates development and maintains functions of trophoblasts
Relaxin	Decidual cells	Makes cervix and fibrocartilage of pubic symphysis more pliable for parturition
Leptin	Syncytiotrophoblasts	Controls maternal nutrient status and facilitates transport of nutrients across the placental barrier
Fibroblast growth factor	Syncytiotrophoblasts	Facilitates proliferation of cytotrophoblasts
Colony-stimulating factor	Syncytiotrophoblasts	Facilitates proliferation of cytotrophoblasts
Platelet-derived growth factor	Syncytiotrophoblasts	Facilitates proliferation of cytotrophoblasts
Interleukin 1	Syncytiotrophoblasts	Facilitates proliferation of cytotrophoblasts
Interleukin 3	Syncytiotrophoblasts	Facilitates proliferation of cytotrophoblasts
Tumor necrosis factor	Syncytiotrophoblasts	Inhibits proliferation of cytotrophoblasts

hCG, human chorionic gonadotropin; hCS, human chorionic somatomammotropin; IGF-I and II, insulin-like growth factors I and II; EGF, endothelial growth factor.

factor, platelet-derived growth factor, tumor necrosis growth factor, relaxin, leptin, and interleukins 1 and 3.
3. It also produces **estrogen** with the assistance of the liver and the adrenal cortex of the fetus.
4. Decidual cells of the stroma produce **prostaglandins** and **prolactin**.

CLINICAL CONSIDERATIONS The polypeptide hormone **prolactin**, manufactured by basophils of the adenohypophysis (anterior pituitary), causes an increase in breast size in the pregnant female and induces milk formation as well as lactation in the mammary glands of the postpartum female. Interestingly, it also causes the feeling of sexual gratification subsequent to the sexual act. Because progesterone has been shown to alleviate the symptoms of multiple sclerosis (MS) in the pregnant female, recent investigations using a mouse model demonstrated that treatment of MS-afflicted mice with prolactin resulted in remyelination of nerve fibers, whose myelin was destroyed by the disease. It is believed that prolactin stimulates the formation of prooligodendrocytes, which differentiate into oligodendrocytes, cells that are responsible for myelination of axons in the central nervous system.

VIII. VAGINA

A. **Overview**
1. The vagina is a **fibromuscular canal** with a wall that is composed of three layers: an inner **mucosa**, a middle **muscularis**, and an external **adventitia**.
2. It is circumscribed by a **skeletal muscle** sphincter at its external orifice.
3. It lacks glands throughout its length and is lubricated by secretions from the cervix and by seepage of the extracellular fluid from the vascular supply of the lamina propria.

B. **The mucosa** is composed of a thick, **stratified squamous nonkeratinized epithelium** and a fibroelastic connective tissue, the **lamina propria**.
1. The **epithelium** contains **glycogen**, which is used by the vaginal bacterial flora to produce **lactic acid**, an acid that lowers the pH during the follicular phase of the menstrual cycle and inhibits invasion by pathogens.
2. The **lamina propria** is a fibroelastic connective tissue that is **highly vascular** in its deeper aspect (which is possibly analogous to a submucosa).

C. **The muscularis** is composed of irregularly arranged layers of **smooth muscle** (thin inner circular layer and a thicker outer longitudinal layer) interspersed with **elastic fibers**.

D. **The adventitia** is composed of **fibroelastic** connective tissue. It attaches the vagina to the surrounding structures.

IX. EXTERNAL GENITALIA (VULVA)

A. **The labia majora** are **fat-laden folds of skin; hair and** secretions of **sebaceous glands** and **sweat glands** are present on their external surfaces.

B. **Labia minora**
1. The labia minora are folds of skin that possess a core of **highly vascular** connective tissue containing elastic fibers.
2. They lack hair follicles, but their dermis contains numerous **sebaceous glands**, which open directly onto the epithelial surface.

C. **The vestibule** is the space between the two labia minora. **Glands of Bartholin (mucus-secreting glands)** and numerous smaller mucus-secreting glands around the urethra and clitoris (**minor vestibular glands**) open into this space.

D. **Clitoris**
   1. The clitoris is composed of two small, cylindrical **erectile bodies**, which terminate in the prepuce-covered **glans clitoridis**.
   2. It contains many sensory nerve fibers and specialized nerve endings (e.g., Meissner corpuscles and pacinian corpuscles).

X. MAMMARY GLANDS

Mammary glands of both genders are identical for the first decade or so of life, but when the female reaches puberty, the flow of estrogens and progesterone as well as lactogenic hormone induces the mammary gland to enlarge and develop a system of lobules and terminal ductules as well as an increase in the connective tissue mass and a deposit of adipose tissue. Each mammary gland of the postpubertal female is composed of numerous **compound tubuloalveolar glands**, each with its own lactiferous sinus and a duct that opens at the apex of the nipple.

CLINICAL CONSIDERATIONS The use of lavender oil and tea tree oil–based products in prepubescent males has been shown to cause gynecomastia, the development of breasts in these individuals. The presence of the breast tissue persisted for several months after the boys stopped using these products, and then slowly regressed to its normal condition. It appears that these oil products are able to imitate estrogens and even inhibit the effects of androgens.

A. **Resting (nonlactating) mammary glands** (in adult, nonpregnant women)
   1. Resting mammary glands are composed of **lactiferous sinuses** and **ducts** lined in most areas by a stratified cuboidal epithelium, with a basal layer consisting of scattered **myoepithelial cells**.
   2. A basal lamina separates the epithelial components from the underlying stroma.

B. **Active (lactating) mammary glands** are enlarged during pregnancy by the development of **alveoli**.
   1. **Alveolar cells** (secretory cells) (Figure 19.6)
      a. Alveolar cells line the alveoli of active mammary glands and are surrounded by an incomplete layer of **myoepithelial cells**.
      b. They are richly endowed with RER and contain several Golgi complexes, numerous mitochondria, lipid droplets, and vesicles containing milk protein (caseins) and lactose.
   2. **Secretion by alveolar cells**
      a. **Lipids** are released into the lumen, perhaps, via the **apocrine** mode of secretion.
      b. **Proteins** and sugars are released into the alveolar lumen via the **merocrine** mode of secretion (exocytosis).

C. **Nipple**
   1. The nipple is composed of dense, irregular collagenous connective tissue interlaced with smooth muscle fibers that act as a **sphincter**.
   2. It contains the openings of the lactiferous ducts.
   3. It is surrounded by pigmented skin (**areola**) that is more deeply pigmented during and subsequent to pregnancy and contains the **areolar glands (of Montgomery)**.

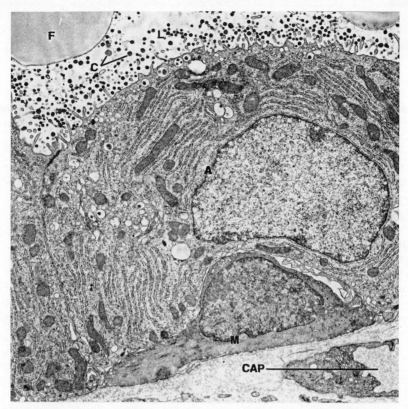

FIGURE 19.6. Transmission electron micrograph showing alveolar epithelial cell (A) from lactating mammary gland and an underlying myoepithelial cell (M). CAP, capillary; L, lumen of alveolus containing milk; F, fat droplet; C, casein. (Reprinted with permission from Strum J. *A Study Atlas of Electron Micrographs*. 3rd ed. Baltimore, MD: University of Maryland School of Medicine; 1992:105.)

CLINICAL CONSIDERATIONS

1. **Breast cancer** may originate from the epithelium lining the ducts (**ductal carcinoma**) or the terminal ductules (**lobular carcinoma**). If breast cancer is not treated early, the tumor cells **metastasize** via lymphatic vessels to the axillary nodes near the affected breast and later via the bloodstream to the lungs, bone, and brain. In the United States, 180,000 new cases of breast cancer are diagnosed annually, and every year 43,000 women die of this disease. **Early detection** by self-examination, mammography, or ultrasound has led to a reduction in the mortality rate associated with breast cancer.

2. Deficiency or mutation in the gene **BRCA1** has been shown to decrease the stability or elevate the incidence of the mutation rate of **tumor suppressor genes** such as **p53**. It appears that **mutations in the BRCA1 gene** result in incapacitation of the checkpoint at G2-M of the cell cycle, and concurrently, the number of centrosomes of these cells is increased. Therefore, these mutated cells have the capability to proliferate unchecked.

D. Secretions of the mammary glands

1. **Colostrum (protein-rich yellowish fluid)**
   a. Colostrum is produced during the first few days after birth.
   b. It is rich in cells (lymphocytes, monocytes), lactalbumin, fat-soluble vitamins, and minerals and contains **immunoglobulin A (IgA)**.

2. **Milk**
   a. Milk begins to be secreted by the third or fourth day after birth.
   b. Milk consists of proteins (caseins, IgA, lactalbumin), many lipid droplets, and lactose.
   c. It is released from the mammary glands via the **milk ejection reflex** in response to a variety of external stimuli related to suckling. The milk ejection reflex involves release of **oxytocin** (from axons in the pars nervosa of the pituitary gland), which induces contraction of the **myoepithelial cells**, forcing milk into the larger ducts and out of the breast.

Review Test

Directions: Each of the numbered items or incomplete statements in this section is followed by answers or completions of the statement. Select the ONE lettered answer that is BEST in each case.

1. Which of the following statements concerning secondary ovarian follicles is true?

(A) They lack liquor folliculi.
(B) They contain a secondary oocyte.
(C) Their continued maturation requires follicle-stimulating hormone.
(D) They lack a theca externa.
(E) They have a single layer of cuboidal follicular cells surrounding the oocyte.

2. Colostrum contains which of the following antibodies?

(A) IgA
(B) IgD
(C) IgE
(D) IgG
(E) IgM

3. Which of the following statements concerning the corpus luteum is true?

(A) It produces LH.
(B) It produces FSH.
(C) It derives its granulosa luteal cells from the theca externa.
(D) It becomes the corpus albicans.
(E) It is derived from atretic follicles.

4. LH exerts which one of the following physiological effects?

(A) It triggers completion of the second meiotic division by secondary oocytes.
(B) It triggers ovulation.
(C) It suppresses release of estrogens.
(D) It induces primary follicles to become secondary follicles.
(E) It induces primordial follicles to become primary follicles.

5. The basal layer of the uterine endometrium

(A) is sloughed during menstruation.
(B) has no glands.
(C) is supplied by coiled arteries.
(D) is supplied by straight arteries.
(E) is avascular.

6. One of the recognized phases of the menstrual cycle is termed the

(A) gestational phase.
(B) active phase.
(C) follicular phase.
(D) resting phase.
(E) anaphase.

7. During the proliferative phase of the menstrual cycle, the functional layer of the endometrium undergoes which of the following changes?

(A) Blood vessels become ischemic.
(B) The epithelium is renewed.
(C) The stroma swells because of edema.
(D) Glands become coiled.
(E) Blood vessels break down.

8. Which of the following statements concerning the vaginal mucosa is true?

(A) It is lined by stratified columnar epithelium.
(B) It is lined by stratified squamous keratinized epithelium.
(C) It possesses no elastic fibers.
(D) It is lubricated by glands in the cervix.
(E) Its cells secrete lactic acid.

9. Which of the following statements concerning the oviduct is true?

(A) It is lined by a simple cuboidal epithelium.
(B) Its epithelium contains peg cells.
(C) It functions in nourishing trilaminar germ discs.
(D) Fertilization most often occurs in its fimbriated portion.
(E) Its epithelium contains goblet cells.

10. Which one of the following teratomas is a malignant, fast-growing tumor?

(A) Mature teratoma
(B) Monodermal teratoma
(C) Immature teratoma
(D) Struma ovarii
(E) Ovarian carcinoid

Answers and Explanations

1. **C.** Secondary follicles depend on follicle-stimulating hormone for their continued development. They are established when liquor folliculi (an ultrafiltrate of plasma and granulosa cell secretions) begins to accumulate among the granulosa cells. Secondary follicles contain a primary oocyte blocked in the prophase of meiosis I (see Chapter 19 II B 1 b).

2. **A.** IgA antibodies are present in colostrum and milk. IgG antibodies are acquired by the fetus by placental transfer from the mother (see Chapter 19 X D 1).

3. **D.** A corpus albicans is formed from a corpus luteum that has ceased to function. LH and FSH are both produced in the anterior pituitary gland. Granulosa luteal cells are derived from the granulosa cells of an ovulated graafian follicle (see Chapter 19 II B 4).

4. **B.** A sudden surge of LH near the middle of the menstrual cycle triggers ovulation (see Chapter 19 II D 1 d).

5. **D.** The basal layer of the uterine endometrium is supplied by the straight arteries and contains the deeper portions of the uterine glands. Cells from these glands reepithelialize the endometrial surface after the functional layer (supplied by the coiled arteries) has been sloughed (see Chapter 19 IV A 1 b).

6. **C.** The recognized phases of the menstrual cycle are the follicular (proliferative), secretory (luteal), and menstrual phases. The mammary glands are characterized by active (lactating) and resting phases. The term *gestational phase* refers to pregnancy (see Chapter 19 IV B 3).

7. **B.** During the proliferative phase of the menstrual cycle, the entire functional layer of the endometrium is renewed, including the epithelium lining the surface and glands. Edema in the stroma and coiled glands is characteristic of the secretory phase of the cycle, and ischemia is responsible for the menstrual phase (see Chapter 19 IV B 2).

8. **D.** The vagina lacks glands and is lubricated by secretions from cervical glands. It is lined by a stratified squamous nonkeratinized epithelium with cells that release glycogen, which is used by the normal bacterial flora of the vagina to manufacture lactic acid (see Chapter 19 VIII A 3).

9. **B.** The oviduct is lined by a simple columnar epithelium composed of ciliated cells and peg cells but no goblet cells. Fertilization most often occurs in the ampulla of the oviduct, not in the infundibulum, where fimbriae are located. Under normal circumstances, the trilaminar germ disk stage occurs after the blastocyst is implanted in the wall of the uterus, and is not present in the oviduct (see Chapter 19 III A 1).

10. **C.** Immature teratomas are fast-growing malignant tumors. The other teratomas listed are usually benign, but even those that do become malignant are slow growing (see Chapter 19 VI B 4).

chapter **20** Male Reproductive System

I. OVERVIEW—MALE REPRODUCTIVE SYSTEM

A. The male reproductive system consists of the **testes, genital ducts**, accessory genital glands (**seminal vesicles, prostate gland**, and **bulbourethral glands**), and the **penis**.

B. Function. The male reproductive system produces **spermatozoa** (sperm), **testosterone**, and **seminal fluid**. Seminal fluid transports and nourishes the sperm as they pass through the excretory ducts. The penis delivers sperm to the exterior and also serves as the conduit for excretion of urine from the body.

II. TESTES

The paired testes develop in the abdominal cavity and later descend into the scrotum, where they are suspended at the ends of the **spermatic cords**. They are the sites of **spermatogenesis** and production of the male **sex hormones**, primarily **testosterone** (Figure 20.1).

CLINICAL CONSIDERATIONS	Cryptorchidism

1. Cryptorchidism is a developmental defect characterized by **failure of one or both testes to descend** into the scrotum. The chance of this happening in full-term births is 1%, whereas it rises to a 30% chance in premature births.
2. This condition results in sterility because the temperature of the undescended testes (i.e., normal body temperature) inhibits spermatogenesis; however, it does not affect testosterone production.
3. It is **associated with** a much higher incidence of **testicular malignancy** than in normally descended testes.
4. It can be **surgically corrected**. In order to avoid complications later on in life, the usual recommendation is that the surgery be performed prior to the age of one, assuming that the child is healthy enough for the procedure.

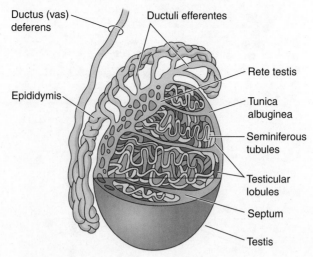

FIGURE 20.1. The testis and epididymis. (Reprinted with permission from Gartner LP, Hiatt JL. *Color Textbook of Histology.* 2nd ed. Philadelphia, PA: Saunders; 2001:488.)

A. **Testicular tunicae** (covering of the testes) are applied to the testes as they descend through the abdominal wall to enter the scrotum.
  1. The **tunica vaginalis** is a **serous sac** derived from the peritoneum that partially covers the anterior and lateral surfaces of each testis.
  2. **Tunica albuginea**
      a. **Tunica albuginea is the thick, fibrous connective tissue capsule** of the testis.
      b. It is lined by a highly vascular layer of loose connective tissue, the **tunica vasculosa**.
      c. It is thickened posteriorly to form the **mediastinum testis**, from which incomplete connective tissue septa arise to divide the organ into approximately 250 compartments (**lobuli testis**). Additionally, the mediastinum testis is the passage way for blood and lymphatic vessels in and out of the testes.

B. **Lobuli testes** (Figure 20.1)
  1. The lobuli testes are pyramidal intercommunicating compartments that are separated by incomplete septa.
  2. Each contains one to four **seminiferous tubules** where spermatozoa are produced. These highly convoluted tubules are embedded in a meshwork of loose connective tissue containing blood and lymphatic vessels, nerves, and interstitial cells of Leydig.

C. **Interstitial cells of Leydig**
  1. Interstitial cells of Leydig are round to polygonal cells in the interstitial regions between seminiferous tubules.
  2. They possess a large central nucleus, numerous mitochondria, a well-developed Golgi complex, and many lipid droplets. The lipid droplets contain cholesterol esters, precursors of testosterone.
  3. They are richly supplied with capillaries and lymphatic vessels.
  4. **Function.** Interstitial cells of Leydig are **endocrine cells** that produce and secrete **testosterone**. Secretion is stimulated by **luteinizing hormone** (LH; interstitial cell–stimulating hormone) produced in the pituitary gland. These cells mature and begin to secrete during puberty.

D. **Seminiferous tubules**
  1. **Overview** (Figure 20.2)
      a. Seminiferous tubules are 30 to 70 cm long, with a diameter of 150 to 250 μm.
      b. They are enveloped by a fibrous connective tissue tunic composed of several layers of fibroblasts and extensive capillary beds.
      c. They form tortuous pathways through the testicular lobules and then narrow into short, straight segments, the **tubuli recti**, which connect with the **rete testis**.

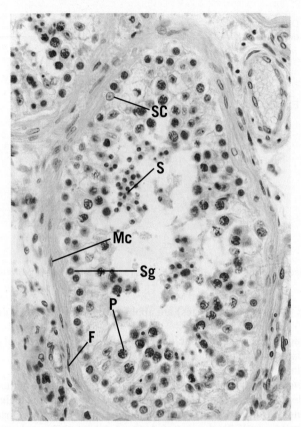

FIGURE 20.2. Light micrograph of the seminiferous tubules in the testis (×132). Observe myoid cells (Mc) and fibroblasts (F) composing the wall of the seminiferous tubules. Spermatogonia (Sg) and the Sertoli cells (SC) lie in the basal compartment. Just superior to this are primary spermatocytes (P). Note that spermatids (S) are located near the lumen.

   d. The lumina of the seminiferous tubules are lined by a thick complex epithelium (**seminiferous** or **germinal epithelium**). This epithelium consists of four to eight cell layers and contains **spermatogenic cells**, from which the germ cells eventually develop (spermatogenesis), and **Sertoli cells**, which have several functions.
2. Sertoli cells (Figures 20.2 and 20.3)
   a. Structure
      (1) Sertoli cells are columnar cells that extend from the basal lamina to the lumen of the seminiferous tubule. They have a pale, oval nucleus that displays frequent indentations; they are highly infolded and possess a large nucleolus. Sertoli cells no longer undergo mitosis after puberty.
      (2) Their lateral plasma membranes have long processes that interdigitate with those of neighboring Sertoli cells enfolding small clusters of developing spermatogenic cells. Their apical cell membranes are highly convoluted, forming finger-like processes where the interstices between these processes are occupied by developing spermatozoa.
      (3) They have a well-developed smooth endoplasmic reticulum (SER), some rough endoplasmic reticulum (RER), an abundance of mitochondria and lysosomes, and an extensive Golgi complex.
      (4) Receptors for follicle-stimulating hormone (FSH) are present on their basal plasma membranes.
      (5) They form **zonulae occludentes** (tight junctions) with adjacent Sertoli cells near their bases, thus dividing the lumen of the seminiferous tubule into a **basal** and an **adluminal compartment**. These tight junctions are responsible for the **blood–testis barrier**, which protects developing sperm cells from autoimmune reactions.

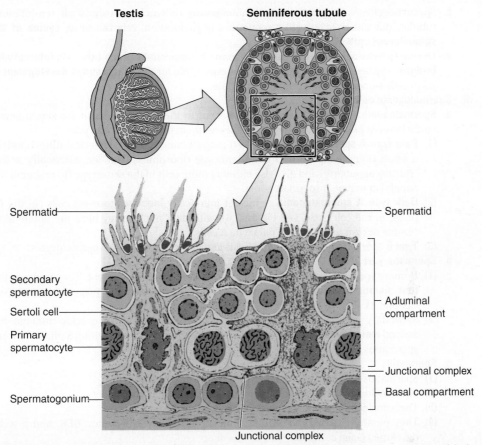

Testis **Seminiferous tubule**

Spermatid — — Spermatid

Secondary spermatocyte —

Sertoli cell —

Primary spermatocyte —

— Adluminal compartment

— Junctional complex

— Basal compartment

Spermatogonium —

Junctional complex

FIGURE 20.3. The seminiferous (germinal) epithelium. Note the intercellular bridges between spermatocytes and the junctional complexes near the bases of adjacent Sertoli cells. These junctional complexes of the Sertoli cells divide the epithelium into an adluminal and a basal compartment. (Reprinted with permission from Krause WJ, Cutts JH. *Concise Text of Histology.* 2nd ed. Baltimore, MD: Williams & Wilkins; 1986:414.)

b. Function

(1) Sertoli cells support, protect, and nourish the spermatogenic cells.

(2) They phagocytose excess cytoplasm discarded by maturing spermatids.

(3) They secrete a fructose-rich fluid into the lumen that nourishes and facilitates the transport of spermatozoa through the seminiferous tubules to the genital ducts.

(4) They synthesize **androgen-binding protein (ABP)** under the influence of FSH. **ABP** assists in maintaining the necessary concentration of testosterone in the seminiferous tubule so that spermatogenesis can progress.

(5) They secrete **inhibin**, a hormone that inhibits the synthesis and release of FSH by the anterior pituitary, as well as the hormone **activin** which boosts FSH release from the anterior pituitary.

(6) They establish a blood–testis barrier.

(7) During fetal development they synthesize and release **antimüllerian hormone**, which determines maleness.

(8) They manufacture and release **testicular transferrin**, a protein that facilitates the transfer of iron from **serum transferrin** to maturing spermatogenic cells.

3. Spermatogenesis

a. Shortly before puberty, the rise in gonadotrophins initiates spermatogenesis, the process of spermatozoon (sperm) formation. It is divided into three phases:

(1) Spermatocytogenesis—differentiation of spermatogonia into primary spermatocytes.

(2) Meiosis—reduction division to reduce the diploid chromosomal complement of primary spermatocytes to form haploid spermatids (see Chapter 2 XI).

(3) Spermiogenesis—transformation of spermatids into spermatozoa.

b. Spermatogenesis does **not** occur simultaneously or synchronously in all seminiferous tubules, but rather in wavelike sequences of maturation, referred to as **cycles of the seminiferous epithelium**.

c. During spermatogenesis, daughter cells remain connected to each other via **intercellular bridges**. The resultant **syncytium** may be responsible for the **synchronous development** of germ cells along **any one** seminiferous tubule.

4. **Spermatogenic cells** (Figure 20.2)
   a. **Spermatogonia** are **diploid** germ cells adjacent to the basal lamina of the seminiferous epithelium. At puberty, testosterone influences them to enter the cell cycle.
      (1) **Pale type A spermatogonia** possess a pale-staining nucleus, spherical mitochondria, a small Golgi complex, and abundant, free ribosomes. They are **mitotically active** (starting at puberty) and give rise either to more cells of the same type (to maintain the supply) or to type B spermatogonia.
      (2) **Dark type A spermatogonia** represent mitotically **inactive** (reserve) cells (in the G_0 phase of the cell cycle, see Figure 2.6), with dark nuclei; they have the potential to resume mitosis and produce pale type A cells.
      (3) **Type B spermatogonia** undergo mitosis and give rise to primary spermatocytes.
   b. **Spermatocytes**
      (1) Primary spermatocytes are large **diploid** cells with 4cDNA content. They undergo the **first meiotic division** (reductional division) to form secondary spermatocytes (see Chapter 2).
      (2) Secondary spermatocytes are **haploid** cells with 2cDNA that quickly undergo the **second meiotic division** (equatorial division), without an intervening S phase, to form spermatids.
   c. **Spermatids**
      (1) Spermatids are small **haploid** cells containing only **1cDNA**.
      (2) They are located near the lumen of the seminiferous tubule.
      (3) Their nuclei often display regions of condensed chromatin.
      (4) They possess a pair of centrioles, mitochondria, free ribosomes, SER, and a well-developed Golgi complex.

5. **Spermiogenesis** is a unique process of **cytodifferentiation**, whereby **spermatids** shed much of their cytoplasm and **transform into spermatozoa**, which are released into the lumen of the seminiferous tubule. Spermiogenesis is divided into four phases.
   a. **Golgi phase**
      (1) The Golgi phase is characterized by the formation of an **acrosomal granule**, enclosed within an **acrosomal vesicle**, which becomes attached to the anterior end of the nuclear envelope of a spermatid.
      (2) In this phase, centrioles migrate away from the nucleus to form the **flagellar axoneme**. Centrioles then migrate back toward the nucleus to assist in forming the **connecting piece** associated with the tail.
   b. The **cap phase** is characterized by expansion of the acrosomal vesicle over much of the nucleus, forming the **acrosomal cap**.
   c. **Acrosomal phase** is characterized by the following:
      (1) The **nucleus** becomes condensed, flattened, and located in the head region.
      (2) Mitochondria aggregate around the proximal portion of the flagellum, which develops into the middle piece of the tail.
      (3) The **spermatid** elongates; this process is aided by a temporary cylinder of microtubules called the **manchette**.
      (4) The acrosomal phase ends as the spermatid is oriented with its acrosome pointing toward the base of the seminiferous tubule.
   d. **Maturation phase is characterized by the following:**
      (1) Loss of excess cytoplasm and intercellular bridges connecting spermatids into a syncytium. The discarded cytoplasm is phagocytosed by Sertoli cells.
      (2) Maturation phase ends when the **nonmotile** spermatozoa are released (tail first) into the lumen of the seminiferous tubule. Spermatozoa remain immotile until they leave the epididymis. They become **capacitated** (capable of fertilizing) in the female reproductive system.

6. **Spermatozoon**
   a. **Head of the spermatozoon** (Figure 20.4)
      (1) The spermatozoon head is flattened and contains a dense, homogeneous nucleus with 23 chromosomes: (22 plus the Y chromosome or 22 plus the X chromosome).
      (2) It also possesses the acrosome, which contains **hydrolytic enzymes** (e.g., acid phosphatase, neuraminidase, hyaluronidase, and proteases) that assist the sperm in penetrating the corona radiata and zona pellucida of the oocyte (see Chapter 19). Release of these enzymes is termed the **acrosomal reaction**.
   b. **Tail of the spermatozoon** includes the neck, middle piece, principal piece, and the end piece.
      (1) The **neck** includes the centrioles and the **connecting piece**, which is attached to the nine **outer dense fibers** of the remainder of the tail.
      (2) The **middle piece** extends from the neck to the **annulus** and contains the axoneme, nine outer dense fibers, and a spirally arranged **sheath of mitochondria**.
      (3) The **principal piece** extends from the annulus to the end piece and contains the axoneme with its surrounding dense fibers, which in turn are encircled by a **fibrous sheath** that has circumferential ribs.
      (4) The **end piece** consists of the axoneme and the surrounding plasma membrane.

CLINICAL CONSIDERATIONS **Testicular cancer**

1. Most often attacks men younger than 40 years of age and is the most common cancer of men between the ages of 20 and 34 years.
2. Usually present as swellings in the scrotum.
3. Those with malignancy typically have elevated blood α-fetoprotein and human chorionic gonadotropin (hCG) levels.
4. Surgical removal of the affected testis is the common treatment.
5. Testicular cancer that has metastasized necessitates radiation therapy and chemotherapy.

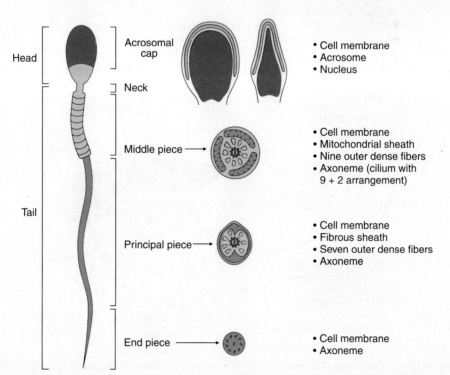

FIGURE 20.4. A human sperm. Regions of the mature sperm are shown on the left. Diagrams of sections through the head and the major segments of the tail are shown on the right. (Reprinted with permission from Henrikson RC, Kaye GI, Mazurkiewicz JE. *Histology National Medical Series for Independent Study.* Baltimore, MD: Williams & Wilkins; 1997:399.)

E. Regulation of spermatogenesis

1. **Critical testicular temperature** is 35°C for spermatogenesis. Testicular arteries that arise from the aorta accompany the testes into the scrotum, providing each testis with a vascular supply. As these convoluted arteries approach the testes, they are surrounded by a **pampiniform plexus of veins** that dissipates the heat of the arterial blood, resulting in its temperature being reduced to 35°C. (See Section II, **Clinical Considerations** in this chapter.)

2. **Hormonal interactions** (Figure 20.5)
   a. **Certain neurons in the hypothalamus** produce luteinizing hormone-releasing hormone (LHRH), also known as gonadotropin-releasing hormone (GnRH). LHRH initiates the release of LH and FSH from the adenohypophysis.
   b. **Stimulation of testicular hormone production** is effected by these two pituitary gonadotropins.
      (1) LH stimulates the interstitial cells of Leydig to secrete **testosterone**.
      (2) FSH promotes the synthesis of **ABP** by Sertoli cells.
   c. **Testosterone** is necessary for the normal development of not only male germ cells but also secondary sex characteristics.
   d. **ABP** binds testosterone and maintains it at a high concentration in the seminiferous tubule to facilitate succession of spermatogonia into spermatozoa; it can also bind estrogens, thus inhibiting spermatogenesis.

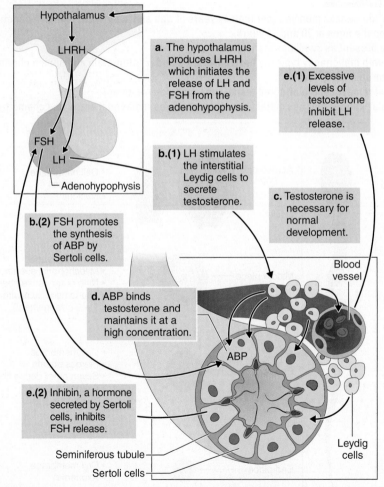

FIGURE 20.5. The hormonal control of testicular function. Note the feedback inhibition of the pituitary by testicular hormones. LHRH, luteinizing hormone–releasing hormone; LH, luteinizing hormone; FSH, follicle-stimulating hormone ABP, androgen-binding protein.

e. Inhibition and stimulation of FSH and LH release

(1) Excessive levels of **testosterone** inhibit LH release.

(2) Inhibin, a hormone secreted by Sertoli cells, inhibits GnRH, and, thereby, FSH release from the hypophysis.

(3) Activin, also secreted by Sertoli cells, stimulates the release of GnRH and, thereby, FSH release.

CLINICAL CONSIDERATIONS   **Hyperthermia** is a major factor that results in sterility in males. Sperm production is heat sensitive. The optimum temperature for sperm production is 35°C. Hence, the testes are housed in the scrotum as opposed to being housed within the body, where the temperature would be around 37°C. It has been reported that males who operate laptop computers situated in their laps for an hour are increasing their intrascrotal temperatures by as much as 2.8°C. Although these studies are not definitive, it might be wise for young males to limit the use of laptop computers in their laps for extended time periods.

III. GENITAL DUCTS (Table 20.1)

A. Intratesticular ducts

1. The continuation of the seminiferous tubules are the **tubuli recti**, short, straight tubules lined by Sertoli cells in their proximal half and lined by a **simple cuboidal epithelium** in their distal half. These cuboidal cells possess **microvilli**, and some display a single **flagellum**.

2. Rete testis is a labyrinthine plexus of anastomosing channels within the mediastinum testis lined by a **simple cuboidal epithelium**; many of the cells possess microvilli as well as a single luminal **flagellum**.

---

t a b l e 20.1   Histology and Functions of the Male Genital Ducts

Duct	Epithelium	Connective Tissue	Muscle Layers	Function
Tubuli recti	Sertoli cells in proximal half; simple cuboidal epithelium in distal half	Loose	No smooth muscle	Conduct spermatozoa from seminiferous tubules to rete testis
Rete testis	Simple cuboidal epithelium	Vascular	No smooth muscle	Conduct spermatozoa from tubuli recti to ductuli efferentes
Ductuli efferentes	Regions of ciliated columnar cells alternating with unciliated cuboidal cells	Thin, loose	Thin layer of circularly arranged smooth muscle cells	Conduct spermatozoa from rete testis to epididymis
Epididymis	Pseudostratified epithelium composed of tall principal cells with stereocilia, short basal cells	Thin, loose	Layer of circularly arranged smooth muscle cells	Conduct spermatozoa from ductuli efferentes to ductus deferens
Ductus (vas) deferens	Pseudostratified stereociliated columnar epithelium	Loose, fibroelastic	Thick three-layer smooth muscle coats: inner and outer longitudinal; middle circular	Deliver spermatozoa from tail of epididymis to ejaculatory duct
Ejaculatory duct	Simple columnar epithelium	Subepithelial; thrown into folds, giving lumen irregular appearance	No smooth muscle	Deliver spermatozoa, seminal fluid to prostatic urethra at colliculus seminalis

B. Extratesticular ducts

  1. Ductuli efferentes

    a. Ductuli efferentes are a collection of 10 to 20 tubules leading from the rete testis to the ductus epididymis. Therefore, the ductuli efferentes begin as intratesticular ducts, leave the testicles, and their distal portions may be considered to be extratesticular ducts.

    b. They possess a thin circular layer of **smooth muscle** beneath the basal lamina of the epithelium, which is responsible for peristaltic movements.

    c. They are lined by a **simple epithelium** composed of **alternating clusters** of **nonciliated cuboidal cells** and **ciliated columnar cells**. The arrangement of epithelial cells of two different heights imparts a characteristic festooned appearance to the luminal outline of the ductuli efferentes.

    d. Function. Ductuli efferentes reabsorb fluid from the semen and form the **head of the epididymis**.

  2. Ductus epididymis (Figure 20.6)

    a. Ductus epididymis, together with the ductuli efferentes, constitutes the **epididymis**.

    b. It is surrounded by **circular layers of smooth muscle** that undergo **peristaltic contractions**, which assist in conveying sperm toward the ductus deferens.

    c. It is lined by a **pseudostratified columnar epithelium**, which is supported by a basal lamina and contains the following two cell types:

      (1) Basal cells are round and, morphologically, appear to be undifferentiated; they serve as precursors of the principal cells.

      (2) Principal cells, which are columnar and possess nonmotile stereocilia (long, irregular microvilli) on their luminal surfaces

        (a) These cells possess a large Golgi complex, RER, lysosomes, and many apical pinocytotic and coated vesicles.

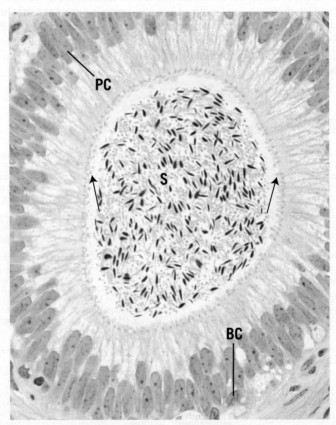

FIGURE 20.6. Light micrograph of the epididymis (×270). Observe the short basal cells (BC) and the columnar principal cells (PC) lining the lumen of the epididymis. Stereocilia (*arrows*) project into the lumen packed with spermatozoa (S).

        (b) Principal cells function, in concert with the ductuli efferentes, to absorb nearly 90% of the testicular fluid.

        (c) They secrete various factors that facilitate sperm maturation; however, they also produce **glycerophosphocholine**, which inhibits **capacitation** (the process whereby a sperm becomes capable of fertilizing an oocyte). Thus, capacitation occurs only after the sperm enters the female genital tract.

3. Ductus (vas) deferens

    a. The ductus deferens, which begins at the tail of the epididymis, has a **thick muscular wall** with inner and outer layers of longitudinal smooth muscle, which are separated from one another by a middle circular layer.

    b. It possesses a narrow, irregular lumen lined by **pseudostratified columnar epithelium** similar to that of the ductus epididymis.

4. Ejaculatory duct

    a. The ejaculatory duct is the straight continuation of the ductus deferens beyond where it receives the duct of the seminal vesicle.

    b. It lacks a muscular wall.

    c. It enters the prostate gland and terminates in a slit on the **colliculus seminalis** located in the prostatic urethra.

CLINICAL CONSIDERATIONS A normal sperm count for a single ejaculate is approximately 50 to 100 million spermatozoa/mL. An individual with a sperm count of less than 20 million spermatozoa/mL. of ejaculate is considered to be **sterile**.

IV. ACCESSORY GENITAL GLANDS

Include the paired seminal vesicles, prostate gland, and the paired bulbourethral glands

A. Seminal vesicles

  1. Epithelium

    a. Epithelium of the seminal vesicles is **pseudostratified columnar**, with a height that varies with testosterone levels; it lines the **extensively folded mucosa**.

    b. It contains many **yellow lipochrome pigment granules** and secretory granules, a large Golgi complex, many mitochondria, and abundant RER.

  2. The **lamina propria** consists of **fibroelastic** connective tissue surrounded by an inner circular and outer longitudinal layer of smooth muscle.

  3. The **adventitia** is composed of **fibroelastic** connective tissue.

  4. The seminal vesicles **secrete** a yellowish, viscous fluid containing substances that **activate sperm** (e.g., fructose providing the energy source for the sperm); this fluid constitutes about 70% of the human ejaculate.

  5. The duct of the seminal vesicle joins the ductus deferens at its ampulla (the enlarged terminal end), thus forming the right and left ejaculatory ducts that enter the prostate gland continuing to the urethra.

B. Prostate gland (Figure 20.7)

  1. Overview

    a. The prostate gland surrounds the urethra as it exits the urinary bladder.

    b. It consists of 30 to 50 discrete **branched tubuloalveolar glands** that empty their contents via excretory ducts into the prostatic urethra. These glands are arranged in three concentric layers (**mucosal, submucosal**, and **main**) around the urethra.

    c. The gland is covered by a **fibroelastic capsule** that contains smooth muscle. Septa from the capsule penetrate the gland and divide it into lobes.

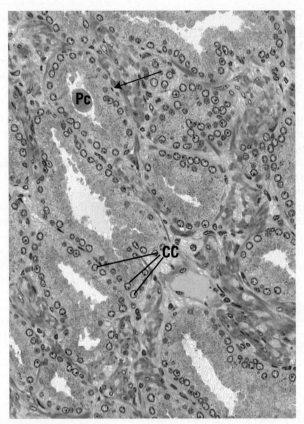

FIGURE 20.7. Light micrograph of the prostate gland (×132). Note the prostrate concretion (Pc), smooth muscle (*arrow*), and the compressed columnar cells (CC) forming the glandular parenchyma.

2. **Epithelium**
   a. The epithelium of the prostate gland is **simple** or **pseudostratified columnar** and lines the individual glands that constitute the prostate.
   b. It is composed of cells that contain abundant RER, a well-developed Golgi complex, numerous lysosomes, and many secretory granules.
3. **Corpora amylacea** are prostatic **concretions**, composed of glycoprotein, which may become calcified; their numbers increase with age.
4. The **prostate secretes** a thin whitish fluid, a part of the semen containing proteolytic enzymes, citric acid, acid phosphatase, fibrinolysin, and lipids. The prostatic secretion serves to liquefy the coagulated semen after it is deposited in the female genital tract. Its synthesis and release are regulated by dihydrotestosterone.

CLINICAL CONSIDERATIONS   Benign prostatic hypertrophy (BPH)

1. BPH most commonly involves only an enlargement of the **mucosal glands**.
2. It is frequently associated with an inability to begin and cease urination because the urethra is partially strangulated by the enlarged prostate.
3. It leads to **nocturia** (urination at night) and sensory urgency (the desire to urinate without having to void).
4. This disease is common in older men, occurring in about 50% of men older than 50 years of age and in 95% of those older than 80 years of age. BPH can be confirmed by a digital rectal examination; however, a biopsy is required to rule out prostatic cancer.

Adenocarcinoma of the prostate gland

1. Adenocarcinoma of the prostate gland may be indicated by palpation through the rectum. However, a biopsy is required for positive identification of the disease.
2. Although this cancer grows slowly, it commonly **metastasizes to bone** via the circulatory system.
3. It occurs in about one-third of men older than 75 years of age and is the second most common form of cancer in men.
4. It is associated with an elevated **prostate-specific antigen (PSA)** level in blood. Men with elevated PSA values are candidates for more aggressive diagnostic tests for prostatic cancer. Surgical removal with or without radiation therapy is the usual treatment, although there may be complications of impotence and/or incontinence. Newer procedures (e.g., brachytherapy) include radioactive seeding within the gland.

C. **Bulbourethral (Cowper) glands**
   1. Bulbourethral glands are adjacent to the membranous urethra.
   2. They empty their viscous, slippery secretions into the lumen of the membranous urethra to lubricate it just prior to the emission of semen.
   3. The glands are lined by a **simple cuboidal** or **columnar epithelium**.
   4. They are surrounded by a **fibroelastic capsule** containing smooth and skeletal muscle.

CLINICAL CONSIDERATIONS **Vasectomy** is the chosen means of permanent contraception by more than 600,000 US males each year. A physician may perform the procedure in the office, where the scrotum is slit open, a portion of the spermatic cord is pulled out, cut, cauterized, and returned to the scrotum. At the conclusion of 6 weeks or so, after the procedure, semen is collected and examined to assure that no spermatozoa are ejaculated. This procedure is nearly 100% effective. The procedure may have a few complications, but they usually dissipate after a short period of time.

V. URETHRA

The urethra conveys urine from the bladder to outside the body. In males, the urethra also carries semen during ejaculation. It has a **two-layered muscularis** consisting of an inner longitudinal and an outer circular layer of smooth muscle. It is surrounded at some point by an **external sphincter of skeletal muscle**, which permits its voluntary closure.

A. The male urethra is about 20 cm long and is divided into **prostatic, membranous**, and **cavernous** portions.

B. It is lined by **transitional epithelium** in the prostatic portion and by **pseudostratified** or **stratified columnar epithelium** in the other two portions. The **fossa navicularis**, located at the distal end of the cavernous urethra, is lined by **stratified squamous epithelium**.

C. It contains mucus-secreting **glands of Littre** in the lamina propria.

VI. PENIS

A. **Corpora cavernosa**
1. Corpora cavernosa are **paired** masses of erectile tissue that contain **irregular vascular spaces** lined by a continuous layer of endothelial cells. These spaces are separated from each other by trabeculae of connective tissue and smooth muscle.
2. The vascular spaces decrease in size toward the periphery of the corpora cavernosa.
3. During erection, the vascular spaces become engorged with blood as a result of **parasympathetic impulses,** which constrict arteriovenous shunts and dilate the helicine arteries, thus increasing flow to the vascular spaces of the two corpora cavernosa and the single corpus spongiosum.

B. **Corpus spongiosum**
1. The corpus spongiosum is a single mass of **erectile tissue** that contains vascular spaces of uniform size.
2. It possesses **trabeculae** that contain more elastic fibers and less smooth muscle than those of the corpora cavernosa.
3. The penile portion of the urethra passes through the length of the corpus spongiosum, opening to the exterior at the tip of the glans penis.

C. **Connective tissue and skin**
1. The **tunica albuginea** is a thick, fibrous connective sheath that surrounds the paired corpora cavernosa and the corpus spongiosum. The arrangement of dense collagen bundles permits extension of the penis during erection.
2. **Glans penis**
   a. The glans penis is the dilated distal end of the corpus spongiosum.
   b. It contains dense connective tissue and longitudinal muscle fibers.
   c. It is covered by retractable skin, the **prepuce,** which is lined by stratified squamous lightly keratinized epithelium.
3. **Glands of Littre** are mucus-secreting glands present throughout the length of the penile urethra.

Review Test

Directions: Each of the numbered items or incomplete statements in this section is followed by answers or by completions of the statement. Select the ONE lettered answer or completion that is BEST in each case.

1. Which one of the following functions is attributed to the Sertoli cells?

(A) Secretion of follicle-stimulating hormone
(B) Secretion of testosterone
(C) Secretion of androgen-binding protein
(D) Secretion of LH
(E) Secretion of ABP

2. Which of the following statements concerning the cells of Leydig is true?

(A) They become functional at puberty.
(B) They are within the seminiferous tubules.
(C) They are stimulated by FSH.
(D) They secrete much of the fluid portion of semen.
(E) They respond to inhibin.

3. Type A spermatogonia are germ cells that

(A) develop from secondary spermatocytes.
(B) undergo meiotic activity subsequent to sexual maturity.
(C) develop through meiotic divisions.
(D) give rise to primary spermatocytes.
(E) may be dark or pale.

4. Which of the following statements is related to the ductus epididymis?

(A) It begins at the rete testis.
(B) It is lined by a pseudostratified columnar epithelium.
(C) It secretes a large volume of fluid into its lumen.
(D) It possesses motile cilia.
(E) It capacitates spermatozoa.

5. Testosterone is produced by

(A) interstitial cells of Leydig.
(B) Sertoli cells.
(C) spermatogonia.
(D) spermatids.
(E) spermatocytes.

6. Spermatozoa are conveyed from the seminiferous tubules to the rete testis via the

(A) ductus epididymis.
(B) tubuli recti.
(C) ductuli efferentes.
(D) ductus deferens.
(E) ejaculatory duct.

7. Manchette formation occurs during which of the following phases of spermiogenesis?

(A) Meiotic phase
(B) Maturation phase
(C) Golgi phase
(D) Cap phase
(E) Acrosomal phase

8. The structural feature that best distinguishes the ductus deferens from the other genital ducts is its

(A) smooth-bore lumen.
(B) thick wall containing three muscle layers.
(C) lining of transitional epithelium.
(D) flattened mucosa.
(E) nonmotile stereocilia.

9. Inhibin, a hormone that inhibits synthesis and release of FSH, is secreted by

(A) prostate gland.
(B) Sertoli cells.
(C) seminal vesicles.
(D) bulbourethral glands.
(E) interstitial cells of Leydig.

10. A 55-year-old man has urinary complications. He complains of difficulty urinating and reduced urinary flow. He also has an elevated prostate-specific antigen (PSA) level, along with palpable hard nodules on the prostate. The possible diagnosis is

(A) benign prostatic hyperplasia.
(B) adenocarcinoma of the prostate.
(C) prostatic concretions.
(D) initiation of impotence.
(E) incontinence.

11. A 33-year-old man detected a swelling in his scrotum. Careful palpation did not reveal whether the swelling was associated with his testis. His physician ordered blood tests, and it was determined that he had increased levels of hCG in his blood. A probable diagnosis is

(A) benign lump.
(B) hematocele.
(C) cryptorchidism.
(D) testicular cancer.
(E) hydrocele.

Answers and Explanations

1. **C.** Sertoli cells have many functions, including the synthesis of ABP. Testosterone is secreted by the interstitial cells of Leydig, whereas FSH and LH (also known as interstitial cell–stimulating hormone) are secreted by the pituitary gland (see Chapter 20 II D 2).

2. **A.** Interstitial cells of Leydig become functional at puberty as a result of the action of LH produced in the pituitary gland (see Chapter 20 II C).

3. **E.** Type A spermatogonia, which may be pale or dark, are primitive germ cells. Pale type A spermatogonia become mitotically active at puberty and give rise to type B spermatogonia, which undergo mitoses, giving rise to primary spermatocytes (see Chapter 20 II D 4).

4. **B.** The ductus epididymidis begins at the termination of the ductuli efferentes and is lined by a pseudostratified columnar epithelium, which has principal cells that possess nonmotile stereocilia. These cells are involved in fluid resorption and secrete glycerophosphocholine, which inhibits capacitation (see Chapter 20 III B 2).

5. **A.** The hormone testosterone is produced by the interstitial cells of Leydig (see Chapter 20 II C).

6. **B.** The seminiferous tubules are connected to the rete testis by the tubuli recti (see Chapter 20 II D).

7. **E.** Spermiogenesis is the process of cytodifferentiation by which spermatids are transformed into spermatozoa. It does not involve cell division. Manchette formation occurs during the acrosomal phase of spermiogenesis (see Chapter 20 II D 5).

8. **B.** The ductus (vas) deferens possesses three layers of smooth muscle in its wall, whereas the other genital ducts do not. Like the ductus epididymidis, the ductus deferens is lined by a pseudostratified columnar epithelium with principal cells that possess nonmotile stereocilia (see Chapter 20 III B 3).

9. **B.** Inhibin is secreted by Sertoli cells (see Chapter 20 II D 2).

10. **B.** Although some of the symptoms are characteristic of benign prostatic hypertrophy, rectal palpation indicating hard nodules, along with an elevated PSA level, indicates probable prostatic adenocarcinoma (see Chapter 20 IV B Clinical Considerations).

11. **D.** Palpable swellings in the scrotum, especially in men younger than 40 years of age, should be seen by a physician. Elevated blood serum levels of hCG and α-fetoprotein are usually associated with testicular cancer (see Chapter 20 II D Clinical Considerations).

I. OVERVIEW—SPECIAL SENSE RECEPTORS

A. Special sense receptors are responsible for the five special senses: **taste, smell, seeing, hearing**, and **feeling** (which includes touch, pressure, temperature, pain, and proprioception). The sense of smell is described in Chapter 15, and the sense of taste is described in Chapter 16. The remaining special senses are described here.

B. **Function.** Special sense receptors **transduce stimuli from the environment into electrical impulses**.

II. SPECIALIZED DIFFUSE RECEPTORS (Figure 21.1)

A. **Overview:** Sensory receptors may be categorized into three groups:
1. Exteroceptors—access information from the outside environment.
2. Proprioceptors—access information from muscles, tendons, and joint structures.
3. Interoceptors—access information from within the internal environment.
Additionally, receptors may be categorized according to the type of stimulus perceived.
1. **Mechanoreceptors**—are activated as the receptor or tissue in which the receptor is located physically is deformed in some manner.
2. **Thermoreceptors**—are activated by either heat or cold.
3. **Nociceptors**, also known as **pain receptors**, are activated by painful stimuli such as extreme temperatures that are hot or cold enough to cause damage to the tissues, pressure or touch that are intense enough to cause damage to the tissues.
   a. Specialized diffuse receptors are **dendritic nerve endings** in the skin, fascia, muscles, joints, and tendons.
   b. They respond to stimuli related to **deep touch, pressure, temperature, pain**, and **proprioception**.
   c. These receptors are specialized to receive only **one** type of sensory stimulus, although they will respond to other types of stimuli provided that the stimulus is sufficiently intense.
   d. They are divided morphologically into **free nerve terminals** and **encapsulated nerve endings**, which are ensheathed in a connective tissue capsule.

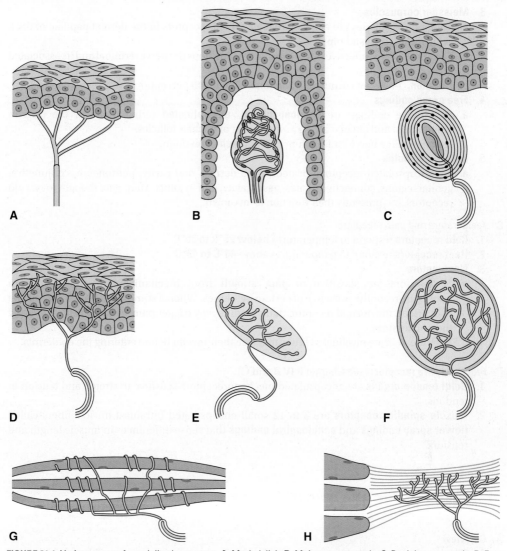

FIGURE 21.1. Various types of specialized receptors. **A.** Merkel disk. **B.** Meissner corpuscle. **C.** Pacinian corpuscle. **D.** Free nerve endings, nociceptors, and thermoreceptors. **E.** Ruffini corpuscle. **F.** Krause end bulb (cold receptor). **G.** Neuromuscular spindle. **H.** Golgi tendon organ.

B. Touch and pressure receptors

1. Pacinian corpuscles

    a. Pacinian corpuscles are large, ellipsoid **encapsulated** receptors in the dermis and hypodermis and in the connective tissue of the mesenteries and joints.

    b. They are especially abundant in the digits and breasts.

    c. They are composed of a **multilayer capsule** consisting of fibroblasts and collagen and bathed in tissue fluid. The capsule surrounds an **inner unmyelinated nerve terminal**.

    d. They **often** resemble a sliced onion in histological sections.

    e. Function. Pacinian corpuscles perceive **pressure, touch**, and **vibration**.

2. Ruffini endings

    a. Ruffini endings are **encapsulated** receptors in the dermis and joints.

    b. They are composed of groups of **branched terminals** from myelinated nerve fibers and are surrounded by a thin connective tissue capsule.

    c. Function. Ruffini endings function in **pressure, stretching**, and **touch** reception.

3. **Meissner corpuscles**
   a. Meissner corpuscles are ellipsoid, **encapsulated** receptors in the dermal papillae of thick skin, eyelids, lips, and nipples.
   b. They possess a connective tissue capsule that envelops the nerve terminal and its associated Schwann cell.
   c. **Function.** Meissner corpuscles function in **fine touch** perception.
4. **Free nerve endings**
   a. Free nerve endings are **unencapsulated, unmyelinated** terminations in the skin in longitudinal and circular arrays around most of the hair follicles.
   b. **Function.** Free nerve endings function in **touch** perception.
5. **Krause end bulbs**
   a. are encapsulated receptors located in the dermis, oral cavity, peritoneum, conjunctiva, genital regions, connective tissues, nasal cavity, and in joints. They were thought to be cold receptors, but presently their function is unknown.

C. **Temperature and pain receptors**
   1. **Cold receptors** respond to temperatures **below 25°C to 30°C**.
   2. **Heat receptors** respond to temperatures above **40°C to 42°C**.
   3. **Nociceptors**
      a. Nociceptors are sensitive to **pain stimuli** from mechanical stress, extremes in temperature, or the presence of certain cytokines. When a stimulus is sufficiently strong to overload the normal receptor, that stimulus may trigger pain sensations by activating the nociceptors.
      b. They are delicate myelinated fibers that lose their myelin before entering the epidermis.

D. **Proprioceptive receptors** (see Chapter 8 IV B and C)
   1. **Golgi tendon organs** are encapsulated mechanoreceptors sensitive to stretch and tension in tendons.
   2. **Muscle spindle receptors** are 3 to 12 small encapsulated intrafusal muscle fibers called **flower spray endings** and **annulospiral endings** that sense differences in muscle length and tension.

III. SENSE OF SIGHT—EYE (Figure 21.2)

A. **Overview**
   1. The eyes, housed in the bony orbits, are the photosensitive organs responsible for vision.
   2. Each eye is composed of three tunics: the **tunica fibrosa** (outer layer), **tunica vasculosa** (middle layer), and **retina**.
   3. It receives **light** through the **cornea**. The light is focused by the **lens** on the **retina**, which contains specialized cells that encode the various patterns of the image for transmission to the brain via the **optic nerve**.
   4. The eye possesses **intrinsic muscles** that adjust the aperture of the iris and alter the lens diameter, permitting **accommodation** for close vision.
   5. The eye also possesses **extrinsic muscles**, attached to the external aspect of the eyeball, which move both eyes in a coordinated manner to perceive the desired visual fields.
   6. The eyeball is continually moistened on its anterior surface with **lacrimal fluid** (tears) secreted by the **lacrimal gland**.
   7. The **eyeball** is covered by the upper and lower eyelids, which protect its anterior surface.

B. **Tunica fibrosa** (see Figure 21.2)
   1. The outermost tunica fibrosa is composed of the sclera and the cornea. The **sclera** (the white of the eye) is an **opaque**, relatively avascular fibrous connective tissue layer that covers the posterior five-sixths of the eyeball. The sclera receives insertions of the extrinsic ocular muscles.

Posterior segment of globe   Anterior segment of globe

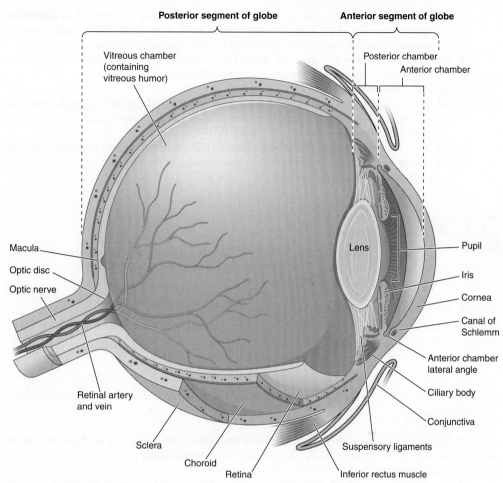

FIGURE 21.2. Anatomy of the eyeball. (Adapted with permission from McConnell TH. *The Nature of Disease.* Baltimore, MD: Lippincott Williams & Wilkins; 2007:680.)

2. The **cornea** is the **transparent**, highly innervated **avascular** anterior one-sixth of the tunica fibrosa. It joins the sclera in a region called the **limbus**. The cornea is composed of five layers.
    a. **Corneal epithelium**
        (1) The corneal epithelium lines the **anterior aspect** of the cornea and is continuous with the **conjunctiva** (a mucous membrane covering the anterior sclera and lining the internal surface of the eyelids).
        (2) It is a **stratified squamous nonkeratinized epithelium**.
        (3) It possesses **microvilli** in its superficial layer that trap moisture, protecting the cornea from dehydration.
        (4) The corneal epithelium is highly innervated with free nerve endings.
    b. **Bowman membrane** is a homogeneous **noncellular** layer that provides form, stability, and strength to the cornea. The basal layer of the corneal epithelium is attached to Bowman membrane via hemidesmosomes.
    c. **Corneal stroma**
        (1) The corneal stroma is the thickest corneal layer. It is composed of about five layers of both **type I** and **V collagen fibers** lying parallel to each other within each row and at oblique angles to each other in adjoining layers, thus forming a lattice. These collagen fibers are embedded in a ground substance composed mostly of chondroitin sulfate and keratan sulfate. A few fibroblasts are located between the laminae of collagen fibers.

     (2) The stroma has channels in the region of the limbus that are lined by **endothelium**, forming the **canal of Schlemm** (see Figure 21.2). This canal drains fluid (aqueous humor) from the anterior chamber of the eye into the venous system.

  d. Descemet membrane is a thick (5–10 μm) basal lamina that is interposed between the endothelium and the connective tissue stroma of the cornea.

  e. Corneal endothelium

    (1) The corneal endothelium lines the **posterior aspect** of the cornea beneath Descemet membrane, where it separates the cornea from the aqueous humor in the anterior chamber of the eye.

    (2) It is a **simple squamous epithelium** with cells that exhibit numerous **pinocytic vesicles**.

    (3) It **resorbs fluid** from the stroma, thus contributing to the transparency of the cornea, contributory to light refraction.

CLINICAL CONSIDERATION

Cornea

Because the cornea is without a blood supply and lymphatics, the cornea may be transplanted without eliciting an immune response that would result in tissue rejection. Thus, it is one of the most frequently donated tissues.

Corneal Reflex (blink response)

A wisp of cotton that has touched the cornea will cause the patient to blink. The blink is a test of the integrity of the ophthalmic division of the trigeminal nerve (Cranial nerve V).

C. Tunica vasculosa (uvea, the middle tunic) is composed of three parts: choroid, ciliary body, and iris. (see Figure 21.2)

  1. Choroid

    a. The choroid is the **highly vascular, pigmented layer** of the eye on the posterior wall of the eyeball; its loose connective tissue contains many **melanocytes**.

    b. It is loosely attached to the tunica fibrosa.

    c. Its deepest layer, **Bruch membrane** extends from the ora serrata to the optic disk and separates the choriocapillary layer from the pigment epithelium. It is composed of two thin layers of collagen fibers with an intervening layer of elastic fibers. Both layers of collagen fibers are covered by basal laminae.

    d. The **choriocapillary layer** contains the blood capillaries derived from the choroid stroma that supply the retina.

  2. Ciliary body

    a. The ciliary body is the wedge-shaped **anterior expansion of the choroid**.

    b. It completely encircles the lens and separates the ora serrata from the iris.

    c. It is lined on its inner surface by two layers of cells: an **outer pigmented columnar epithelium** rich in melanin and an **inner nonpigmented simple columnar** epithelium.

    (1) Ciliary processes

      (a) are radially arranged extensions (about 70) of the ciliary body.

      (b) have a connective tissue core containing many **fenestrated capillaries**.

      (c) are covered by two epithelial layers. The **nonpigmented inner layer** transports components from the plasma filtrate in the posterior chamber and thus forms the **aqueous humor**, which flows to the anterior chamber via the pupillary aperture (see Figure 21.2).

      (d) possess **suspensory ligaments** (zonulae) that arise from the processes and insert into the capsule of the lens, serving to anchor it in place.

    (2) Ciliary muscle

      (a) is attached to the sclera and ciliary body in such a manner that its contractions stretch the ciliary body and release tension on the suspensory ligament and lens. Ciliary muscle contraction permits the lens to become more convex, allowing the eye to focus on nearby objects (**accommodation**). With advancing age, the lens loses its elasticity, thereby gradually losing the ability to accommodate.

(b) The ciliary muscle is innervated via **parasympathetic fibers** of the **oculomotor nerve** (cranial nerve III).

3. **Iris**
   a. **Overview**
      (1) The iris is the most anterior extension of the choroid, separating the anterior and posterior chambers of the eyeball (see Figure 21.2).
      (2) It incompletely covers the anterior surface of the lens, forming an aperture called the **pupil** that is continually adjusted by intrinsic pupillary muscles.
      (3) The iris is covered by an incomplete layer of pigmented cells and fibroblasts on its anterior surface.
      (4) It has a wall composed of loose vascular connective tissue containing melanocytes and fibroblasts.
      (5) The iris is covered on its deep surface by a two-layered epithelium **possessing** pigmented cells that block light from entering the interior of the eye except via the pupil.
   b. **Eye color** is blue only if few melanocytes are present. Increasing amounts of pigment impart darker colors to the eye.
   c. **Dilator pupillae muscle**
      (1) Dilator pupillae muscle is a **smooth muscle** with fibers that radiate from the periphery of the iris toward the pupil.
      (2) It contracts upon stimulation by **sympathetic** nerve fibers, **dilating the pupil**.
   d. **Sphincter pupillae muscle**
      (1) Sphincter pupillae muscle is **smooth muscle** arranged in concentric rings around the pupillary orifice.
      (2) It contracts upon stimulation by **parasympathetic** nerve fibers of the oculomotor nerve (cranial nerve III), **constricting the pupil**.

D. **Refractive media of the eye**
   1. **Aqueous humor**
      a. Aqueous humor is a **plasmalike fluid** in the anterior compartment of the eye that is **formed by epithelial cells lining the ciliary processes**.
      b. It is constantly secreted into the posterior chamber of the eye and then flows into the anterior chamber of the eye via the pupillary aperture; from there it enters the venous system via the canal of Schlemm (Figure 21.2).

CLINICAL CONSIDERATIONS **Glaucoma**

1. Glaucoma is a condition of abnormally **high intraocular pressure**. It is caused by obstructions that prevent drainage of aqueous humor from the eye via the canal of Schlemm. Glaucoma is the leading cause of blindness in African Americans in the United States, and worldwide, it is the second leading cause of blindness after cataracts. Since it is an age-related condition, about 1 in 10 persons 80 years of age have glaucoma.
2. **Chronic glaucoma**, the most common form of glaucoma, may be associated with few symptoms except for a gradual loss of peripheral vision. However, usually, this condition can be controlled with medication in the form of eye drops.

---

2. The **lens** is a biconvex **transparent** flexible structure composed of the lens capsule, subcapsular epithelium, and lens fibers (Figure 21.3).
   a. The **lens capsule** is a thick basal lamina that envelops the entire lens epithelium.
   b. The **subcapsular epithelium** (on the anterior and lateral lens surfaces only) is composed of a single layer of cuboidal cells that communicate with each other via **gap junctions** and interdigitate with lens fibers.

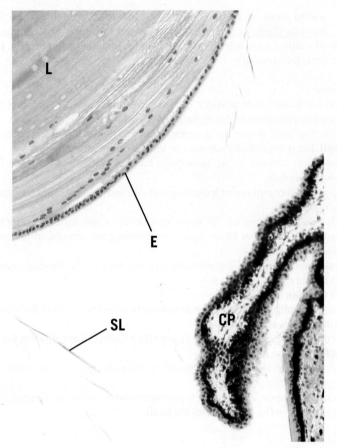

FIGURE 21.3. Light micrograph of the lens of the eye (×132). Observe the lens (L), epithelium (E), suspensory ligament (SL) of the lens, and the ciliary process (CP).

         c. **Lens fibers** represent highly differentiated, elongated cells that when mature **lack** both nuclei and organelles. Lens fibers are filled with a group of proteins called **crystallins**.

         d. The **suspensory ligament** stretches between the lens and the ciliary body, keeping tension on the lens and **enabling it to focus on distant objects**.

    3. The **vitreous body** is a **refractile gel** composed mainly of water, collagen, and hyaluronic acid. This gel fills the interior of the globe posterior to the lens (Figure 21.2).

CLINICAL CONSIDERATIONS   **Cataract**

    1. A cataract is an **opacity of the lens** resulting from the accumulation of pigment or other substances in the lens fibers that scatter the light entering the lens, thus preventing sharp focusing of the light on the retina.

    2. This condition is often associated with **aging**.

    3. If untreated, it leads to a gradual loss of vision.

    4. When the opacity becomes severe, an ophthalmologist may remove and replace the affected lens with a man-made lens restoring clear vision.

Presbyopia

Presbyopia is the inability of the eye to focus on close objects (accommodation). This is usually associated with aging, since it is related to decreasing elasticity of the lens, which prevents it from assuming a spherical shape. This condition can usually be corrected with eyeglasses.

Eye Floaters (vitreous opacities)

Age-related changes with the gel-like vitreous body becoming more liquid cause debris within it to clump, and as light passes through the vitreous body, the debris forms shadows on the retina that appear as black spots, streaks, strings, spiderwebs, etc., which move about in the visual fields. These are called **eye floaters**, which can become an annoyance; however, most people learn to disregard them. Usually, they resolve in a few weeks or so. When eye floaters are accompanied by bright flashes of light or fuzzy vision, an ophthalmologist should be consulted as this may indicate a tear in the retina.

E. **Retina** (Figures 21.4 and 21.5)
1. **Overview**
    a. The retina is the innermost of the three tunicae of the eye and is responsible for **photoreception**. It is interposed between the choroid and the vitreous humor.
        (1) It is composed of two layers—a photosensitive layer containing rods and cones and several interneurons, and a nonsensitive pigmented layer housing melanin producing cells.
        (2) The photosensitive (visual) portion of the retina ends at the ora serrata, whereas the nonsensitive (pigmented) portion continues anteriorly to cover the ciliary body and the posterior surface of the iris.
    b. The retinal layer has a shallow depression in its posterior wall that contains only cones; this is an avascular region, called the **fovea centralis**, whose central region, the **macula**, exhibits the greatest visual acuity (Figure 21.2).

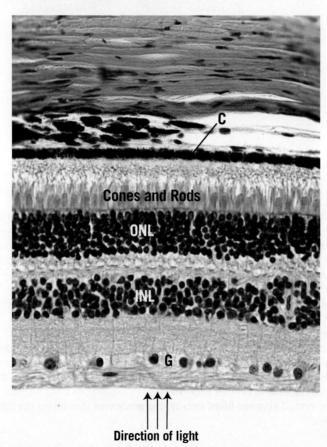

FIGURE 21.4. Light micrograph of the retina (×132). Observe the choroids superior to the pigmented epithelial layer (C), the rods and cones, outer nuclear layer (ONL), the inner nuclear layer (INL), and the ganglion layer (G).

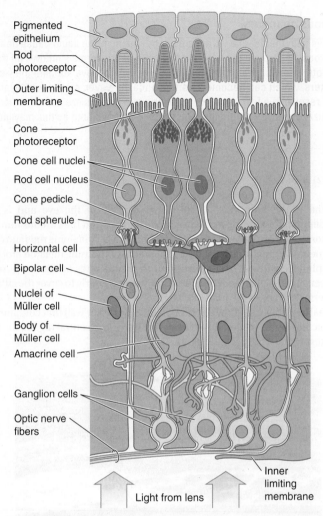

Pigmented epithelium
Rod photoreceptor
Outer limiting membrane
Cone photoreceptor
Cone cell nuclei
Rod cell nucleus
Cone pedicle
Rod spherule
Horizontal cell
Bipolar cell
Nuclei of Müller cell
Body of Müller cell
Amacrine cell
Ganglion cells
Optic nerve fibers
Inner limiting membrane
Light from lens

FIGURE 21.5. The layers of the retina. (Adapted with permission from Gartner LP, Hiatt JL. *Color Textbook of Histology.* 2nd ed. Philadelphia, PA: Saunders; 2001:518.)

 c. The retina displays **10 distinct layers**; later in the chapter, they are discussed in order from the outermost to the innermost.

 d. Only certain of these 10 cell layers are composed of neurons that receive, integrate, and relay or transmit impulses to the brain for processing. These include photoreceptor rods and cones, bipolar cells, and ganglion cells. Cells of the remaining layers function in supporting the architecture of the retina.

2. The **retinal pigment epithelium** is a layer of **columnar cells** firmly attached to the **Bruch membrane**.

 a. Structure

  (1) Retinal pigment epithelial cells have **junctional complexes** and **basal invaginations** that contain mitochondria, suggesting the involvement of these cells in ion transport.

  (2) They contain smooth endoplasmic reticulum (SER) and many **melanin granules** located apically in cellular processes.

  (3) They extend **pigment-filled microvillus processes** that invest the tips of the rods and cones.

 b. Function

  (1) Retinal pigment epithelial cells **esterify vitamin A** (used in the formation of visual pigment by rods and cones).

(2) They **phagocytize** the shed tips of the outer segments of rods.

(3) They **synthesize melanin**, which absorbs light after the rods and cones have been stimulated.

(4) serve as the blood–retinal barrier.

3. The photoreceptor layer consists of neurons (photoreceptor cells) called rods and cones.

   a. **Rods (sensitive to light of low intensity)** (Figure 21.5)

      (1) Overview

         (a) Rods possess four regions—**outer and inner segments**, a **nuclear region**, and a **synaptic region**.

         (b) They may synapse with bipolar cells, giving rise to **summation**.

         (c) They possess an **incomplete cilium** terminating in a basal body within the inner segment.

      (2) Outer segments of rods

         (a) consist mainly of hundreds of **flattened membranous disks** that contain **rhodopsin**, the visual pigment located in the discs of rods and discs of cones.

         (b) eventually shed their disks, which are subsequently phagocytized by the pigment epithelial cells.

      (3) Inner segments of rods possess mitochondria, glycogen, polyribosomes, and proteins, which migrate to the outer segments to be incorporated into the membranous disks.

      (4) Photoreception by rods is initiated by the interaction of **light** with **rhodopsin (visual purple)**, which is composed of the integral membrane protein **opsin** bound to **retinal**, the aldehyde form of vitamin A.

         (a) The retinal moiety of rhodopsin **absorbs light** in the visible range.

         (b) Retinal dissociates from opsin. This reaction, called **bleaching**, eventually closes the Na^+ channels, thus permitting diffusion of bound Ca^{2+} **ions** into the cytoplasm of the outer segment of a rod cell.

         (c) Excess Ca^{2+} acts to **hyperpolarize** the cell because Na^+ is prevented from entering the cell.

         (d) Ionic alterations in the rod generate electrical activity, which is relayed to other rods via gap junctions.

         (e) Dissociated retinal and opsin **reassemble** by an active process in which Müller and pigment epithelial cells also participate.

         (f) Ca^{2+} is recaptured by the membranous disks, leading to reopening of the Na^+ channels and **reestablishment** of the normal resting membrane potential.

   b. **Cones (sensitive to light of high intensity)** (Figure 21.5)

      (1) Cones are **much less numerous than rods**, but produce **greater visual acuity** than do rods; thus, the macula is populated only by cones.

      (2) They are generally similar in structure to rods and mediate photoreception in the same way, with the following exceptions:

         (a) The membranous disks in the outer segments of cones are invaginations of the plasma membrane, whereas in rods they are not.

         (b) The proteins synthesized in the inner segments of cones are passed to the entire outer segment, whereas in rods they are added only to newly forming disks.

         (c) Cones possess **iodopsin** in their disks. The amount of this photopigment varies in different cones, making them differentially sensitive to red, green, or blue light.

         (d) Each cone synapses with a **single** bipolar neuron, whereas each rod may synapse with several bipolar neurons.

CLINICAL CONSIDERATIONS Age-related macular degeneration (AMD) is a disease of the retina located in the central region of the macula, hence affecting central vision. As its name implies, it is a disease of aging, occurring usually after the age of 50 years. There are two forms: dry and wet AMD. **Dry macular degeneration**, the most common, is where the central vision is affected so that objects become very blurred. This is caused by cellular debris (drusen) that appears as yellow spots deposited between the choroids and the retina. **Wet macular degeneration**, the most severe, results when small blood vessels, formed between the choroid and the retina, leak into this space causing the retina to die; as a result, a blind spot forms in the center of the visual field. Wet macular degeneration exhibits a quick onset with a small blind spot that may quickly progress to a larger blind spot. Although an AMD patient may be unable to recognize a face in the center of vision, it is interesting to note that peripheral vision is unaffected by macular degeneration. While there is no cure, certain vitamins and high doses of antioxidants and zinc may be of some benefit for dry AMD, whereas laser surgery and injections of antiangiogenesis drugs are used to manage wet AMD.

4. **External limiting membrane**
   a. The external limiting membrane is not a true membrane, but an area where **zonulae adherentes** (belt desmosomes) are located between the photoreceptor cells and the retinal Müller cells (glial cells).
   b. This membrane also contains microvilli that project from the Müller cells.
5. The **outer nuclear layer** consists primarily of the **nuclei of the rods and cones**.
6. **Outer plexiform layer**
   a. The outer plexiform layer contains **axodendritic synapses** between the axons of photoreceptor cells and the dendrites of bipolar and horizontal cells.
   b. It displays **synaptic ribbons** within the rod and cone cells at synaptic sites.
7. The **inner nuclear layer** contains the **cell bodies of bipolar neurons**, horizontal cells, amacrine cells, and the nuclei of Müller cells.
8. **Inner plexiform layer**
   a. The inner plexiform layer contains **axodendritic synapses** between the axons of bipolar cells and the dendrites of ganglion cells.
   b. The processes of amacrine cells are located in this layer.
9. The **ganglion cell layer** contains the **somata of ganglion cells**, which form the final link in the retina's neural chain. There are two types of ganglion cells: the majority (about 97% of ganglion cells) are those that function in vision and a very small minority that function in the diurnal rhythm by projecting, *indirectly*, to the pineal body, informing that gland whether it is daylight or night (see Chapter 13 Section VII 2). Only the ganglion cells that function in the sensation of vision are described here.
   a. **Structure—Ganglion cells**
      (1) Ganglion cells are typical neurons that project their axons to a specific region of the retina called the **optic disk**.
      (2) These cells are **midget, diffuse**, and **stratified ganglion cells**.
   b. **Function—Ganglion cells.** Ganglion cells are activated by **hyperpolarization of rods and cones** and generate an **action potential**, which is transmitted to horizontal and amacrine cells and carried to the visual relay system in the brain.
10. The **optic nerve fiber layer** consists primarily of the **unmyelinated axons** of ganglion cells, which form the fibers of the **optic nerve**. As each fiber pierces the sclera, it acquires a myelin sheath.
11. The **inner limiting membrane** consists of the terminations of Müller cell processes and their basement membranes.

CLINICAL CONSIDERATIONS   **Detachment of the retina**

1. Retinal detachment occurs when the neural and pigmented layers separate from each other, for example, as a result of a sudden hard jolt.
2. This condition can sometimes be treated successfully by laser surgery. But extensive separation requires cryosurgery to produce successful adhesion of the two layers. If retinal detachment is left untreated, blindness may occur, and often even with treatment, the rods and cones die, leaving blind spots in the visual field.

F. **Accessory structures of the eye**
   1. **Conjunctiva (transparent mucous membrane)**
      a. The conjunctiva lines the eyelids and is reflected onto the anterior portion of the eyeball to the cornea, where it becomes continuous with the corneal epithelium.
      b. It is a **stratified columnar epithelium** possessing many **goblet cells**.
      c. It is separated by a basal lamina from an underlying lamina propria of loose connective tissue.

CLINICAL CONSIDERATIONS **Conjunctivitis**

1. Conjunctivitis is an inflammation of the conjunctiva producing red sclera and a discharge.
2. It may be caused by bacteria, viruses, parasites, and allergens.
3. Some forms are contagious and may cause blindness if left untreated.

---

   2. **Eyelids**
      a. The eyelids are lined internally by conjunctiva and externally by skin that is elastic and covers a supportive framework of **tarsal plates**.
      b. Eyelids contain highly modified **sebaceous glands** (meibomian glands), smaller **modified sebaceous glands** (glands of Zeis), and **sweat glands** (glands of Moll).
   3. **Lacrimal apparatus** (Figure 21.6)
      a. **Lacrimal gland**
         (1) The lacrimal gland is a compound **tubuloalveolar gland** with secretory units that are surrounded by an incomplete layer of **myoepithelial cells**.
         (2) **Lacrimal fluid (tears)** is mostly water, and contains **lysozyme**, an antibacterial enzyme. Tears drain from the lacrimal gland via 6 to 12 ducts into the conjunctival **fornix**, from

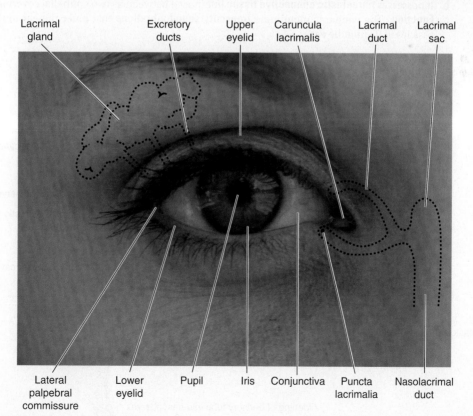

FIGURE 21.6. External anatomy of the eye. (Reprinted with permission from Hiatt JL, Gartner LP: *Textbook of Head and Neck Anatomy.* 4th ed. Baltimore, MD: Lippincott Williams & Wilkins; 2010:164.)

which the tears flow over the cornea and conjunctiva, keeping them moist. Tears then enter the lacrimal puncta, leading to the lacrimal canaliculi.

   b. **Lacrimal canaliculi** are lined by a **stratified squamous epithelium** and unite to form a common canaliculus, which empties into the lacrimal sac.

   c. The **lacrimal sac** is lined by a **pseudostratified ciliated columnar epithelium**.

   d. The **nasolacrimal duct** is the inferior continuation of the lacrimal sac and is also lined by a **pseudostratified ciliated columnar epithelium**. The duct empties into the floor of the nasal cavity.

IV. SENSE OF HEARING—EAR (VESTIBULOCOCHLEAR APPARATUS)

The ear consists of three parts: the **external ear**, which receives sound waves; the **middle ear**, through which sound waves are transmitted; and the **internal ear**, where sound waves are transduced into nerve impulses. The vestibular organ, responsible for equilibrium, is also located in the inner ear.

A. **External ear** (Figure 21.7)

   1. The **auricle (pinna)** is composed of irregular plates of **elastic cartilage** covered by **thin skin**.

   2. The **external auditory meatus** is lined by **skin** containing hair follicles, sebaceous glands, and **ceruminous glands**, which are modified sweat glands that produce **earwax (cerumen)**.

   3. **Tympanic membrane (eardrum)**

     a. The tympanic membrane is covered by **skin** on its external surface and by a **simple cuboidal epithelium** on its inner surface.

     b. It possesses **fibroelastic connective tissue** interposed between its two epithelial coverings.

     c. **Function.** The tympanic membrane **transmits sound vibrations** that enter the ear to the ossicles in the middle ear.

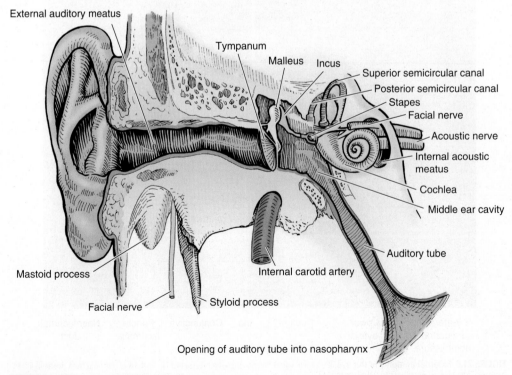

FIGURE 21.7. The external, middle, and inner ears. (Reprinted with permission from Hiatt JL, Gartner LP. *Textbook of Head and Neck Anatomy.* 2nd ed. Baltimore, MD: Williams & Wilkins; 1987:309.)

B. **Middle ear (tympanic cavity)** (Figure 21.7)
   1. The tympanic cavity contains the three bony **ossicles** (**malleus, incus**, and **stapes**), which **transmit movements of the tympanic membrane (eardrum) to the oval window** (a membrane-covered opening in the bony wall of the **cochlea**).
      a. The bony ossicles, **malleus, incus**, and **stapes**, are attached to each other in a chain-like formation between the tympanic membrane and the oval window, a membrane-covered opening in the bony labyrinth. The malleus is attached to the tympanic membrane, whereas the stapes is attached to the membrane of the oval window. The middle ossicle, the incus, is interposed between the malleus and the stapes. Small ligaments interconnect the ossicles. Two separate muscles, innervated by branches of individual cranial nerves, serve to control the functioning of these ossicles. The **tensor tympani muscle** maintains tension on the tympanic membrane and is innervated by a branch of the trigeminal nerve (cranial nerve V). The **stapedius muscle** dampens the movement of the stapes on the membrane covering the oval window. It is innervated by a branch of the facial nerve (cranial nerve VII).
      b. The bony ossicles, as a group, function in modulating movements of the tympanic membrane and in amplifying the sound waves by applying pressure on the membrane covering the oval window in the cochlea.
   2. The middle ear is connected to the nasopharynx via the **auditory tube (eustachian tube)**.
      a. It is lined by a **simple squamous epithelium**, which changes to **pseudostratified ciliated columnar epithelium** near its opening to the auditory tube.
      b. It has a **lamina propria** composed of dense connective tissue tightly adherent to the bony wall.

CLINICAL CONSIDERATIONS **Conductive hearing loss**

1. Conductive hearing loss results from a defect in the conduction of sound waves in the external or middle ear.
2. It may be caused by **otitis media**, a common inflammation of the middle ear; **obstruction** by a foreign body; or **otosclerosis** of the middle ear.

C. **Internal ear (a bony labyrinth within the temporal bone)** (Figure 21.7)
   1. The **bony labyrinth**, composed of the semicircular canals, vestibule, and cochlea, is filled with **perilymph**, and houses the **membranous labyrinth**, which is filled with **endolymph**.
      a. **Semicircular canals** house the **semicircular ducts** of the membranous labyrinth.
      b. The **vestibule** houses the **saccule** and **utricle**.
      c. **Cochlea**
         (1) The cochlea winds two and a half times around a bony core (the **modiolus**), which contains blood vessels and the spiral ganglion.
         (2) It is subdivided into three spaces: the **scala vestibuli** and **scala tympani**, which are both filled with perilymph, and the **scala media**, or cochlear duct, which is filled with endolymph.
   2. The **membranous labyrinth** is filled with **endolymph** and possesses various **sensory structures** that are **specializations of the epithelium**.
      a. **Saccule and utricle** (within the vestibule)
         (1) Overview
            (a) The saccule and utricle are saclike bodies composed of a thin sheath of connective tissue lined by **simple squamous epithelium**.
            (b) Each gives rise to a duct; the two ducts join, forming the **endolymphatic sac**.
            (c) They possess small, specialized regions, called **maculae**, which contain **type I and type II neuroepithelial hair cells**, supporting cells, and a gelatinous layer (**otolithic membrane**).
         (2) Vestibular hair cells
            (a) These **neuroepithelial cells** contain many mitochondria and a well-developed Golgi complex.

(b) They possess 50 to 100 elongated, **rigid stereocilia** (sensory microvilli) arranged in rows and a single cilium (**kinocilium**). These cilia extend from the apical surface of the hair cells into the otolithic membrane. They function in the **detection of linear acceleration**.

(c) Types of vestibular hair cells include the following:

1. **Type I hair cells** (bulbar), which are almost completely surrounded by a **cup-shaped afferent nerve ending**
2. **Type II hair cells** (columnar), which make contact with **small afferent terminals** containing synaptic vesicles

(3) Supporting cells are generally columnar and possess a round basal nucleus, many microtubules, and an extensive terminal web.

(4) The **otolithic membrane** is a **gelatinous layer** of glycoprotein that contains small calcified particles called **otoliths** or **otoconia**.

b. Semicircular ducts are continuous with and arise from the utricle. The three semicircular ducts are perpendicular to each other so that they can **detect angular acceleration** of the head in three-dimensional space (see Figure 21.7).

(1) The **ampullae** are dilated regions of the semicircular ducts near their junctions with the utricle.

(2) Cristae ampullares

(a) are specialized **sensory regions** within the ampullae of the semicircular ducts.

(b) are similar to maculae but have a thicker, conical glycoprotein layer (**cupula**), which does not contain otoliths.

c. The **endolymphatic duct** ends in the expanded endolymphatic sac.

d. Endolymphatic sac

(1) The endolymphatic sac has an epithelial lining containing **electron-dense** columnar cells, which have an irregularly shaped nucleus, and **electron-lucent** columnar cells, which possess long microvilli, many pinocytic vesicles, and vacuoles.

(2) It contains **phagocytic cells** (macrophages, neutrophils) in its lumen.

(3) Function. The endolymphatic sac may function in **resorption of endolymph**.

e. Cochlear duct (Figures 21.8 and 21.9)

(1) Overview

(a) The cochlear duct is a specialized diverticulum of the saccule that contains the **spiral organ of Corti**.

(b) It is bordered above by the **scala vestibuli** and below by the **scala tympani** of the bony cochlea. These scalae, which contain perilymph, communicate with each other at the **helicotrema** at the apex of the cochlea.

(2) Vestibular membrane

(a) is composed of two layers of flattened squamous epithelium separated by an intervening basement membrane.

(b) helps maintain the high ionic gradients between the perilymph in the scala vestibuli and the endolymph in the cochlear duct.

(3) Stria vascularis

(a) is a **vascularized** pseudostratified epithelium that lines the lateral aspect of the cochlear duct.

(b) is composed of basal, intermediate, and marginal cells.

(c) may **secrete endolymph**.

(4) Spiral prominence

(a) The spiral prominence is an epithelium-covered protuberance that extends the length of the cochlear duct. This epithelium is continuous with that of the stria vascularis and is reflected onto the basilar membrane, where it follows an indentation to form the **external spiral sulcus**.

(b) Its cells become cuboidal and continue onto the basilar membrane, where they are known as the **cells of Claudius**, which overlie the polyhedral **cells of Boettcher**.

(5) Basilar membrane

(a) is a thick layer of amorphous material containing **keratin-like fibers**.

(b) extends from the spiral ligament to the tympanic lip of the limbus spiralis.

(c) has two zones: the medial **zona arcuata** and the lateral **zona pectinata**.

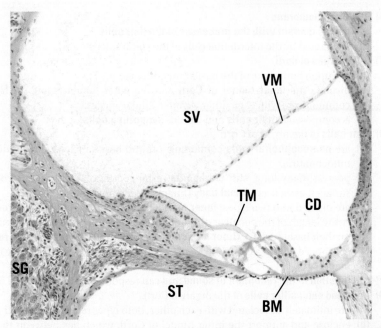

FIGURE 21.8. Light micrograph of the cochlea (×132). Note the spiral ganglion (SG), scala tympani (ST), basilar membrane (BM), scala vascularis (SV), vestibular membrane (VM), tectorial membrane (TM), and the cochlear duct (CD).

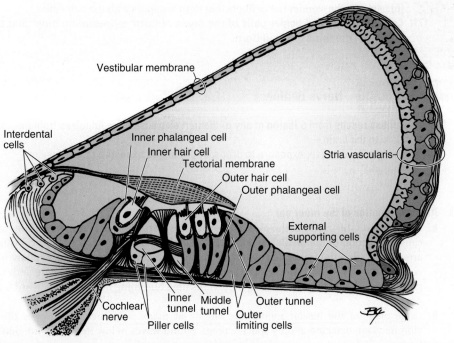

FIGURE 21.9. The cochlear duct and the spiral organ of Corti. (Adapted with permission from Dellmann HD. *Textbook of Veterinary Histology.* 4th ed. Baltimore, MD: Williams & Wilkins; 1993:332.)

(6) Tectorial membrane
- **(a) makes contact with the processes of the hair cells**.
- **(b)** is secreted by the interdental cells of the spiral sulcus.

(7) Spiral organ of Corti
- **(a)** lies upon both parts of the basilar membrane.
- **(b)** displays the **inner tunnel of Corti** and the **outer tunnel (space of Nuel)**, which communicate with each other via intercellular spaces.
- **(c)** is composed of **hair cells** and various **supporting cells**.

(8) Hair cells of the organ of Corti
- **(a)** are **neuroepithelial cells** containing a round basal nucleus surrounded by many mitochondria.
- **(b)** possess many long, **stiff stereocilia** (arranged in a "W" formation) on their free surfaces, as well as a **basal body** (but no kinocilium).
- **(c)** are divided into two types: **Inner hair cells** are organized in a **single row** along the entire length of the cochlear duct and receive numerous afferent synaptic terminals on their basal surface. **Outer hair cells** are organized in **three or more rows** and are ensconced within a cup-shaped afferent nerve ending, where synaptic contacts are made.
- **(d) function** in the **reception of sound** and can respond to different sound frequencies.

(9) Inner and outer pillar cells of the organ of Corti
- **(a)** are intimately associated with each other; both types rest on the basilar membrane.
- **(b)** enclose and support the inner tunnel of Corti, which lies between the inner and outer pillar cells.
- **(c)** possess a wide base and have elongated processes, which contain microtubules, intermediate filaments, and actin filaments.

(10) Inner and outer phalangeal cells of the organ of Corti
- **(a)** are intimately associated with the inner and outer hair cells, respectively.
- **(b)** support the slender nerve fibers that form synapses with the hair cells.

(11) Cells of Hensen and border cells of the organ of Corti delineate the inner and outer borders of the spiral organ of Corti.

CLINICAL CONSIDERATIONS   Nerve deafness

1. Nerve deafness results from a **lesion** in any of the nerves transmitting impulses from the spiral organ of Corti to the brain.
2. It may be caused by disease, exposure to drugs, or prolonged exposure to loud noises.

---

3. **Auditory function of the inner ear**
   a. Movement of the stapes at the oval window causes disturbances in the perilymph, which cause deflection of the **basilar membrane**. Oscillations set in motion at the oval window are dissipated at the secondary tympanic membrane covering the **round window** of the cochlea. (At a very loud concert, the amount of energy absorbed is very high, and it may take up to 72 hours for it to be dissipated. A residual humming noise may be heard for 2–3 days.)
   b. Large areas of the basilar membrane vibrate at many frequencies. However, optimal vibrations are detected at only specific areas. Sound waves of low frequency are detected farther away from the oval window.
   c. The **pillar cells** attached to the basilar membrane move laterally in response to this deflection, in turn causing a lateral shearing of the stereocilia of the sensory hair cells of the organ of Corti against the tectorial membrane.
   d. **Movement of the stereocilia** is transduced into electrical impulses that travel via the **cochlear nerve** to the brain.

4. **Vestibular function of the inner ear**
   a. A change in the position of the head causes a flow of the endolymph in the semicircular ducts (**circular movement**) or in the saccules and utricles (**linear movement**).
   b. Movement of the endolymph in the semicircular ducts displaces the cupula overlying the **cristae ampullares**, causing bending of the stereocilia of the sensory hair cells.
   c. Movement of the endolymph in the saccules and utricles displaces the **otoliths**. This deformation is transmitted to the **maculae** via the overlying gelatinous layer, causing bending of the stereocilia of the sensory hair cells.
   d. In both cases, **movement of the stereocilia** is transduced into **electrical impulses**, which are transmitted to the brain via **vestibular nerve fibers**.

CLINICAL CONSIDERATIONS   **Ménière disease**

1. **Ménière disease** is an inner ear disorder causing hearing loss, vertigo, nausea, tinnitus, and vomiting. It is related to excess fluid in the endolymphatic duct.
2. Drugs are used to treat the vertigo and nausea, but in severe cases, surgery may be required for vestibular neurectomy.

Review Test

Directions: Each of the numbered items or incomplete statements in this section is followed by answers or by completions of the statement. Select the ONE lettered answer or completion that is BEST in each case.

1. Which of the following specialized receptors exhibits a large ovoid capsule consisting of many concentric lamellae, each separated by a space containing tissue fluid?

(A) Cold receptors
(B) Pacinian corpuscles
(C) Ruffini endings
(D) Meissner corpuscles
(E) Krause end bulb

2. Aqueous humor drains from the eye by passing

(A) into the ciliary processes.
(B) from the anterior chamber into the posterior chamber.
(C) through the canal of Schlemm.
(D) into the vitreous body.
(E) through the pupil.

3. Which of the following statements is characteristic of the choroid?

(A) It is avascular.
(B) It is the posterior portion of the tunica fibrosa.
(C) It is tightly attached to the sclera.
(D) It contains many melanocytes.
(E) It is not pigmented.

4. Communication of the scala vestibuli and scala tympani occurs at the

(A) round window.
(B) oval window.
(C) helicotrema.
(D) endolymphatic sac.
(E) inner tunnel.

5. The bony ossicles of the middle ear cavity are arranged in a series bridging the tympanic cavity beginning at the tympanic membrane and ending at the

(A) endolymphatic duct.
(B) round window.
(C) helicotrema.
(D) oval window.
(E) cochlear duct.

6. Which of the following cells in the inner ear are involved in detecting movements of the head?

(A) Hair cells in the maculae
(B) Outer pillar cells
(C) Inner pillar cells
(D) Cells of Hensen
(E) Hair cells in the organ of Corti

7. Rods and cones form synapses with which of the following cells?

(A) Amacrine
(B) Bipolar
(C) Ganglion
(D) Müller
(E) Pigmented epithelium

8. Which of the following statements is characteristic of the cornea?

(A) It represents the anterior portion of the tunica vasculosa.
(B) It is composed of three layers.
(C) It forms the anterior boundary of the posterior chamber of the eye.
(D) It is devoid of nerve endings.
(E) It is the anterior transparent portion of the tunica fibrosa.

9. A patient exhibiting a high intraocular pressure in both eyes is symptomatic for

(A) cataract.
(B) detached retina.
(C) glaucoma.
(D) conjunctivitis.
(E) presbyopia.

10. Aqueous humor is produced by

(A) the corneal epithelium.
(B) the canal of Schlemm.
(C) ciliary epithelium.
(D) conjunctiva.
(E) ora serrata.

11. Which one of the following is related to an overabundance of fluid in the endolymphatic duct?

(A) Glaucoma
(B) Vertigo
(C) Otis media
(D) Conductive hearing loss
(E) Nerve deafness

Answers and Explanations

1. **B.** Pacinian corpuscles are usually macroscopic. Their capsules are composed of several lamellae containing fibroblasts and collagen fibers. The lamellae are separated by sparse amounts of tissue fluid. Pacinian corpuscles respond to vibrations and pressure that distort the lamellae. Meissner corpuscles, responsible for touch, are tapered terminals at the tips of dermal papillae. Ruffini endings, which are sensitive to mechanical stresses, possess a thin connective tissue capsule that surrounds a fluid-filled space. Cold receptors are naked nerve endings that respond to temperatures below 25°C to 30°C (see Chapter 21 II B).

2. **C.** Aqueous humor exits the eye by passing into the canal of Schlemm. The vitreous body is a refractile gel that fills the chamber of the globe posterior to the lens and is not related to the aqueous humor (see Chapter 21 III D 1).

3. **D.** The choroid is the vascular tunic of the eye that loosely adheres to the sclera of the tunica fibrosa. It contains many melanocytes, which impart a dark pigment to the eye (see Chapter 21 III C 1).

4. **C.** The scala vestibuli and the scala tympani are actually one perilymphatic space separated by the cochlear duct (scala media). The scala vestibuli and tympani communicate with each other at the helicotrema (see Chapter 21 IV C 2 e).

5. **D.** The bony ossicles of the middle ear cavity articulate in a series from the tympanic membrane to the oval window (see Chapter 21 IV B).

6. **A.** Neuroepithelial hair cells in the maculae of the saccule and the utricle detect linear movement of the head. These cells are connected to the vestibular portion of the acoustic nerve (see Chapter 21 IV C 2).

7. **B.** Rods and cones synapse with bipolar cells and horizontal cells (see Chapter 21 III E 3).

8. **E.** The cornea is the transparent anterior portion of the tunica fibrosa, the outer covering of the eye; thus it forms the anterior wall of the anterior chamber of the eye. It is also rich in sensory nerve endings. The sclera is the posterior portion of the tunica fibrosa. The tunica vasculosa (middle coat) is composed of the choroid and ciliary body and the iris (see Chapter 21 III B).

9. **C.** High intraocular pressure is a symptom of glaucoma. This condition prohibits the aqueous humor from escaping from the anterior chamber of the eye via the canal of Schlemm. If it is left untreated, a gradual loss of peripheral sight occurs; over time, blindness results. People with cataract have opacity of the lens that blurs the vision. Conjunctivitis is an inflammation of the conjunctiva of the eye with severe reddening of the sclera and the conjunctival surface of the lids, perhaps with a discharge. This condition may be contagious, and if left untreated, blindness may occur (see Chapter 21 III D Clinical Consideration).

10. **C.** The ciliary epithelium that lines the ciliary processes secretes the aqueous humor into the posterior chamber of the eye between the iris and the lens. The aqueous humor then flows through the pupil and into the anterior chamber of the eye and finally leaves the anterior chamber by entering the venous system via the canal of Schlemm (see Chapter 21 III D 1).

11. **B.** An overabundance of endolymph in the endolymphatic duct causes vertigo, nausea, hearing loss, tinnitus, and vomiting, all symptoms of **Ménière disease** (see Chapter 21 IV C 4 Clinical Consideration).

Comprehensive Examination

Directions: Each of the numbered items or incomplete statements in this section is followed by answers or by completions of the statement. Select the ONE lettered answer or completion that is BEST in each case.

1. Which of the following statements concerning ribonucleic acid (RNA) synthesis is true?

(A) RNA synthesis does not require deoxyribonucleic acid to act as a template.

(B) Syntheses of ribosomal RNA, messenger RNA, and transfer RNA are all catalyzed by the same RNA polymerase.

(C) To yield messenger ribonucleoproteins, introns are excised, whereas exons are spliced together.

(D) Protein moieties are removed from messenger ribonucleoproteins within the nucleolus, yielding functional messenger RNAs to exit via the nuclear pores.

(E) The start codon for RNA synthesis is UAG.

2. Which of the following factors is primarily responsible for causing osteoporosis in older women?

(A) Decreased bone formation
(B) Lack of physical exercise
(C) Diminished estrogen secretion
(D) Calcium deficiency
(E) Increased bone formation

3. Which of the following bases that make up deoxyribonucleic acid and ribonucleic acid (RNA) is unique to RNA?

(A) Thymine
(B) Adenine
(C) Cytosine
(D) Guanine
(E) Uracil

4. The centroacinar cells of the pancreas secrete

(A) an alkaline enzyme-poor fluid.
(B) pancreatic digestive enzymes.
(C) secretin.
(D) cholecystokinin.
(E) glucagon.

5. The zona fasciculata of the adrenal cortex synthesizes and secretes

(A) mineralocorticoids.
(B) glucagon.
(C) epinephrine.
(D) aldosterone.
(E) glucocorticoids.

6. Which of the following statements about bony joints is true?

(A) Long bones are generally united by synarthroses.

(B) Diarthroses are classified as synovial joints.

(C) Type A cells of the synovial membrane secrete synovial fluid.

(D) Type B cells of the synovial membrane are phagocytic.

(E) Synarthroses are usually surrounded by a two-layered capsule.

7. All of the following characteristics can be used to distinguish neutrophils and basophils histologically except one. Which one is the exception?

(A) Size of specific granules
(B) Shape of the nucleus
(C) Number of azurophilic granules
(D) The presence or absence of peroxidase
(E) The presence of mitochondria

8. A long-time user of chewing tobacco noticed several whitish, thick, painless patches on the lining of his cheeks. The most probable diagnosis is

(A) aphthous ulcers.
(B) adenocarcinoma.
(C) keloids.
(D) oral leukoplakia.
(E) epidermolysis bullosa.

9. Primordial follicles of the ovary possess

(A) a layer of cuboidal follicular cells.
(B) an oocyte arrested in prophase of meiosis I.
(C) an oocyte arrested in metaphase of meiosis II.
(D) well-defined thecae interna and externa.
(E) a thick zona pellucida.

10. All of the following statements regarding the membranous labyrinth of the inner ear are true except for one. Which is that exception?

(A) It contains the saccule and utricle.
(B) Maculae contain neuroepithelial cells, which possess numerous stereocilia and a single kinocilium.
(C) Cristae ampullares in the semicircular canals detect angular acceleration of the head.
(D) The otolithic membrane contains small calcified particles.
(E) It contains the vestibular membrane.

11. Which of the following statements concerning euchromatin is true?

(A) It constitutes about 90% of the chromatin.
(B) It appears as basophilic clumps of nucleoprotein when seen under the light microscope.
(C) It is concentrated near the periphery of the nucleus.
(D) It is transcriptionally active.
(E) It is transcriptionally inactive.

12. Intercalated disks function in which one of the following?

(A) End-to-end attachments of smooth muscle cells
(B) Intercellular movement of large proteins
(C) Ionic coupling of cardiac muscle cells
(D) Storage of Ca^{2+}
(E) Release of neurotransmitters

13. Release of thyroid hormones from the follicular cells of the thyroid gland depends on thyroid-stimulating hormone (TSH). TSH stimulation involves

(A) binding of TSH to receptors on the apical plasma membrane.
(B) formation of apical microvilli.
(C) exocytosis of colloid droplets.
(D) change in cell shape from flattened to columnar.
(E) secretion of lysosomes from the basal cell surface.

14. Which one of the following statements about the development of the tooth crown is true?

(A) The enamel organ is derived from ectomesenchyme (neural crest).
(B) The dental papilla is derived from the epithelium.
(C) The four-layer enamel organ appears during the cap stage.
(D) Dentin and enamel are formed during the appositional stage.
(E) Cementum is formed at the same time as enamel.

15. Which one of the following statements concerning liver sinusoids is true?

(A) Their lining includes Ito cells (fat-storing cells).
(B) They receive bile from the hepatocytes.
(C) They are lined by nonfenestrated endothelial cells.
(D) The space of Disse is located between sinusoidal cells and hepatocytes.
(E) Sinusoids convey blood from the central vein to the portal vein.

16. A young college student had nausea, vomiting, visual disorders, and muscular paralysis after eating canned tuna fish. The probable diagnosis is botulism, caused by ingestion of the *Clostridium botulinum* toxin. The physiological effect of this toxin is to

(A) inactivate acetylcholinesterase.
(B) bind to and thus inactivate acetylcholine receptors at myoneural junctions.
(C) prevent release of calcium ions from the sarcoplasmic reticulum, thus inhibiting muscle contraction.
(D) inhibit release of acetylcholine from presynaptic membranes.
(E) inhibit hydrolysis of adenosine triphosphate during the contraction cycle.

17. Which of the following statements about nucleosomes is true?

(A) Histones form the nucleosome core around which the double helix deoxyribonucleic acid is wound.
(B) Nucleosomes without histones form the structural unit of the chromosome.
(C) Nucleosomes are composed of ribonucleic acid (RNA) molecules and two copies each of four different histones.
(D) Histone H1 forms the core of the nucleosome.
(E) Nucleosomes are linked together with RNA.

18. A high school student complains of fatigue and a sore throat. She has swollen, tender lymph nodes and a fever. Blood test results show an increased white blood cell count with many atypical lymphocytes; the number and appearance of the erythrocytes are normal. This student is likely to have

(A) AIDS.
(B) pernicious anemia.
(C) infectious mononucleosis.
(D) Hodgkin disease.
(E) factor VIII deficiency.

19. Which one of the following statements about the gallbladder is true?

(A) The gallbladder dilutes bile.
(B) Bile enters the gallbladder via the common bile duct.
(C) Bile leaves the gallbladder via the cystic duct.
(D) The gallbladder is lined by a simple squamous epithelium.
(E) Secretin stimulates the wall of the gallbladder to contract, forcing bile from its lumen.

20. Which one of the following statements concerning mitochondria is true?

(A) They change from the orthodox to the condensed form in response to the uncoupling of oxidation from phosphorylation.
(B) They are unable to divide.
(C) They possess the enzymes of the Krebs cycle in their cristae.
(D) They contain elementary particles in their matrix.
(E) They do not contain deoxyribonucleic acid.

21. Which one of the following components is present in muscular arteries but absent from elastic arteries?

(A) Fenestrated membranes
(B) Vasa vasorum
(C) Factor VIII
(D) A thick, complete internal elastic lamina
(E) Smooth muscle cells

22. Which one of the following statements concerning the pancreas is true?

(A) Islets of Langerhans secrete enzymes.
(B) It possesses mucous acinar cells.
(C) The endocrine pancreas has more β-cells than δ-cells.
(D) Its α-cells secrete insulin.
(E) Its δ-cells secrete amylase.

23. Which one of the following stimulates the production of hydrochloric acid in the stomach?

(A) Somatostatin
(B) Gastrin
(C) Secretin
(D) Cholecystokinin
(E) Urogastrone

24. A deficiency or an excess of which of the following vitamins results in short stature?

(A) Vitamin A
(B) Vitamin C
(C) Vitamin D
(D) Vitamin K
(E) Vitamin B

25. The intercellular spaces in the stratum spinosum of the epidermis contain lipid-containing sheets that are impermeable to water. This material is released from

(A) keratohyalin granules.
(B) Langerhans cells.
(C) membrane-coating granules.
(D) sebaceous glands.
(E) melanosomes.

26. Which of the following statements concerning basophilic erythroblasts is true?

(A) The nucleus has a fine chromatin network.
(B) The nucleus is in the process of being extruded.
(C) The cytoplasm contains specific granules.
(D) The cytoplasm is pink and reveals a dense reticulum.
(E) The nucleus is bilobed.

27. The ileum includes which of the following structures?

(A) Rugae
(B) Peyer patches
(C) Brunner glands
(D) Parietal cells
(E) Chief cells

28. A 25-year-old woman complains about a frequently recurring painful lesion on her upper lip that exudes a clear fluid. She probably has

(A) oral leukoplakia.
(B) herpetic stomatitis.
(C) aphthous ulcer.
(D) bullous pemphigoid.
(E) malignant melanoma.

29. Which of the following statements concerning the functions of the skin is true?

(A) Infrared radiation, necessary for synthesis of vitamin D, is absorbed by the skin.
(B) The skin provides no protection against desiccation.
(C) The skin contains temperature receptors and plays a role in regulating body temperature.
(D) Melanin is synthesized by melanocytes, which are located in the dermis.
(E) Sunscreen with a sun protection factor rating of 15 or higher protects the skin from harmful effects caused by ultraviolet light.

30. A person with glomerulonephritis will have which of the following signs or symptoms?

(A) Hypotonic urine
(B) Polyuria
(C) Proteinuria
(D) Dehydration
(E) Polydipsia

31. Stratified squamous keratinized epithelium is always present in the

(A) rectum.
(B) esophagus.
(C) pyloric stomach.
(D) jejunum.
(E) anus.

32. Which of the following properties is exhibited in all three types of cartilage?

(A) It is involved in bone formation.
(B) It possesses type II collagen.
(C) It possesses type I collagen.
(D) It grows interstitially and appositionally.
(E) It has an identifiable perichondrium.

33. Which of the following is a receptor for fine touch?

(A) Pacinian corpuscle
(B) Crista ampullaris
(C) Ruffini ending
(D) Krause end bulb
(E) Meissner corpuscle

34. A premature infant has labored breathing, which is eventually alleviated by administration of glucocorticoids. The most probable diagnosis is

(A) immotile cilia syndrome.
(B) emphysema.
(C) hyaline membrane disease.
(D) asthma.
(E) chronic bronchitis.

35. Which of the following statements concerning the cribriform plate is true?

(A) It is the inner layer of the alveolar bone.
(B) It lacks Sharpey fibers.
(C) It is also known as the spongiosa.
(D) It is composed of cancellous bone.
(E) Normally, it is fused with cementum.

36. Which one of the following substances is synthesized in the pituitary gland?

(A) Oxytocin
(B) Antidiuretic hormone
(C) Somatotropin
(D) Neurophysin
(E) Vasopressin

37. Which one of the following is true in breast cancer cells that involve the BRCA1 gene?

(A) Mutated cells are unable to divide because of increased expression of the BRCA1 gene.
(B) Mutated cells fail to reach the G1-S checkpoint.
(C) Mutated cells have an abnormal number of endosomes.
(D) Mutated cells lose their G2-M cell cycle checkpoint.
(E) Mutated cells become haploid owing to the interaction of the BRCA1 and p53 genes.

Questions 38 to 40

A 42-year-old man arrives in the emergency department with a rash over much of his face, hands, and arms. He states that he was gardening and pulled out a number of weeds. On questioning the patient, the physician realized that the patient inadvertently came in contact with poison ivy.

38. Which of the following cells is responsible for the release of the pharmacological agents that caused the rash?

(A) Diffuse neuroendocrine system cells
(B) Myofibroblasts
(C) Mast cells
(D) Pericytes
(E) Plasma cells

39. Which of the following is a secondary mediator produced by the cell in question 38?

(A) Histamine
(B) Chondroitin sulfate
(C) Neutral protease
(D) Bradykinin
(E) Aryl sulfatase

40. Which of the following white blood cells can also participate in the reaction of this patient to poison ivy?

(A) T cells
(B) B cells
(C) Neutrophils
(D) Basophils
(E) Eosinophils

41. A 26-year-old woman goes to the dentist because of a toothache. On examination, the dentist notes that the patient has a carious lesion that involves not only the enamel but also the dentin and the cementum of the tooth. Which of these substances cannot repair itself?

(A) Dentin
(B) Enamel
(C) Cementum
(D) Dentin and cementum
(E) Dentin, cementum, and enamel

42. Lisa is small and thin in stature. She spends her days indoors and rarely eats dairy products. When she became pregnant at 25 years of age, she had severe lower back and leg pain and tenderness when pressure was applied over bony regions of her body. Radiographs revealed excessive amounts of poorly mineralized osteoid in both femurs. Beneficial treatment of her condition involved high doses of vitamin D, calcium, and phosphorus, a regimen that continued after successful delivery of her baby. Which of the following describes Lisa's disease?

(A) Osteogenesis imperfecta
(B) Osteoporosis
(C) Osteomalacia
(D) Osteopetrosis
(E) Osteopenia

43. Michael had visual problems within a day after being hit in the head with a ball during a soccer game. He saw large floaters and noticed that a dark film was blocking part of the vision in his right eye. An examination by an oph-thalmologist revealed that he had a detached retina, and emergency surgery was done to save the vision in that eye. Which of the following retinal layers were separated from one another to cause Michael's condition?

(A) Layer 1 from layer 2
(B) Layer 2 from layer 3
(C) Layer 3 from layer 4
(D) Layer 5 from layer 6
(E) Layer 6 from layer 7

44. Blood coagulation entails a cascade of reactions that occur in two interrelated pathways, the extrinsic and intrinsic. All of the following are associated with the intrinsic pathway of blood coagulation *except*

(A) conversion of fibrinogen to fibrin.
(B) platelet aggregation.
(C) release of tissue thromboplastin.
(D) von Willebrand factor.
(E) calcium.

45. A scientist spent a summer in a remote region of Africa, where he studied exotic plants. On returning to the United States, he developed a cough and fever that would not go away. Laboratory tests revealed that he had contracted a roundworm, *Ascaris lumbricoides*. Which of the following cells would be expected to be significantly elevated in a differential count of his blood?

(A) Erythrocytes
(B) Lymphocytes
(C) Monocytes
(D) Eosinophils
(E) Neutrophils

46. A 45-year-old musician who played the guitar for 26 years in a rock band noticed he was having difficulty hearing. An otolaryngologist confirmed his loss of hearing and associated it with prolonged exposure to loud sounds. Which of the following structures would show degenerative changes that would account for this man's hearing loss?

(A) The epithelium lining the inner portion of the tympanic membrane
(B) Hair cells in the ampullae of the semicircular ducts
(C) The auditory (eustachian) tube extending to the middle ear cavity
(D) Hair cells of the organ of Corti
(E) Ossicles in the middle ear

47. Which of the following is a protein circulating in the blood that functions in wound healing?

(A) Chondronectin
(B) Plasma fibronectin
(C) Osteonectin
(D) Matrix fibronectin
(E) Laminin

48. Which of the following is an adhesive glycoprotein that forms fibrils in the extracellular matrix?

(A) Chondronectin
(B) Plasma fibronectin
(C) Osteonectin
(D) Matrix fibronectin
(E) Laminin

49. Which of the following is a multifunctional protein that attaches chondrocytes to type II collagen?

(A) Laminin
(B) Plasma fibronectin
(C) Osteonectin
(D) Matrix fibronectin
(E) Chondronectin

50. Which of the following cells in the connective tissue is an antibody-manufacturing cell?

(A) Pericytes
(B) Macrophages
(C) T lymphocytes
(D) Plasma cells
(E) Mast cells

51. Principal phagocytes of connective tissue are the

(A) pericytes.
(B) macrophages.
(C) T lymphocytes.
(D) plasma cells.
(E) mast cells.

52. Cells in the connective tissue that can bind immunoglobulin E antibodies and mediate immediate hypersensitivity reactions are

(A) pericytes.
(B) macrophages.
(C) T lymphocytes.
(D) plasma cells.
(E) mast cells.

53. Connective tissue cells responsible for initiating cell-mediated immune responses are

(A) pericytes.
(B) macrophages.
(C) T lymphocytes.
(D) plasma cells.
(E) mast cells.

54. Pluripotential cells located primarily along capillaries in the connective tissue are

(A) pericytes.
(B) macrophages.
(C) T lymphocytes.
(D) plasma cells.
(E) mast cells.

55. Which of the following functions in activation of secondary messenger systems?

(A) Phospholipid
(B) Glycocalyx
(C) Carrier protein
(D) Band 3 protein
(E) G protein

56. Which of the following is primarily responsible for establishing the potential difference across the plasma membrane?

(A) K^+ leak channel
(B) Glycocalyx
(C) Carrier protein
(D) Band 3 protein
(E) G protein

57. Which of the following is an amphipathic molecule?

(A) Phospholipid
(B) Glycocalyx
(C) Carrier protein
(D) Band 3 protein
(E) G protein

58. Which of the following is a carbohydrate-containing covering associated with the outer leaflet of the plasma membrane?

(A) Phospholipid
(B) Glycocalyx
(C) Carrier protein
(D) Band 3 protein
(E) G protein

59. Which of the following functions in antiport transport?

(A) Phospholipid
(B) Glycocalyx
(C) Carrier protein
(D) Band 3 protein
(E) G protein

60. Which of the following is a surface marker on T killer cells (CTL)?

(A) CD4
(B) CD8
(C) Interleukin 1
(D) Interleukin 2
(E) Perforin

61. Which of the following is a surface marker on T helper cells?

(A) CD4
(B) CD8
(C) Interleukin 1
(D) Interleukin 2
(E) Perforin

62. Which of the following mediates lysis of tumor cells?

(A) CD4
(B) CD8
(C) Interleukin 1
(D) Interleukin 2
(E) Perforin

63. Which of the following is released by macrophages and stimulates activated T helper cells?

(A) CD4
(B) CD8
(C) Interleukin 1
(D) Interleukin 2
(E) Interferon-γ

64. Which of the following stimulates activation of natural killer cells?

(A) CD4
(B) Interferon-γ
(C) Interleukin 1
(D) Interleukin 2
(E) Perforin

65. Identify the cells that replicate their deoxyribonucleic acid during the S phase of the cell cycle and undergo meiosis.

(A) Sertoli cells
(B) Primary spermatocytes
(C) Secondary spermatocytes
(D) Interstitial cells of Leydig
(E) Spermatids

66. Identify the cells that form a temporary cylinder of microtubules called the manchette.

(A) Sertoli cells
(B) Primary spermatocytes
(C) Secondary spermatocytes
(D) Interstitial cells of Leydig
(E) Spermatids

67. Identify the cells that possess receptors for luteinizing hormone (LH) and produce testosterone in response to binding of LH.

(A) Sertoli cells
(B) Primary spermatocytes
(C) Secondary spermatocytes
(D) Interstitial cells of Leydig
(E) Spermatids

68. Identify the cells that are responsible for formation of the blood–testis barrier.

(A) Sertoli cells
(B) Primary spermatocytes
(C) Secondary spermatocytes
(D) Interstitial cells of Leydig
(E) Spermatids

69. Identify the cells that synthesize androgen-binding protein when stimulated by follicle-stimulating hormone.

(A) Sertoli cells
(B) Primary spermatocytes
(C) Secondary spermatocytes
(D) Interstitial cells of Leydig
(E) Spermatids

70. Which of the following organelles possesses mixed-function oxidases that detoxify phenobarbital and other drugs?

(A) Rough endoplasmic reticulum
(B) Smooth endoplasmic reticulum
(C) Mitochondrion
(D) Annulate lamella
(E) Lysosome

71. Which of the following organelles contains ribophorins?

(A) Rough endoplasmic reticulum
(B) Smooth endoplasmic reticulum
(C) Mitochondrion
(D) Polyribosome
(E) Lysosome

72. Which of the following is the site where degradation of foreign material ingested by the cell takes place?

(A) Rough endoplasmic reticulum
(B) Smooth endoplasmic reticulum
(C) Mitochondrion
(D) Annulate lamellae
(E) Lysosome

73. Which of the following organelles contains adenosine triphosphate synthase?

(A) Rough endoplasmic reticulum
(B) Smooth endoplasmic reticulum
(C) Mitochondrion
(D) Annulate lamellae
(E) Lysosome

74. Which of the following stimulates secretion of pepsinogen?

(A) Gastrin
(B) Somatostatin
(C) Motilin
(D) Secretin
(E) Lysozyme

75. Which of the following is produced by Brunner glands and inhibits hydrochloric acid secretion by parietal cells?

(A) Gastrin
(B) Somatostatin
(C) Urogastrone
(D) Pepsinogen
(E) Lysozyme

76. Which of the following functions as an antibacterial agent?

(A) Gastrin
(B) Somatostatin
(C) Motilin
(D) Pepsinogen
(E) Lysozyme

77. Which of the following stimulates contraction of smooth muscle in the wall of the digestive tract?

(A) Gastrin
(B) Somatostatin
(C) Motilin
(D) Pepsinogen
(E) Lysozyme

78. Which of the following inhibits secretion by nearby enteroendocrine cells?

(A) Gastrin
(B) Somatostatin
(C) Motilin
(D) Pepsinogen
(E) Lysozyme

79. Which of the following is involved in forming cross-links between adjacent tropocollagen molecules?

(A) Lysine
(B) Desmosine
(C) Hydroxyproline
(D) Arginine
(E) Proline

80. Which of the following cross-links elastin molecules to form an extensive network?

(A) Lysine
(B) Fibrillin
(C) Hydroxyproline
(D) Arginine
(E) Proline

81. Inadequate amounts of iodine in the diet lead to which one of the following conditions?

(A) Simple goiter
(B) Exophthalmic goiter
(C) Graves disease
(D) Addison disease
(E) Hyperparathyroidism

82. Which of the following conditions is associated with the destruction of the adrenal cortex?

(A) Simple goiter
(B) Exophthalmic goiter
(C) Graves disease
(D) Addison disease
(E) Hyperparathyroidism

83. Which of the following hydrolyzes adenosine triphosphate?

(A) Troponin C
(B) Globular head (S1 fragment) of myosin
(C) Myoglobin
(D) Actin
(E) Tropomodulin

84. Which of the following binds oxygen?

(A) Troponin C
(B) Globular head (S1 fragment) of myosin
(C) Myoglobin
(D) Actin
(E) Tropomodulin

85. Which of the following binds Ca^{2+}?

(A) Troponin C
(B) Globular head (S1 fragment) of myosin
(C) Myoglobin
(D) Actin
(E) Tropomodulin

86. Which of the following is a rare form of skin cancer that may be fatal?

(A) Epidermolysis bullosa
(B) Basal cell carcinoma
(C) Malignant melanoma
(D) Psoriasis
(E) Warts

87. Which of the following is a hereditary skin disease characterized by blister formation after minor trauma?

(A) Epidermolysis bullosa
(B) Basal cell carcinoma
(C) Malignant melanoma
(D) Psoriasis
(E) Warts

88. Which of the following regions of the respiratory system would concern a patient with an adenoid?

(A) Trachea
(B) Nasopharynx
(C) Terminal bronchiole
(D) Alveolar duct
(E) Intrapulmonary bronchi

89. Which of the following possesses C-shaped rings of hyaline cartilage?

(A) Trachea
(B) Nasopharynx
(C) Terminal bronchiole
(D) Alveolar duct
(E) Intrapulmonary bronchi

90. Which of the following contains smooth muscle at the openings into alveoli?

(A) Trachea
(B) Nasopharynx
(C) Terminal bronchiole
(D) Alveolar duct
(E) Intrapulmonary bronchi

91. Which of the following is lined by an epithelium containing ciliated cells and Clara cells?

(A) Trachea
(B) Nasopharynx
(C) Terminal bronchiole
(D) Alveolar duct
(E) Intrapulmonary bronchi

92. Which of the following is associated with rupture of the oviduct and hemorrhaging into the peritoneal cavity?

(A) Endometriosis
(B) Cervical cancer
(C) Ectopic tubal pregnancy
(D) Breast cancer
(E) Teratomas

93. Which of the following may be classified as lobular carcinoma?

(A) Endometriosis
(B) Cervical cancer
(C) Ectopic tubal pregnancy
(D) Breast cancer
(E) Teratomas

94. Which of the following may be detected by a Papanicolaou smear?

(A) Endometriosis
(B) Cervical cancer
(C) Ectopic tubal pregnancy
(D) Breast cancer
(E) Teratomas

95. Which of the following commonly results in hemorrhaging into the peritoneal cavity dependent on the stage of the menstrual cycle?

(A) Endometriosis
(B) Cervical cancer
(C) Ectopic tubal pregnancy
(D) Breast cancer
(E) Teratomas

96. Which of the following facilitates the absorption of vitamin B_{12}?

(A) Pepsin
(B) Enzyme associated with the glycocalyx of the intestinal striated border
(C) Lipase
(D) Chylomicron
(E) Gastric intrinsic factor

97. Which of the following functions in the digestion of carbohydrates?

(A) Pepsin
(B) Enzyme associated with the glycocalyx of the intestinal striated border
(C) Lipase
(D) Chylomicron
(E) Gastric intrinsic factor

98. Which of the following functions in the digestion of proteins?

(A) Pepsin
(B) Enzyme associated with the glycocalyx of the intestinal striated border
(C) Lipase
(D) Chylomicron
(E) Gastric intrinsic factor

99. Which of the following functions in the transport of triglycerides into lacteals?

(A) Pepsin
(B) Enzyme associated with the glycocalyx of the intestinal striated border
(C) Lipase
(D) Chylomicron
(E) Gastric intrinsic factor

100. Which of the following is manufactured and released by parietal cells?

(A) Pepsin
(B) Enzyme associated with the glycocalyx of the intestinal striated border
(C) Lipase
(D) Chylomicron
(E) Gastric intrinsic factor

Answers and Explanations

1. **C.** To yield messenger ribonucleoproteins (mRNPs), introns are excised, whereas exons are spliced together. Deoxyribonucleic acid does act as the template for the synthesis of ribonucleic acid (RNA). Three RNA polymerases (I, II, and III) are needed to synthesize ribosomal RNA, messenger RNA, and transfer RNA, respectively. Protein moieties are removed from the mRNPs as they leave the nucleus to yield functional mRNAs outside the nucleus. (See Chapter 2 VIII A.)

2. **C.** The most common cause of osteoporosis in older women is diminished estrogen secretion. (See Chapter 7 II J Clinical Consideration.)

3. **E.** Although adenine, cytosine, and guanine are found in both deoxyribonucleic acid (DNA) and ribonucleic acid (RNA), uracil is found only in RNA. Uracil substitutes for the base thymine in DNA. (See Chapter 2 VIII.)

4. **A.** Pancreatic centroacinar cells form the initial segment of the intercalated duct and are part of the exocrine pancreas. They secrete an enzyme-poor alkaline fluid when stimulated by secretin. Pancreatic digestive enzymes are synthesized by the acinar cells of the exocrine pancreas; their release is stimulated by cholecystokinin. Glucagon is produced in the endocrine pancreas (islets of Langerhans). (See Chapter 17 III A 2.)

5. **E.** The zona fasciculata, the largest region of the adrenal cortex, produces glucocorticoids (cortisol and corticosterone). The zona glomerulosa produces mineralocorticoids, primarily aldosterone. Epinephrine is produced in the adrenal medulla. Glucagon is produced in the pancreas, not in the adrenal gland. (See Chapter 13 VI A 2.)

6. **B.** Diarthroses, the type of joint connecting two long bones, are classified as synovial joints, which are surrounded by a two-layered capsule housing a synovial membrane. Type A cells of the synovial membrane are phagocytic, whereas type B cells secrete the synovial fluid. Synarthrosis joints are those found joining the bones of the skull, which are immovable. (See Chapter 7 III B.)

7. **E.** Neutrophils have a nucleus with three or four lobes, many azurophilic granules, and small specific granules that lack peroxidase. In contrast, basophils have an S-shaped nucleus, few azurophilic granules, and large specific granules that contain peroxidase. Both neutrophils and basophils possess mitochondria. (See Table 10.2.)

8. **D.** Oral leukoplakia, which results from epithelial hyperkeratosis, is usually of unknown etiology, but is often associated with the use of chewing tobacco. Although the characteristic painless lesions are benign, they may transform into squamous cell carcinoma. Aphthous ulcers are painful lesions of the oral mucosa that are surrounded by a red border. Adenocarcinoma is a form of cancer arising in glandular tissue. Keloids are swellings in the skin that arise from increased collagen formation in hyperplastic scar tissue. Epidermolysis bullosa is a group of hereditary skin diseases characterized by blister formation after minor trauma. (See Chapter 16 II.)

9. **B.** A primordial follicle is composed of a flattened layer of follicular cells surrounding a primary oocyte, which is arrested in prophase of meiosis I. Well-defined thecal layers and a thick zona pellucida are found in growing follicles. A graafian (mature) follicle possesses a secondary oocyte, which becomes arrested in metaphase of meiosis II just before ovulation. (See Chapter 19 II B 1.)

10. **E.** The first four statements are true. Linear acceleration of the head is detected by the neuroepithelial hair cells of the maculae, which are specialized regions of the saccule and utricle. However, the vestibular membrane is a part of the organ of Corti. (See Chapter 21 IV C 2.)

11. **D.** Euchromatin, the transcriptionally active form of chromatin, represents only about 10% of the chromatin. In the light microscope, it appears as a light-staining, dispersed region of the nucleus. (See Chapter 2 V 2.)

12. **C.** Large protein molecules cannot move across intercalated disks (the steplike junctional complexes present in cardiac, not smooth, muscle). These junctional structures possess three specializations: desmosomes, which provide end-to-end attachment of cardiac muscle cells; fascia adherentes, to which the thin myofilaments attach; and gap junctions, which permit intercellular movement of small molecules and ions (ionic coupling). (See Chapter 8 V B 6.)

13. **D.** Flattened squamous cells are characteristic of an unstimulated, inactive thyroid gland. TSH binds to G protein–linked receptors on the basal surface of follicular cells. Under TSH stimulation, thyroid follicular cells become columnar and form pseudopods, which engulf colloid. Lysosomal enzymes split thyroxine and triiodothyronine from thyroglobulin; the hormones are then released basally. (See Chapter 13 IV B 2.)

14. **D.** The enamel organ is epithelially derived, whereas the dental papilla comes from ectomesenchyme. The bell, not the cap, stage of odontogenesis is characterized by possessing a fourth layer in its enamel organ. Formation of dentin and enamel occurs during the appositional stage of tooth development. Cementum is located on the root and is formed only after the crown is complete and enamel ceases to be elaborated. (See Chapter 16 II C 3.)

15. **D.** Liver sinusoids convey blood to the central vein. Their endothelial cells are fenestrated, and material from the sinusoids may enter the space of Disse through the fenestrae, where it may be endocytosed by hepatocytes. The space of Disse houses Ito cells (fat-storing cells). Because bile is the exocrine secretion of hepatocytes, it does not enter the sinusoids. (See Chapter 17 IV B 2.)

16. **D.** The toxin from *Clostridium botulinum* inhibits the release of acetylcholine, the neurotransmitter at myoneural junctions. As a result, motor nerve impulses cannot be transmitted across the junction, and muscle cells are not stimulated to contract. (See Chapter 8 IV 2 Clinical Considerations.)

17. **A.** The nucleosome, the structural unit of chromatin packing, does not contain ribonucleic acid. In extended chromatin, two copies each of histones H2A, H2B, H3, and H4 form the nucleosome core around which a deoxyribonucleic acid molecule is wound. Condensed chromatin contains additional histones (H1), which bind to nucleosomes, forming the condensed 30-nm chromatin fiber. (See Chapter 2 VI A.)

18. **C.** Only infectious mononucleosis is characterized by all of the signs and symptoms indicated. AIDS is associated with a decreased lymphocyte count, particularly of T helper cells. Pernicious anemia is associated with a decreased red blood cell count. Hodgkin disease is associated with fatigue and enlarged lymph nodes, but the nodes are not painful, and the presence of Reed–Sternberg cells is diagnostic of this disease. Factor VIII deficiency, a coagulation disorder, is not associated with any of these signs and symptoms. (See Chapter 10 II B 2 Clinical Considerations.)

19. **C.** The gallbladder, which concentrates and stores bile, is lined by a simple columnar epithelium. Cholecystokinin stimulates contraction of the gallbladder wall, forcing bile from the lumen into the cystic duct; this joins the common hepatic duct to form the common bile duct, which delivers bile to the duodenum. (See Chapter 17 III A 2.)

20. **A.** Uncoupling of oxidation from phosphorylation induces mitochondria to change from the orthodox to the condensed form. Condensed mitochondria are often present in brown fat cells, which produce heat rather than adenosine triphosphate. Mitochondria possess circular deoxyribonucleic acid, and they reproduce (divide) by fission. (See Chapter 3 II 6 e.)

21. **D.** Muscular (distributing) arteries have a thick, complete internal elastic lamina in the tunica intima, whereas elastic (conducting) arteries have an incomplete internal elastic lamina. Both types of arteries have vasa vasorum, factor VIII, and smooth muscle cells in their walls. Muscular arteries possess numerous layers of muscle cells in the tunica media, but elastic arteries do not. Only elastic arteries possess fenestrated (elastic) membranes in the tunica media, in which smooth muscle cells are dispersed. (See Chapter 11 I B 1 b.)

22. **C.** In the endocrine pancreas, β-cells account for about 70% of the secretory cells; α-cells about 20%; and δ-cells less than 5%. Polypeptide hormones are synthesized by and released from the islets of Langerhans (endocrine pancreas). The exocrine pancreas possesses serous (not mucous) acinar cells. Insulin is produced by β-cells. (See Chapter 17 III B 3.)

23. **B.** Somatostatin and urogastrone both inhibit the production of hydrochloric acid, whereas gastrin enhances it. Secretin and cholecystokinin act on the pancreas to facilitate secretion of buffer and pancreatic enzymes, respectively. (See Chapter 16 III B 2.)

24. **A.** A deficiency of vitamin A inhibits bone formation and growth, whereas an excess stimulates ossification of the epiphyseal plates, thus leading to premature closure of the plates. Both conditions result in short stature. A deficiency of vitamin D reduces calcium absorption from the small intestine and results in soft bones, whereas an excess of vitamin D stimulates bone resorption. A deficiency of vitamin C results in poor bone growth and fracture repair. Vitamin K plays no role in bone formation. (See Chapter 7 II I.)

25. **C.** Membrane-coating granules are present in keratinocytes in the stratum spinosum (and stratum granulosum). The contents of these granules are released into the intercellular spaces to help waterproof the skin. Keratinocytes in the stratum granulosum also possess keratohyalin granules; these contain proteins that bind keratin filaments together. (See Chapter 14 II B 2.)

26. **A.** The nucleus of erythroblasts is not in the process of being extruded and is round with a very fine chromatin network. The cytoplasm is blue and possesses no granules. (See Chapter 10 VI C.)

27. **B.** The ileum includes Peyer patches. Rugae, parietal cells, and chief cells are located in the stomach. Brunner glands are present in the submucosa of the duodenum. (See Table 16.1.)

28. **B.** Herpetic stomatitis is characterized by painful fever blisters on the lips or near the nostrils. These blisters exude a clear fluid. Aphthous ulcers (canker sores) do not exude fluid. Bullous pemphigoid is an autoimmune disease marked by chronic generalized blisters in the skin. (See Chapter 16 II B Clinical Considerations.)

29. **C.** The skin, which consists of the epidermis and dermis, is important in the regulation of body temperature and contains temperature receptors in the dermis. Ultraviolet (not infrared) radiation absorbed by the skin is necessary for the synthesis of vitamin D. Protection against desiccation is provided by the contents of the membrane-coating granules of the epidermis. Melanocytes are located in the deepest layer of the epidermis (stratum basale). Sunscreen with sun protection factor rating of 15 or higher offers no protection against ultraviolet light of longer wavelengths, that is, in the UVA spectrum. (See Chapter 14 I E.)

30. **C.** Patients with glomerulonephritis excrete protein in their urine. All of the other symptoms are characteristic of patients with diabetes insipidus, who are incapable of producing adequate amounts of antidiuretic hormone and therefore have polyuria (large volume of hypotonic urine production), polydipsia, and dehydration. (See Chapter 18 III A Clinical Considerations.)

31. **E.** The anus is lined by stratified squamous keratinized epithelium. The rectum, jejunum, and pyloric stomach are lined by simple columnar epithelium. The esophagus is lined by stratified squamous (nonkeratinized) epithelium. (See Chapter 16 III D 4.)

32. **D.** Hyaline cartilage, elastic cartilage, and fibrocartilage all exhibit both interstitial and appositional growth. Hyaline cartilage and elastic cartilage have type II collagen in their matrix and are surrounded by a perichondrium, whereas fibrocartilage has type I collagen and lacks an identifiable perichondrium. Only hyaline cartilage is involved in endochondral bone formation. (See Chapter 7 I A, B, C.)

33. **E.** Meissner corpuscles, in the papillary layer of the dermis, are fine touch receptors. Pacinian corpuscles perceive pressure, touch, and vibration; they are located in the dermis, hypodermis, and connective tissue of mesenteries and joints. Cristae ampullares are special regions of the semicircular canals that detect circular movements of the head. Ruffini endings, in the dermis and joints, function in pressure and touch perception. Krause end bulbs are cold and pressure receptors in the dermis. (See Chapter 14 III A.)

34. **C.** Hyaline membrane disease, which results from inadequate amounts of pulmonary surfactant, is characterized by labored breathing and is typically observed in premature infants. Glucocorticoids stimulate synthesis of surfactant and can correct the condition. (See Chapter 15 VIII D Clinical Considerations.)

35. **A.** The cribriform plate, the inner layer of the alveolar bone, is composed of compact bone. It is attached to the principal fiber groups of the periodontal ligament via Sharpey fibers. The outer layer of the alveolar bone is the cortical plate. The spongiosa is the region of cancellous (spongy) bone enclosed between the cortical and cribriform plates. (See Chapter 16 II D 3.)

36. **C.** Somatotropin (growth hormone) is synthesized by cells called somatotrophs, which are acidophils located in the pars distalis of the anterior lobe of the pituitary gland. Oxytocin and antidiuretic hormone (also called vasopressin) are produced in the hypothalamus and transported to the pars nervosa of the pituitary. Neurophysin, a binding protein, aids in this transport. (See Chapter 13 III A 1 a.)

37. **D.** Mutations in the BRCA1 gene, a breast tumor suppressor gene, are the major cause of breast cancer. In most breast cancers involving this gene, deoxyribonucleic acid synthesis proceeds, indicating that the G1-S checkpoint is not affected; however, the mutated cells cannot control the transition between G2 and M. Moreover, the mutated cells had abnormal centrosome numbers, and their nuclear division did not proceed normally, leading to aneuploidy and genetic instability of the daughter cells. (See Chapter 19 X C Clinical Considerations.)

38. **C.** The patient has an immediate (type I) hypersensitivity reaction. The cells responsible for releasing the primary and secondary mediators are the mast cells. (See Chapter 6 III D.)

39. **D.** Bradykinins are the only listed pharmacological agents that are produced via the arachidonic acid pathway. All of the others are primary mediators because they are stored in the storage granules of mast cells. (See Chapter 6 III D.)

40. **D.** Basophils are very similar in function to mast cells. They also participate in the immediate (type I) hypersensitivity reaction. (See Chapter 6 III H 3.)

41. **B.** The only hard tissue of the tooth that cannot be repaired by the body is enamel because ameloblasts, the cells that manufacture enamel, are eliminated as the tooth emerges into the oral cavity. (See Chapter 16 II C 2.)

42. **C.** Osteomalacia, or adult rickets, is Lisa's disorder. It is characterized by a failure of newly formed osteoid to calcify because there is a lack of calcium, vitamin D, and phosphorus. The bones gradually soften and bend, and pain accompanies the condition, which often becomes severe during pregnancy as the fetus removes calcium from the mother's body. Osteogenesis imperfecta is a genetic condition affecting the synthesis of type I collagen in the bone matrix and results in extreme bone fragility and breakage. Osteoporosis is a disease characterized by low bone mineral density and structural deterioration, making bone more susceptible to fracture, and osteopenia is reduced bone mass caused by inadequate osteoid synthesis. Osteopetrosis is the excessive formation of bone, which obliterates the marrow cavities and thus impairs the formation of blood cells. (See Chapter 7 II I Clinical Consideration.)

43. **A.** The pigmented epithelium (layer 1) was separated from the layer of rods and cones (layer 2), which make up the light-sensitive part of the neural retina. (See Chapter 21 III E Clinical Consideration.)

44. **C.** The extrinsic pathway is initiated by the release of tissue thromboplastin after trauma to extravascular tissue. Platelet aggregation is promoted by von Willebrand factor, which is associated with the intrinsic pathway only. Calcium is required in both pathways, and the final reaction—the conversion of fibrinogen to fibrin—is the same in both. (See Chapter 10 III D 1.)

45. **D.** Eosinophils are increased in parasitic infections and allergic reactions. Both eosinophils and basophils have receptors for immunoglobulin E, which seems to be important in the destruction of parasites. Both neutrophils and monocytes lack immunoglobulin E receptors. (See Table 10.2.)

46. **D.** The inner ear is where sound waves are transduced into nerve impulses that convey auditory information to the brain, and the hair cells of the organ of Corti play a key role in this process. Sound waves are initially received by the outer ear and transmitted via the tympanic membrane (eardrum) to the middle ear, where ossicles transmit the vibrations to the inner ear. The inner ear has an auditory system for hearing (the organ of Corti) and a vestibular system of semicircular ducts that control equilibrium and spatial orientation. (See Chapter 21 IV C e 8.)

47. **B.** Plasma fibronectin functions in wound healing, blood clotting, and phagocytosis of material from the blood. (See Chapter 4 II C 1.)

48. **D.** Matrix fibronectin mediates cell adhesion to the extracellular matrix by binding to fibronectin receptors on the plasma membrane. (See Chapter 4 II C 1.)

49. **E.** Chondronectin has binding sites for type II collagen, proteoglycans, and chondrocyte cell-surface receptors. (See Chapter 4 II C 5.)

50. **D.** Plasma cells, which arise from antigen-activated B lymphocytes, produce antibodies and are thus directly responsible for humoral-mediated immunity. (See Chapter 6 III G.)

51. **B.** Macrophages, the principal phagocytes of connective tissue, remove large particulate matter and assist in the immune response by acting as antigen-presenting cells. (See Chapter 6 III E.)

52. **E.** Mast cells (and basophils) have receptors for immunoglobulin E antibodies on their surface. These cells release histamine, heparin, leukotriene C (slow-reacting substance of anaphylaxis), and eosinophil chemotactic factor, which have effects that constitute immediate hypersensitivity reactions. (See Chapter 6 III D.)

53. **C.** T lymphocytes initiate cell-mediated immune responses. (See Chapter 6 III F.)

54. **A.** Pericytes are smaller than fibroblasts and are located along capillaries. When necessary, they assume the pluripotential role of embryonic mesenchymal cells. (See Chapter 6 III B.)

55. **E.** G proteins are membrane proteins that are linked to certain cell-surface receptors. Upon binding of a signaling molecule to the receptor, the G protein functions as a signal transducer by activating a secondary messenger system that leads to a cellular response. (See Chapter 1 IV B 2 c.)

56. **A.** K^+ leak channels are ion channels that are responsible for establishing a potential difference across the plasma membrane. (See Chapter 1 III C 1.)

57. **A.** The term "amphipathic" refers to molecules, such as phospholipids, that possess both hydrophobic (nonpolar) and hydrophilic (polar) properties. The plasma membrane contains two phospholipid layers (leaflets), with the hydrophobic tails of the molecules projecting into the interior of the membrane and the hydrophilic heads facing outward. (See Chapter 1 II A 2.)

58. **B.** The glycocalyx (cell coat) is associated with the outer leaflet of the plasma membrane. It is composed primarily of proteoglycans, which possess polysaccharide side chains. (See Chapter 1 II C 1.)

59. **C.** Membrane carrier proteins are highly folded transmembrane proteins that undergo reversible conformational alterations, resulting in transport of specific molecules across the membrane. The Na^+-K^+ pump is a carrier protein that mediates antiport transport, the transport of two molecules concurrently in opposite directions. (See Chapter 1 II B 1.)

60. B. T killer cells (cytotoxic T lymphocytes) have CD8 marker molecules on their surfaces. (See Chapter 12 II B 3.)

61. A. T helper cells have CD4 marker molecules on their surfaces. (See Chapter 12 II B 3.)

62. E. Perforin, which is released by cytotoxic T cells, mediates lysis of tumor cells and virus-infected cells. (See Chapter 12 II B 3.)

63. C. Interleukin 1, which is produced by macrophages, stimulates activated T helper cells. In turn, activated T helper cells produce interleukin 2 and other cytokines involved in the immune response. (See Chapter 12 II E 2.)

64. B. Interferon-γ (macrophage-activating factor) stimulates activation of natural killer cells and macrophages, thereby increasing their cytotoxic and/or phagocytic activity. (See Chapter 12 II D 3.)

65. B. Primary spermatocytes undergo the first meiotic division following deoxyribonucleic acid replication in the S phase. The resulting secondary spermatocytes undergo the second meiotic division, without an intervening S phase, forming spermatids. (See Chapter 20 II D 4 b.)

66. E. During spermiogenesis, the manchette is formed. This temporary structure aids in elongation of the spermatid. (See Chapter 20 II D 5 c.)

67. D. Interstitial cells of Leydig produce testosterone when they are stimulated by LH. (See Chapter 20 II C 4.)

68. A. Sertoli cells are columnar cells that extend from the basal lamina to the lumen of the seminiferous tubules. Adjacent Sertoli cells form basal tight junctions, which are responsible for the blood–testis barrier, thus protecting the developing sperm cells from autoimmune reactions. (See Chapter 20 II D 2.)

69. A. Sertoli cells produce androgen-binding protein, which binds testosterone and maintains it at a high level in the seminiferous tubules. (See Chapter 20 II D 2.)

70. B. Smooth endoplasmic reticulum possesses mixed-function oxidases that detoxify phenobarbital and certain other drugs. (See Chapter 3 II 4.)

71. A. The membrane of the rough endoplasmic reticulum contains ribophorins, receptors that bind the large ribosome subunit. (See Chapter 3 II A 3.)

72. E. The lysosome is the organelle where the degradation of foreign material takes place in the cell. The term "heterophagy" refers to the ingestion and degradation of foreign material, in contrast to autophagy, where parts of the cell itself are digested and degraded. (See Chapter 3 III C 2.)

73. C. The inner membrane of the mitochondrion contains adenosine triphosphate synthase, a special enzyme consisting of a head portion and a transmembrane H^+ carrier; as H^+ passes through adenosine triphosphate synthase, the enzyme uses the energy of the proton flow to drive the production of adenosine triphosphate. (See Chapter 3 II A 6 d.)

74. A. Gastrin, a paracrine hormone secreted in the pylorus and duodenum, stimulates pepsinogen secretion by chief cells in the gastric glands. (See Chapter 16 III B 2.)

75. C. Urogastrone, produced by Brunner glands in the duodenum, inhibits gastric hydrochloric acid secretion and enhances division of epithelial cells. (See Chapter 16 III C 4.)

76. E. Lysozyme, manufactured by Paneth cells in the crypts of Lieberkühn, is an enzyme that has antibacterial activity. (See Chapter 16 III C 3 b (3) a.)

77. C. Motilin, a paracrine hormone secreted by cells in the small intestine, increases gut motility by stimulating smooth muscle contraction. (See Table 16.2.)

78. B. Somatostatin, produced by enteroendocrine cells in the pylorus and duodenum, inhibits secretion by nearby enteroendocrine cells. (See Table 16.2.)

79. A. Lysine and hydroxylysine residues within and between tropocollagen molecules form cross-links with each other or with other lysines or hydroxylysines. These covalent links add great tensile strength to the newly formed fibril. (See Chapter 4 III A 1.)

80. A. Lysine cross-links elastin molecules, forming a network. Fibrillin is the glycoprotein that organizes elastin into fibers. (See Chapter 4 III B 1.)

81. A. Simple goiter is an enlargement of the thyroid gland resulting from inadequate dietary iodine ($<$10 μg/d). It is common where the food supply is low in iodine. (See Chapter 13 IV D Clinical Considerations.)

82. D. Addison disease is most commonly caused by an autoimmunity that destroys the adrenal cortex. As a result, inadequate amounts of glucocorticoids and mineralocorticoids are produced. Unless these are replaced by steroid therapy, the disease is fatal. (See Chapter 13 VI A Clinical Considerations.)

83. B. The globular head of the myosin molecule has adenosine triphosphatase (ATPase) activity, but interaction with actin is required for the non-covalently bound reaction products adenosine diphosphate (ADP) and P_i to be released. This ATPase activity is retained by the S1 fragment resulting from digestion of myosin with proteases. (See Chapter 8 II F 2.)

84. C. Myoglobin, a sarcoplasmic protein, like hemoglobin, can bind and store oxygen. The myoglobin content of red (slow) muscle fibers is higher than that of white (fast) muscle fibers. (See Chapter 8 II B 2.)

85. A. Troponin C is one of the three subunits of troponin that along with tropomyosin binds to actin (thin) filaments in skeletal muscle. Binding of Ca^{2+} by troponin C results in unmasking of the myosin-binding sites on thin filaments. (See Chapter 8 II F 2.)

86. C. Malignant melanoma, a relatively rare form of skin cancer, arises from melanocytes. It is aggressive and invasive. Surgery and chemotherapy are usually necessary for successful treatment of this cancer. (See Chapter 14 II B Clinical Considerations.)

87. A. Epidermolysis bullosa is a group of hereditary skin diseases characterized by the separation of the layers in skin with consequent blister formation. (See Chapter 14 II D Clinical Considerations.)

88. B. The nasopharynx is the site of the pharyngeal tonsil; when enlarged and infected, this tonsil is known as an adenoid. (See Chapter 15 II B.)

89. A. The trachea and extrapulmonary (primary) bronchi have walls supported by C-shaped hyaline cartilages (C-rings), whose open ends face posteriorly. (See Chapter 15 II D.)

90. D. The alveolar duct has alveoli with openings that are rimmed by sphincters of smooth muscle. Alveoli more distal than these have only elastic and reticular fibers in their walls. (See Chapter 15 III B.)

91. C. Terminal bronchioles are lined by a simple cuboidal epithelium containing ciliated cells and Clara cells. Clara cells can divide and regenerate both cell types. (See Chapter 15 II F 2.)

92. C. An ectopic tubal pregnancy occurs when the embryo implants in the wall of the oviduct (rather than in the uterus). Because the oviduct cannot support the developing embryo, the duct eventually bursts, causing hemorrhaging into the peritoneal cavity. (See Chapter 19 VI B Clinical Considerations.)

93. D. Breast cancer that originates from the epithelium lining the terminal ductules of the mammary gland is classified as lobular carcinoma. (See Chapter 19 X C Clinical Considerations.)

94. B. Abnormal cells associated with cervical cancer are revealed in a Papanicolaou smear, providing a simple method for the early detection of this cancer. (See Chapter 19 V E Clinical Considerations.)

95. **A.** Endometriosis is a condition in which uterine endometrial tissue is located in the pelvic peritoneal cavity. The misplaced endometrial tissue undergoes cyclic hormone-induced changes, including menstrual breakdown and bleeding. (See Chapter 19 IV A 1 c Clinical Considerations.)

96. **E.** Gastric intrinsic factor, which is produced by parietal cells in the gastric glands, is necessary for absorption of vitamin B_{12} in the ileum. (See Chapter 16 III B 2.)

97. **B.** Disaccharidases in the glycocalyx of the striated border hydrolyze disaccharides to monosaccharides. (See Chapter 16 IV A 2.)

98. **A.** Digestion of proteins begins with the action of pepsin in the stomach, forming a mixture of polypeptides. Activation of pepsinogen to pepsin only occurs at a low pH. (See Chapter 16 IV B 1.)

99. **D.** After free fatty acids and monoglycerides in micelles enter the surface absorptive cells of the small intestine, they are reesterified to form triglycerides. These are complexed with proteins, forming chylomicrons, which are released from the lateral cell membrane and enter lacteals in the lamina propria. (See Chapter 16 IV C 2.)

100. **E.** Parietal cells are responsible for establishing the low pH of the stomach by manufacturing hydrochloric acid. Another function of parietal cells is the synthesis and release of gastric intrinsic factor, necessary for the absorption of vitamin B_{12} in the ileum. (See Chapter 16 III B 2 a.)

Index

Note: Page numbers followed by f denote figure; those followed by t denote table.